The Crucial Principles
in Care of the Knee

The Crucial Principles in Care of the Knee

Editors

■■ JOHN A. FEAGIN, JR., MD

Col. US Army (Retired)
Associate Professor Emeritus, Duke University, Durham, North Carolina
Clinical Professor, Department of Surgery, Uniformed Services University of Health
    Sciences, F. Edward Hebert School of Medicine, Bethesda, Maryland
Fellow Mentor, Steadman Hawkins Research Foundation, Vail, Colorado

■■ J. RICHARD STEADMAN, MD

Chairman, Medical Group, and Chief Physician, US Ski and Snowboard Team
Team Physician, Denver Broncos
Clinical Professor, University of Texas Southwestern Medical School, Dallas, Texas
Managing Partner, Steadman Hawkins Clinic, Vail, Colorado
Chairman & Founder, Steadman Hawkins Research Foundation, Vail, Colorado

KAREN BRIGGS
Authors' Editor

NANCY PLACE
Medical Illustrator

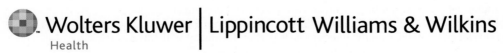

Wolters Kluwer | Lippincott Williams & Wilkins
Health

Philadelphia • Baltimore • New York • London
Buenos Aires • Hong Kong • Sydney • Tokyo

Acquisitions Editor: Robert A. Hurley
Managing Editor: Dave Murphy
Developmental Editor: Karen Briggs and Lottie Applewhite
Project Manager: Rosanne Hallowell
Manufacturing Manager: Benjamin Rivera
Marketing Manager: Sharon Zinner
Design Coordinator: Teresa Mallon
Cover Designer: Joseph DePinho
Production Services: Aptara, Inc.

© 2008 by Lippincott Williams & Wilkins, a Wolters Kluwer business
530 Walnut Street
Philadelphia, PA 19106
LWW.com

Printed in China

Library of Congress Cataloging-in-Publication Data

The crucial principles in care of the knee / [edited by] John A. Feagin Jr., J. Richard Steadman.
     p. ; cm.
  Includes bibliographical references and index.
  ISBN-13: 978-0-7817-7250-1
  ISBN-10: 0-7817-7250-8
 1. Knee—Surgery.   I. Feagin, John A., 1934–   II. Steadman, J. Richard.
 [DNLM: 1. Knee Injuries—therapy.   2. Athletic Injuries—therapy.   WE 870 C9556 2008]
 RD561.C783 2008
 617.5'82089—dc22

                                                           2007050293

10 9 8 7 6 5 4 3 2 1

The Crucial Principles in Care of the Knee is a distillation of our life's work in the treatment of the knee, including surgery and rehabilitation.

We dedicate this book to those who have joined in the journey with us: our families, our partners, our colleagues in sports medicine and rehabilitation, our friends, and especially, our patients.

The Crucial Principles shows where we have been and where we are going. Our love and appreciation to each of you for the help and inspiration you have given us, which has led us to this work, and made our lives of service possible.

Contents

Contributors ix
Foreword xi
Preface xiii
Acknowledgments xv
How to Use This Book xvii

The ACL-Deficient Knee 3
John A. Feagin, Jr., MD

PART I

THE BASICS: PHYSICAL EXAMINATION AND THREE CLASSIC CASE STUDIES 5

1 The Crucial Principles and the Care of the Knee-Injured Patient 7
John A. Feagin, Jr., MD

2 Principles of Diagnosis and Treatment 11
John A. Feagin, Jr., MD

3 Case Studies 27
John A. Feagin, Jr., MD

Classic Bibliography 44
John A. Feagin, Jr., MD

4 The Envelope of Function 51
Scott F. Dye, MD

5 Anterior Cruciate Ligament Injury Prevention: Concepts, Strategies, and Outcomes 59
Allston J. Stubbs, MD, and Mininder S. Kocher, MD, MPH

Appendix: The Physical Examination of the Knee 72
John A. Feagin, Jr., MD

PART II

APPLIED SURGICAL CARE: MICROFRACTURE, HEALING RESPONSE, AND "THE PACKAGE" 83

6 Philosophy of Knee Care 85
J. Richard Steadman, MD

7 Imaging of the Knee 87
Charles P. Ho, PhD, MD

8 Anterior Cruciate Ligament Reconstruction 117
J. Richard Steadman, MD

9 Microfracture 129
J. Richard Steadman, MD

10 The Healing Response Technique: A Minimally Invasive Procedure to Stimulate Healing of Anterior Cruciate Ligament Injuries Using the Microfracture Technique 153
J. Richard Steadman, MD, and William G. Rodkey, DVM

11 Arthrofibrosis of the Knee: Diagnosis and Management 163
Peter J. Millett, MD

12 Arthroscopic Treatment of the Degenerative Knee 177
J. Richard Steadman, MD

13 Joint Preservation: Care of the Older Athlete 185
William I. Sterett, MD, Mark Adickes, MD, and Karen Briggs, MPH

14 A Look Beyond the Horizon 197
William G. Rodkey, DVM

15 Rehabilitation Principles 203
Steve Stalzer, MSPT, John Atkins, MS, ATC, and Gene Hagerman, PhD

16 The Horse-Human Relationship: Research and the Future 221
C. Wayne McIlwraith, BVSc, PhD, DSc, FRCVS and William G. Rodkey, DVM

17 Functional Biomechanics of Healthy, Anterior Cruciate Ligament-Deficient and -Reconstructed Knees 229
Kevin B. Shelburne, PhD, Marcus G. Pandy, PhD, and Michael R. Torry, PhD

The Pursuit of the Crucial Principles 246
John A. Feagin, Jr., MD, and J. Richard Steadman, MD

Index 247

Contributors

MARK S. ADICKES, MD Roger Clemons Institute for Sports Medicine, Houston, Texas

JOHN ATKINS, MS, ATC Howard Head Sports Medicine Center, Vail, Colorado

KAREN K. BRIGGS, MPH Steadman Hawkins Research Foundation, Director of Clinical Research, Vail, Colorado

SCOTT F. DYE, MD Associate Clinical Professor of Orthopaedic Surgery and Co-Director, Sports Injury Clinic, University of California, San Francisco; Department of Orthopaedic Surgery, California Pacific Medical Center, Davies Campus, San Francisco, California

JOHN A. FEAGIN, JR., MD, FACS Col. US Army (Retired); Associate Professor Emeritus, Duke University, Durham, North Carolina; Clinical Professor, Department of Surgery, Uniformed Services University of Health Sciences, F. Edward Hebert School of Medicine, Bethesda, Maryland

GENE "TOPPER" HAGERMAN, PHD Howard Head Sports Medicine Center, Vail, Colorado

CHARLES P. HO, PHD, MD Medical Director, National Orthopedic Imaging Associates, California Advanced Imaging, Atherton, California

MININDER S. KOCHER, MD, MPH Associate Director, Division of Sports Medicine, Department of Orthopaedic Surgery, Children's Hospital; Associate Professor of Orthopaedic Surgery, Harvard Medical School, Harvard School of Public Health; Team Physician, Boston Public Schools, Babson College, Boston Ballet, and Boston Marathon, Boston, Massachusetts

C. WAYNE MCILWRAITH, BVSc, PHD, DSc, FRCVS Barbara Cox Anthony University Chair, Professor and Director, Orthopaedic Research Center, Colorado State University, Fort Collins, Colorado

PETER J. MILLETT, MD, MSC Consultant Montreal Canadians, United States Ski Team Physician, Steadman Hawkins Clinic, Steadman Hawkins Research Foundation, Vail, Colorado

MARCUS G. PANDY, PHD Professor and Chair of Mechanical and Biomedical Engineering, Department of Mechanical Engineering, The University of Melbourne, Victoria, Australia

WILLIAM G. RODKEY, DVM Diplomate, American College of Veterinary Surgeons Director, Basic Science Research, Steadman Hawkins Research Foundation; Vice President Scientific Affairs, ReGen Biologics, Inc., Vail, Colorado

KEVIN B. SHELBURNE, PHD Senior Scientist and Assistant Director, Biomechanics Research Laboratory, Steadman Hawkins Research Foundation, Vail, Colorado

STEVE STALZER, MSPT, SCS Clinic Director, Howard Head Sports Medicine Centers, Vail Valley Medical Center, Vail, Colorado

J. RICHARD STEADMAN, MD Chairman, Medical Group, and Chief Physician, US Ski and Snowboard Team; Team Physician, Denver Broncos; Clinical Professor, University of Texas Southwestern Medical School; Managing Partner, Steadman Hawkins Clinic; Chairman & Founder, Steadman Hawkins Research Foundation, Vail, Colorado

WILLIAM I. STERETT, MD Chief of Surgery, Vail Valley Medical Center; Head Physician, US Women's Alpine Ski Team; Steadman Hawkins Clinic, Vail, Colorado

ALLSTON J. STUBBS, MD The North Carolina Sports Medicine Institute, Winston-Salem, North Carolina

MICHAEL R. TORRY, PHD Director, Biomechanics Research Laboratory, Steadman Hawkins Research Foundation, Vail, Colorado

Foreword

Sports today has become an important part of our civilization as well as of our social life. With the multitude of sports activities available, the number of injuries has increased tremendously. This evolution in sports activities especially affects the knee. The knee—with its special joint congruence, not given by the configuration of the bones but by the ligaments and the menisci—has its own functional congruence that allows the most differentiated function in six degrees of freedom within the individual envelope of motion.

Our goal is to enable the patient to regain normal function after serious knee trauma. It is easier to fix a fracture back into anatomic position than to restore critical function when the key ligaments are disrupted. The knowledge of the usual macrobiomechanics is no longer sufficient: we have to go deeply into the micro- and nanobiomechanics as well as the molecular field for better understanding the consequences of the trauma and the possibilities of repair of all the involved tissues.

Because 10% to 20% of the estimated 175,000 yearly anterior cruciate ligament reconstructions end up with a suboptimal and unsatisfying result, the American Orthopaedic Society for Sports Medicine (AOSSM) initiated a multicenter study in 78 centers. This indicates that there is a need to look more closely at the pathomechanics of the injury, the types of lesions, and the physical possibilities of tissue healing and restoration.

Our teacher, Carl Henschen, Professor of Surgery at the Basel University, stated more than 60 years ago: "Do not disturb the intelligence of the tissues!" This is essential for the body's own healing and repair under anatomically and biomechanically correct conditions. All that we now know from macro- to micro- to nanobiomechanics, and even downsized to the molecular processes, does not allow us to neglect the clinical basis of care with a classic anamnesis including the patient's history, the mechanism of trauma, and the physical examination under the principles of "Listen, Look, Examine." And who could be a better teacher for the art of examining and evaluating the patient's findings than the first main author, John A. Feagin? This was already shown in his first two very successful books on the crucial ligaments. For the final decision-making, he discusses the actual technical possibilities of imaging with x-rays and magnetic resonance imaging as well as arthroscopy, if necessary. When it comes to the treatment, either nonoperative or operative, good knowledge about anatomy and biomechanics, based on scientific research, is mandatory.

The second main author, J. Richard Steadman, with his great experience over many years in nonoperative and operative treatment, guarantees a therapeutic overview of the highest standard. Dr. Steadman also shows how the intelligence of the tissues can be stimulated in order to use the potency of natural restoration.

Besides anatomically correct positioning of an anterior cruciate ligament (ACL) graft, the possibilities of biological stimulation with microfracture for the activation of the healing response in special cases of proximal ACL rupture and for cartilage regeneration are explained and the techniques meticulously described. All 17 chapters are written in the best didactic manner by the most competent experts in the different involved fields of knee repair. The latter part of the book deals with the degenerative knee, followed by a rehabilitation section with the very well-adapted procedures for the different lesions, repairs, and patient conditions.

After all the years during which many ACL graft placements have not been anatomically correct because of misguidance resulting from inappropriate instrumentation and biomechanically wrong theories, quite a few people began to believe that the double-bundle technique is now the solution. The authors of this book show that the correct anatomic placement of the ACL graft, even as one strong bundle alone with a corresponding and adequate operative technique, leads to a highly sufficient functional result. All this well-documented knowledge will help to us come to a better and more successful treatment for the injured knee, to the benefit of the patient.

Werner Müller, Prof. Med
Basel, Switzerland

Preface

The Crucial Principles in Care of the Knee is written to bring the essence and essentials of modern knee surgery to you—the forward-thinking knee surgeon.

The text is a distillation of nearly 75 years of experience in the ever-progressive arena of knee surgery. Our quest throughout this experience has been to improve the care of the active athlete as well as our aging population. The "crucial principles" are those principles that have improved the care of our patients and made our careers enjoyable and successful.

We have not only covered the basics of physical examination and rehabilitation but also addressed in detail Dr. Steadman's contributions of microfracture, healing response, joint contracture, and care of the aging athlete. We are grateful to our other colleagues and contributors:

Drs. Adickes, Dye, Hagerman, Ho, Kocher, McIlwraith, Millett, Pandy, Rodkey, Shelburne, Sterett, Stubbs, and Torry, and also to Karen Briggs, John Atkins, and Steve Stalzer, who complement our experience with special areas of expertise and experience of their own.

We believe *The Crucial Principles in Care of the Knee* will serve you well in your practice, your community, and your teaching. Our every effort is to help you as you strive for better care of the knee and the very best for your patients. May these *Principles* guide you as they have guided us.

Godspeed!

John A. Feagin, Jr., MD
J. Richard Steadman, MD
Vail, Colorado, July 2007

Acknowledgments

For special help in preparing *The Crucial Principles:*

Karen Briggs and Lottie B. Applewhite, authors' editors, without whom this book would not have been possible.

Nancy Place and Marsha Dohrmann, whose illustrations brighten this text and whose professional expertise adds so much to our science

The staff at Lippincott, Bob Hurley, David Murphy, and all who have contributed so much to the quality we expected and enjoy in *The Crucial Principles*.

I especially would like to thank my wife, Gay, whose editing help and ideas contributed so much to my chapters in this text. I am grateful, as well, to my children, Lyon and Liddy, for their love and support, and for paying me the supreme compliment of also choosing to work in the field of orthopaedics.—JRS

Our Partners: William I. Sterett, MD, Randy W. Viola, MD, Donald S. Corneman, MD, DC, Marc J. Philippon, MD, David C. Karli, MD, Tom Hackett, MD, and Peter J. Millett, MD, Msc.

The Clinic and Foundation Staff, especially: Cristal, Shirley, Lyon, Mona, Mike Egan, Marc Prisant, John McMurtry, Norm Waite, Karen Briggs, Mike Torry, and Dr. William Rodkey.

The Scientific Advisory Committee: Steven P. Arnoczky, DVM, Richard J. Hawkins, MD, Charles Ho, MD, PhD, Mininder Kocher, MD, C. Wayne McIlwraith, DVM, PhD, Peter Millett, MD, Msc, Marcus G. Pandy, PhD, Marc Philippon, MD, William G. Rodkey, DVM, Juan J. Rodrigo, MD, Theodore Schlegel, MD, William I. Sterett, MD, and Savio Lau-Yuen Woo, PhD, Sc (Hon).

The Steadman Hawkins Research Foundation Board: Adam Aron, Harris Barton, Howard Berkowitz, Robert Bourne, Michael J. Egan, Julie Esrey, Jack Ferguson, George Gillett, Earl G. Graves, Ted Hartley, Richard J. Hawkins, MD, H. Mike Immel, The Honorable Jack Kemp, Arch J. McGill, John G. McMillian, Betsy Nagelsen–McCormack, Cynthia L. Nelson, Mary K. Noyes, Al Perkins, Marc J. Philippon, MD, Cynthia S. Piper, Steven Read, Damaris Skouras, Gay L. Steadman, William I. Sterett, MD, Stewart Turley, Norm Waite, and HM King Juan Carlos I of Spain.

The Fellows, 1983–2008

The Vail Valley Hospital and Staff: Mr. Greg Repetti, Ron Davis, Art Kelton, and the Hospital Board, Ed O'Brien, and the Vail Valley Medical Center Foundation.

The Operating Room and Outpatient Surgical Staffs

Our Major Commercial Support: Arthrex, Ossur, Smith & Nephew, Vail Valley Medical Center.

Special Donors: Mr. Herb Allen, Mr. and Mrs. Earl G. Graves, Sr., Mr. Kenneth G. Griffin, Mr. and Mrs. John W. Jordan, Mr. Jim Kennedy and the James M. Cox Jr. Foundation, Charles G. Koch Charitable Foundation, Glen Nelson, MD, Starvos S. Niarchos Foundation, Mr. and Mrs. Alan W. Perkins, and Mr. and Mrs. Steven Read.

Special Orthopaedic Mentors and Friends: My late uncles, John Ellis, MD, and Paul Ellis, MD, whose worthy example led me to the field of medicine, and James Weilbaecher, MD, my Chief during residency in New Orleans (JRS), the late Irving Cohen, MD, from residency days, Paul Fry, MD, my partners at the Tahoe Clinic, Bob Larson, MD, the late Jack Hughston, MD, Jay Rodrigo, MD, Werner Mueller, Dr med, Hans Mueller-Wohlfahrt, Dr med, the late Frank Bassett, MD, the late John Marshall, DVM, Stephen Arnocsky, DVM, Savio Woo, PhD, Van Mow, PhD, Richard J. Hawkins, MD, and so many more.

Dr. Wayne McIlwraith, Dr. Dave Frisbie, and Research Staff at Colorado State University

Dr. Charles Ho and the Imaging Team

The U.S. Ski Team and Snowboard Association: Bill Marolt, and all the medal winners and other skiers who helped us learn so much about the successful treatment and recovery from potentially career ending knee injuries.

Our Rehabilitation Team: The Howard Head Sports Medicine Center and Marty Head, John Atkins, Topper Hagerman, Steve Stalzer, Luke, and so many more.

Our colleagues in the American Orthopaedic Society for Sports Medicine and the European Society for Knee Surgery and Arthroscopy.

Special Friends in Life and the Vail Valley:

JRS: Rose and George Gillett: Through their vision and generosity the Steadman Hawkins Clinic and Research Foundation were created. Special thanks to the late President and Mrs. Gerald R. Ford, Mayor Rod Slifer and the Vail community, Dr. Jack Eck, Sheika and Pepi Gramshammer, Sally and Bill Hanlon, the Vail Ski Patrol, Bill Jensen and the entire Vail Resorts team, and the Vail Valley Foundation.

JAF: Drs. Dean Taylor and Tom Debererdino, Joachim Tenuta, Curt Alitz, Steve Svoboda, Jane Reddington, and the West Point Staff, and the John A. Feagin Jr. Sports Medicine Fellows.

Duke and Dr. Ralph Coonrad, Tony and Judy Seaber, William Garrett, "T." Moorman, Clyde Helms, Nancy Majors, Bryan Casey, Kevin Waters, Coach "K" staff and family, Mrs. Mary D. B. Semans, and so many more.

Patients and partners from the Army, Jackson, Wyoming, and Duke.

Venna Sparks, Andy Chambers, Peter Stiegler, Ken Lambert, Ray Cunningham, and the Jackson Team.

Reverend and Mrs. Dick Camp and The Christian Ministry in the National Parks.

Dr. and Mrs. William Stetson, Dr. and Mrs. Rodrigo Alvarez, and our Cuban colleagues.

John Logan and my fellow pilots.

Younger colleagues who have inspired me: Drs. Michel Berend, Ed Lilly, Tad Vail, Julian Feller, Walt Curl, Carl Savory, Champ Baker, Scott Dye, and so many more.

My West Point classmates and friends.

Fellow Army Orthopaedic Surgeons: Sterling Mutz, A.A. "Gus" White, Jerry Sisler, Bob Arciero, Jack Ryan, John Uhorchek, Winston Warme, John Dietz, and a host of others.

Dr. Stanley Hoppenfeld, who "planted" and nourished the idea for a "book."

Trudi and Raissa Wilkes and the Staff at 325 Mill Creek. Jack and Kathleen Eck, Dr. Ron Losee, Steve Oordt, Bill Bue, and Breg.

My Family: Marty my love and her family for their role in my life and loving support. Randle, Robert, Nancy, Jonathan, Connor, Katherine, and Jack Jeter, and all the extended family over all the years.

And to Gay and Richard Steadman for putting "the package together."

Most of All, Our Patients and Our Families

"If we have been able to see further it is because we have stood on the Shoulders of Giants."

—*adapted from Sir Isaac Newton*

How to Use This Book

A RECIPE AND A PHILOSOPHY

The Crucial Principles in Care of the Knee was conceived as a manual to define the principles and practice of knee care. Although intended primarily for the knee surgeon, it is also meant for the student who aspires to improve his or her physical examination technique, patient care, and understanding of the pathophysiology and rehabilitation of the knee-injured patient. These aspects are important because the knee is a frequently injured joint and is seldom forgiving. An early and precise diagnosis is desirable to patient and physician alike; it is cost-effective as well. This manual is for all who aspire to be better students, counselors, caregivers, teachers, and surgeons.

The text is divided into two parts:

Part 1. The crucial principles in the diagnosis and treatment of knee injuries with three case studies is intended to review the basics of knee examination and to integrate the art and science of diagnosis and treatment into the more complex issues of knee care that are presented in Part 2.

Part 1 is, in large part, adopted from *The Crucial Ligaments* and emphasizes the fundamentals of knee care and interaction with the patient.

Part 2. The crucial principles are applied to advanced surgical care of the knee. The life's work of Dr. Steadman as evidenced by examination of the topics of microfracture, healing response, joint contracture, and care of the aging athlete are presented and discussed in detail with emphasis on basic science, the pathophysiology, and research applied to these difficult, but often encountered, knee problems.

Rehabilitation, the crown jewel of orthopaedics and knee surgery, is discussed in detail for each operation included. As our surgery becomes more complex, our rehabilitation must become science-based.

A specific advantage of Part 2 of *The Crucial Principles* is that the database of more than 8,000 cases from the Steadman-Hawkins Clinic has been used extensively to present the elements of treating the knee. This database has proved invaluable in developing our principles and practice of knee care.

We hope you enjoy *The Crucial Principles in Care of the Knee*. Also, we hope you find these principles and experiences beneficial to you as you care for the knee-injured patient.

We are deeply indebted to our co-authors and our many colleagues around the world who have shared their experiences and enriched our lives with their teachings.

JAF
JRS

The Crucial Principles
in Care of the Knee

The ACL-Deficient Knee: Some Thoughts—Past and Future

John A. Feagin, Jr.

Problems left unattended within the knee do not become easier with the passage of time. . . Technology is an essential adjunct to our surgical management of the knee. Today we are appropriately selective in our choice of techniques; tomorrow we must be precisely selective in our use of technological advances. We are in the dawn of greatly improved treatment of the knee.

The Crucial Ligaments,
second edition, 1994, page 4

NATURAL HISTORY OF THE ACL-DEFICIENT KNEE

The natural history of the anterior cruciate ligament (ACL)-deficient knee is still imperfect. The patient plays a critical role and partners with the surgeon in establishing the unique natural history of the knee. Sometimes the surgeon can harness the patient's ability and energy to enhance the end result, but sometimes the patient is not in concert with the optimum treatment plan. Thus, the art and science of knee surgery and the lessons learned through experience are presented in this text.

Patient Selectivity

Not all patients need an ACL. Partial tears of the ACL are common. The ACL is a proprioceptive neural tube. The question often is: Does sufficient strength and function remain after ACL injury to provide adequate function and protect against further knee damage? What are the biomechanical demands?

Does the patient depend on the knee for enjoyment and participation in cutting sports or was this injury incidental to an unusual activity? The Tegner scale is helpful in establishing the past and expected level of activity. Dale Daniel believed that an athlete committed to 1 hour of exercise daily needed an ACL (D. Daniel, personal communication, Jan. 1976). I have found that asking the patient if he/she exercised for an hour each day is useful.

The surgeon must guide the patient to the successful selection of the best treatment regimen for that patient and his or her unique demands.

Surgical Methodology

The multiplicity of successful surgical solutions for today's knee-injured patient has amazed me. Bone-patella-bone replacement, hamstring grafts, allografts, primary repair, healing response, and even prostheses have all been successful in selected patients with appropriate demands. For sure, we have learned that accurate anatomic restoration and adequate fixation are more important than graft selection. Every effort made toward anatomic restoration, functional competence, fixation, and reproducibility is worthwhile. This is the essence of our surgical competence today.

Rehabilitation

I am not sure we fully understand rehabilitation and the ACL-compromised knee. Certainly we can show that particular regimens are less stressful to the ACL, that joint contracture is reduced by early motion, and that our patients are able to return to their desired activities at an earlier time, but this is problematic and programmatic progress, not scientific progress. The ACL is a complex neural ligament with proprioceptive feedback to both quadriceps and hamstrings controlling six degrees of freedom. Does our rehabilitation acknowledge the neural elements of ligamentous and supporting capsular structures? I think not; certainly not well enough or often enough. We should optimize our functional rehabilitation and seek more science.

Our Surgical Future

Neither the patient nor the surgeon will accept compromised function or prolonged disability. Patients' expectations are always on the increase. A return to "normal" or preinjury level is their goal. They demand more and more of us and more and more they impose their goals on our standards. This is a desirable partnership. No member of the team should accept less than the best. "We are not there yet" but we have come a long way. The future is not for the faint but for the committed, that is, the team leaders like yourselves.

I

The Basics: Physical Examination and Three Classic Case Studies

The Crucial Principles and the Care of the Knee-Injured Patient

1

John A. Feagin, Jr.

■ **INTRODUCTION: THE EVOLUTION AND APPLICATION OF THE CRUCIAL PRINCIPLES 7**

■ **PRINCIPLE I. THREE-DIMENSIONAL ANATOMIC DIAGNOSIS 8**
Anatomic Diagnosis of ACL Deficiency or
    ACL Ruptures 8
Kinematic Competence 8
Anatomic Diagnosis, Prognosis, and Kinematic
    Competence of the Knee 8

■ **PRINCIPLE II. TREATMENT PROGRAM AIMED AT OPTIMIZING FUNCTION 8**
The Process Behind Diagnosis 8
Return of Function within Realistic Expectations 9

■ **PRINCIPLE III. SURGERY MAXIMIZING THE BODY'S POTENTIAL 9**

■ **PRINCIPLE IV. REHABILITATION AIMED AT RETURN TO ACTIVITY WITHIN THE ENVELOPE OF REALISTIC FUNCTION 9**
Rehabilitation 9
"Within an Envelope of Realistic Function" 9

■ **PRINCIPLE V. COMMUNICATION BETWEEN PATIENT AND TEAM 9**
Communication Skills 9
Communicating with the Team 10

■ **PRINCIPLE VI. MAINTENANCE OF A DATABASE THAT VALIDATES THE CRUCIAL PRINCIPLES 10**

INTRODUCTION: THE EVOLUTION AND APPLICATION OF THE CRUCIAL PRINCIPLES

As we grow in experience, we try to simplify and codify for those who follow. Sometimes that becomes a mantra, strikes a familiar chord, or gives the reader the "ah-ha" phenomenon. I cannot claim an experience of this magnitude for the six crucial principles but, on the other hand, surely we have enjoyed enough science in knee surgery to give structure to our thought process.

For me, the six principles—anatomic diagnosis; treatment aimed at optimizing function; surgery maximizing the body's healing potential; rehabilitation within the envelope of realistic function; communication between patient, surgeon, and team; and maintenance of a database—capture the essence and expertise in the care of the knee. These six principles are not meant to be exclusive; they are meant to challenge you and encourage you to reformulate and improve these principles to meet your expanding knowledge of the knee.

The principles espoused are perhaps overdistilled and "overdidactic," but the "longest journey begins with a single step" and they are a stepping-off point into the craft of knee care for master or novice.

I encourage you to visit these principles now with an eye toward your practice skills and to revisit them as your experience and skills grow. You will then amplify and improve these principles and the quest will have been worth your effort and mine.

The Crucial Principles

Principle I. Three-dimensional anatomic diagnosis

Principle II. Treatment program aimed at optimizing function

Principle III. Surgery maximizing the body's potential

Principle IV. Rehabilitation aimed at return to activity within the envelope of realistic function

Principle V. Communication between patient and team

Principle VI. Maintenance of a database that validates the crucial principles

Principle I. A Three-Dimensional Anatomic Diagnosis with an Understanding of the Requisites for Kinematic Competence

Anatomic Diagnosis of ACL Deficiency or ACL Ruptures

Accurate anatomic diagnosis has always been our quest and a right of the patient. The past three decades emphasize the progress we have made in this quest. The biomechanical principles of primary and secondary restraints were established by Butler et al.[1] The concepts of rotatory laxity and the pivot shift were promulgated by Slocum and Larson,[2] Liorzou,[3] Losee,[4] Losee et al.,[5] and Kocher et al.[6] Documentation as directed by the International Knee Documentation Committee, direct view by arthroscopy and imaging by magnetic resonance imaging, computed axial tomographic scanning, and technetium scanning have empowered us with the ability to make a three-dimensional anatomic diagnosis of the highest order of accuracy at both macroscopic and microscopic levels. We should expect no less.

Kinematic Competence

Too long, we have been "hung up" on form. We have not been precise enough in considering functional competence. A patient who did not complain was considered functionally intact. We now see many patients who had reconstructed anterior cruciate ligaments (ACLs) 15 to 20 years previously and who returned to a high level of function and are now showing degenerative changes with an excess of medial compartment loading.

We do need to integrate into the rather static equation, a dynamic understanding of which way the pathologic process is heading and how fast, that is, is Mother Nature doing her utmost to heal the insult of overuse or has the

process played out and a ~~biologic stimulus~~, such as microfracture, is needed? Certainly when we look at fracture imaging, this is uppermost in our minds. Should it not be the same where soft tissue and the knee are involved? Is postoperative osteoarthrosis a concomitant of surgical intervention, or have we failed to restore kinematic competence? I wish I knew the answer with certainty. I suspect both are implicated and related. On postoperative physical examination, if I can elicit some anatomic flaw that affects kinematic competence, whether this will be in limited mobility of the patellofemoral joint or as a subtle pivot glide with increased varus-valgus laxity, I know these are related to a less-than-perfect ACL construct.

~~Our goal should be to seek kinematic competence as well as anatomic form.~~ Our methods of measurement have improved so that we are now able to measure restoration of anatomic form. We can now demand much more from our kinematic knowledge base. The best example of past failures that exemplifies this concept is our extra-articular repairs,[7] which featured so prominently in our surgical techniques of the 1980s.

Anatomic Diagnosis, Prognosis, and Kinematic Competence of the Knee

Patients with ligamentous injuries deserve ~~accurate anatomic diagnosis and restoration of kinematic~~ competence. The concept of diagnosis as a dynamic process, that leads us also to a prognosis is important. This is what we mean by three-dimensional anatomic diagnosis: juxtaposition of the anatomic, the pathophysiologic, and the temporal considerations. We should strive for a prognosis as well as a diagnosis, for the patient's consideration as well as our own discipline.

Principle II. A Treatment Program Aimed at Optimizing Return of Function within Realistic Expectations

The Process Behind the Diagnosis

~~A diagnosis is but a moment in time; a point of departure.~~ Diagnoses are simple enough now with the aid of magnetic resonance imaging. Patients expect a buzzword, "You blew out your ACL."

Yet, the buzzword is not enough for either the surgeon or the patient. The joy comes with the understanding of the process behind the diagnosis: the mechanism of injury, the body's reaction to the injury, the direction and rate of change at the cellular level, and the prognosis. Sharing this knowledge with the patient enhances the patient's understanding, and this new-found knowledge will enhance the healing process. Sharing the injury process with the patient will enhance the bond between patient and physician and will send the signal that this is an interactive, cooperative, team process, a work in progress. The necessity for a comprehensive program is based on an infinite number of factors. Too often, the patient "factors" are left out of the plan or the program. The expectations, the time framework, the work implications, the emotional context, the past experiences, trust, compliance, cooperation, and commitment are essential. *Never, never end up with just the diagnosis.* Garner every bit of success you and the patient deserve from the plan and process, the successful resolution of the pathophysiologic process. A review of Chapter 2 and its discussion of physical examination will help you understand my thoughts on this matter and how physical examination and anatomic diagnosis lead to a plan, prognosis, and a program, all of which are equally as important as the diagnosis.

Return of Function within Realistic Expectations

Too much too soon can sometimes be as inappropriate as too little too late. To be in step and in sync with the healing process is essential. The second step is to determine the biomechanics of the functional demands of the patient and of the end result. Of course, our goal is to return the patient to normal, to their best, and to their preinjury level of function, however almost every elite athlete's career terminates because of the limitations of injury, whether it is one severe blow or a series of minor injuries. Therefore, dealing with the ultimate limitations of the pathophysiologic process is, in itself, an art and a science. Scott Dye[8] has written eloquently on this subject and encourages us to understand and apply the concept of the envelope of function and load acceptance to our healing art. He is so right.

Principle III. Surgery Maximizing the Body's Healing Potential Through Anatomic Restoration and Restoration of Kinematic Competence

Much of our philosophy regarding the crucial principles is included in Principles I and II. Because we are surgeons, heart and soul, we think surgically. This is understandable and acceptable, provided that we think within the foregoing pathologic process and are certain that surgery is the best and fastest solution to restore function and long-term kinematic competence. We also must be certain that our timing of surgery is appropriate for the healing process and that the force and discipline of rehabilitation have been maximized. Easy to verbalize, not easy to teach, and often difficult to conceptualize. The judgment that is implicit—when to apply our hard-earned, hard-won, highly effective surgical techniques—is the crux of this principle and the essence of this text.

Principle IV. Rehabilitation Aimed at Return of Activity within the Envelope of Realistic Function

Rehabilitation

So often I see rehabilitation applied in rote or cookbook fashion. One size fits all. Too often the communication process between surgeon and rehabilitation specialist, whether it be preoperative or postoperative, is such that "this is the best that can be done." A thinking surgeon who applies Principles I, II, and III, in concert with a thinking rehabilitation specialist and a concerned patient, are one of the most powerful forces and teams we have in medicine. The application of this teamwork to patient care has been the hallmark of the Steadman Clinic for more than 20 years. The database and patient loyalty reflect the advantages and efforts of this teamwork.

The critical component to this principle is *timely and effective communication. The time you spend in application of Principle IV is probably the crucial principle through which you achieve the most progress and the most satisfaction from your practice and patient care (see Chapter 13). Always be "building your team" and always include the patient.*

"Within an Envelope of Realistic Function"

Sometimes realistic function must be arrived at over a span of time with the patient. Certainly, one does not want to counsel a patient on a career-ending injury at the instant of injury. Return of realistic function takes time to ascertain. The patient and the physician must be in concert on this matter. *They must define return of realistic function in the appropriate time framework requisite to the needs of the patient.*

Principle V. Communication with the Patient and Team that Engenders Confidence and Success and Promotes a Sense of Well-Being

Communication Skills

One-way directed communication in medicine is no longer the norm. The communication skills essential to the teacher, the team leader, and family are equally as essential to the physician. Our words and our body language must soothe, engender confidence, transmit information, promote well-being, and muster the team. *The acquisition of appropriate effective communication skills is a lifelong quest.* Your patients will appreciate your concern for this vital area of your profession and your days will grow in grace. Clinic becomes an ideal time and place to develop and practice these skills. Effective communication with the patient will save you both time and frustration. ~~To carry this one step further, I have made a practice of dictating the note on my new patient in the form of a letter to the patient that reiterates the symptoms, the diagnostic studies, the diagnosis, and the plan. These letters stood me in good stead many~~ times during many years.

Communicating with the Team

The nurse, the rehabilitation specialist, and your operating room technician are seldom there at the same time. Yet, your team-building skills and communication are time-sensitive. The solution is twofold. First, secure an administrative assistant who is by your side in the clinic and understands that he or she is your communication arm. Second, regular postoperative rounds with the rehabilitation team and the patient facilitates communication.

The "by-your-side administrative assistant" can be of any discipline, but I have found that a rehabilitation specialist (athletic trainer or physical therapist) is the most effective. They are best able to facilitate your diagnostic efforts and the preoperative and postoperative care for each patient. Their thinking, as a result of their training, is more parallel to your own. Athletic trainers and operating room nurses with some exposure to physical therapy have also worked well for me in this role. These critical support personnel facilitate communications, make the patient feel inclusive, and rally the team. They add a joy to your day, purpose to your work, and often "save the bacon."

Regular postoperative rounds with the rehabilitation specialists are the second essential of organization in your professional life. Your patients and your team appreciate this critical time during which progress is recorded, problems can be addressed, and adjustments effected. Your administrative assistant is there too—coordinating, complementing, and facilitating; generally "picking up the pieces." The team is humming. They understand you are committed to the best and they want the best. Their strength comes from you, the patient, and their pride. This is your "finest hour." Almost all the "greats" I have known in orthopaedics use such a format.

Principle VI. The Maintenance of the Database that Validates the Crucial Principles

---

Principle VI is neither as obvious as the foregoing principle nor as well-defined. We say in academia that "He who has the best database usually wins," but we are not all in academia nor do we care to be. A database does not have to implicate a huge computer effort. A database denotes respon-

sible patient management. A visual analog scale or the SANE (subjective assessment numeric evaluation) index reference is helpful. We should know where our patients come from. Do we lose track of our patients, are they satisfied with our office procedures, are they comfortable with the quality of their care, is the outcome of the surgery what they expected, and were they able to optimize their return to function through rehabilitation? In other words, are we available and able!

The database provides guidelines of value to patient, physician, and the team.

Principle VI, perhaps more than any other, requires thought and management on a regular basis to ensure quality in matches quality out. The "database" cannot consume us, but must serve us to manage our time, our practice, and our patients more effectively and efficiently.

SUMMARY

We have discussed six crucial principles. I am sure there are many more awaiting our discovery. This is not meant to be an end-all or a be-all, it is merely meant to emphasize that knee surgery has come a long way, and we can now be principle-based. When I started performing knee surgery, it was definitely "anecdote"-based and the foundation was uncertain. Nevertheless, those great surgeons of yesteryear pointed the way and knew the direction. They were great leaders and motivators and paved the way for the scientist. Enjoy these principles, apply them, critique them, amplify them, and move forward to the next level. Bring your patients and team along on the journey.

REFERENCES

1. Butler DL, Noyes FR, Grood ES. Ligamentous restraints to anterior-posterior drawer in the human knee. A biomechanical study. *J Bone Joint Surg Am* 1980;62:259–270.
2. Slocum DB, Larson RL. Rotatory instability of the knee. Its pathogenesis and a clinical test to demonstrate its presence. *J Bone Joint Surg Am* 1968;50:211-255.
3. Liorzou F. *Le Genou Ligamentaire* [Knee Ligaments, Clinical Examination]. Heidelberg: Springer-Verlag, 1990.
4. Losee RE. Diagnosis of chronic injury to the anterior cruciate ligament. *Orthop Clin North Am* 1985;16:83-97.
5. Losee RE, Johnson TR, Southwick WO. Anterior subluxation of the lateral tibial plateau. A diagnostic test and operative repair. *J Bone Joint Surg Am* 1978;60:1015-1030.
6. Kocher MS, Steadman JR, Briggs KK, Sterett WI, Hawkins RJ. Relationships between objective assessment of ligament stability and subjective assessment of symptoms and function after anterior cruciate ligament reconstruction. *Am J Sports Med* 2004;32:629-634.
7. Andrews JR, Sander R. A "mini-reconstruction" technique in treating anterolateral rotatory instability (ALRI). *Clin Orthop* 1983;172:93-96.
8. Dye SF. An evolutionary prospective. In: Feagin JA, ed. *The Crucial Ligaments*, 2nd ed. New York: Churchill Livingston, 1994;223-234.

Principles of Diagnosis and Treatment

2

John A. Feagin, Jr.

■ **INTRODUCTION 11**

■ **HISTORY AND MECHANISMS OF TRAUMA 12**
History of Previous Injury 12
Mechanism of Injury 12
Pain 12
Pop 12
Onset of Swelling 13

■ **PRINCIPLES OF PHYSICAL EXAMINATION 13**
Inspection—Look! 13
Palpation—Feel! 13
Movement—Move! 13
Flexion/Extension 13
Varus/Valgus Angulation 14
Anteroposterior Glide—The Lachman or
   Drawer Test 14
Rotation 15
Combined Anteroposterior Glide and Rotation 15
Patella 15

■ **PHYSICAL EXAMINATION TESTS 15**
Lachman Test 15
Pivot Shift Tests 18

■ **ADJUNCT TESTS 18**

■ **EXAMINATION UNDER ANESTHESIA 20**

■ **IMAGING 20**
Radiographic Standard Views 20
Stress Radiographs 20
Magnetic Resonance Imaging 20

■ **ARTHROSCOPY 22**

■ **DECISION-MAKING 22**

■ **REHABILITATION 24**

■ **COMMENT 24**

Part I of *The Crucial Principles* is devoted to principles of diagnosis and treatment of the knee-injured patient. These principles are illustrated in three key case studies (see Chapter 3).

The skills necessary for the diagnosis and treatment of knee ligament injuries are hard-earned and are the result of a never-ending quest for excellence. These skills are passed from generation to generation, perhaps more through the spoken word than through our texts. These skills form the basis of good judgment and become sources of unending pride.

One of the great teachers of orthopaedics had this to say:

> Accurate diagnosis, the essential preliminary to appropriate treatment, is difficult because the diagnostic pathway is beset by tripwires. A detailed history of the injury is seldom obtainable; the most complete ligamentous and capsular disruptions are often the least painful because the sensory nerve fibers also are torn, and sometimes they are the least swollen (because the torn capsule allows the effusion to leak away). Moreover, even an innocent radiograph can be misleading, because a ligament whose substance is torn is more difficult to repair than that which has avulsed its bony attachment. For all these reasons and because the initial physical assessment may determine the entire future athletic life of the patient, the initial examination must be both meticulous and systematic.*

---

*A. Graham Apley, FRCS, MB, MRCS, editor emeritus of the British issue of the *Journal of Bone and Joint Surgery* (personal communication, Jackson, Wyoming, May 1986).

It would be impossible to acknowledge all who, like A. Graham Apley, have guided me with their wisdom and philosophy. Readers will get to know these mentors of mine in this book or in the selected bibliography. The bibliography is a collection of readings from colleagues the world over whose contributions form the core of science and experience that is fundamental to the care of the knee.

The information and philosophy presented under this chapter title, "Principles of Diagnosis and Treatment," should be kept in mind while reading the case studies. References accompany each case study. Also, within the case study, the reader may be referred to other chapters within the text.

HISTORY AND MECHANISMS OF TRAUMA

In athletic trauma, the history is usually quite straightforward and the patient usually is aware of the details and circumstances. This is a luxury not always found in the other fields of trauma. In obtaining the history, the physician should elicit from the patient the history of previous injury or dysfunction and the mechanism of injury. Also, the patient may tell the physician about the swelling (immediate or delayed), the pain, and the ability to continue participation in daily activities or athletics.

History of Previous Injury

Is the injury truly acute or was there a previous laxity or disability? Too often, the athlete "forgets" that the knee was previously injured. Once reminded, the athlete can usually offer the details. These details take on added meaning when the radiographic films are reviewed, as one seeks evidence of old injuries through osteophyte formation.

Simple as it is, the history can be a useful diagnostic tool. In fact, in my experience, deceleration, cutting injuries that are associated with a pop and with the gradual onset of effusion during the ensuing 24 hours will prove in 85% of cases to be an anterior cruciate ligament (ACL) injury. Because an ACL tear is seldom an isolated injury, the examiner's task is to verify the ACL tear and seek out associated injuries through the physical examination.

Mechanism of Injury

The mechanism of injury alerts the physician to which ligaments were at risk in the knee. In Case Study 2, the mechanism of injury is a change of direction involving deceleration with the foot fixed and contact with another player. This classic injury of American football is often called the O'Donoghue triad—a tear of the ACL, the medial collateral ligament (MCL), and the medial meniscus.

As shoe/turf and ski/boot fixation devices have become more efficient, we now often see injuries caused by deceleration and change of direction that do not involve contact with another player. This type of injury is associated with a "pop," the inability to continue "play," and the onset during the next 24 hours of a relatively tense effusion. This mechanism was initially associated with the "isolated tear of the ACL," but with time and sophistication, it has become clear that there is seldom an isolated ligamentous injury to the knee. *The knee is a harmonius symphony of ligaments, in which no ligament stands alone.*

Another mechanism of injury, which occurs predominantly in the skier, is an abrupt contraction by the quadriceps to regain balance—similar to a powerful Lachman test—which pulls the tibia forward on the femur and tears the ACL. This injury may not even be associated with a fall.

There are other mechanisms of injury, but these three predominate and will serve the clinician well:

- Contact with another player and change of direction and deceleration with fixed foot.
- No contact with a player, but change of direction and deceleration.
- Abrupt contraction of the quadriceps to regain balance.

Pain

Many patients are able to walk off the field or ski down a slope after a severe ligamentous injury. Pain is certainly a characteristic of these injuries, but perhaps the feeling of subluxation is more ominous and limiting to the patient. *A tried-and-true dictum of ligament injury is that the more pain, the less severe the injury.* It is probable that a complete tear so disrupts the nerve fibers that the pain is less severe. Certainly, in a complete tear, one can "open" the joint more readily with less discomfort to the patient.

Pop

The pop is characteristic of a tear of the ACL. We know from Biomechanical studies that the helicoid arrangement of the ACL allows it to store considerable energy before its elastic limit is reached. As a result, when the elastic limit is reached, the ligament bursts convulsively, and the patient defines this sensation as "a pop."

The pop is the part of the history that most reliably indicates an ACL tear. Neither the MCL nor the capsuloligamentous structures tear with this pop, perhaps because they have broader origins and insertions and are generally flattened rather then helicoid. At any rate, the pop is characteristic of a tear of the ACL. It has been my experience that few people will continue to play after sustaining a complete ACL tear. If they do continue, a more extensive injury may result, that is, subluxation of the tibia on the femur with increased structural damage.

Onset of Swelling

The onset and amount of swelling is an important diagnostic clue. Swelling that can be appreciated by physical examination is often delayed 6 to 24 hours. In the case of the ACL, the artery, a branch of the posterior geniculate, is not substantial and is easily tamponaded. In the surgical care of acute cases, blood has been seen to "drip much like a leaky faucet." This explains the slow accumulation of the effusion. If the effusion is contained by the capsular mechanism, then it will reach maximum within 12 to 24 hours. If, however, a lesion of the capsule coexists with the ACL injury, the effusion may be slight because the fluid escapes through a rent in the capsuloligamentous structure.

If effusion develops immediately after injury, one should suspect an osteochondral fracture. Bleeding into the joint is more brisk with an osteochondral fracture than with a torn ACL; this distinction is a subtle diagnostic clue. The fluid is usually aspirated because its character and the presence or absence of fat are important diagnostic signs.

PRINCIPLES OF PHYSICAL EXAMINATION

The specific ligamentous injury is sought primarily by comparing the excursion of the tibia on the femur in the injured and uninjured knee. This is done by imparting stress through a range of motion. This can be quite precise, particularly if the clinician can get the patient to relax while the well leg is examined first. *Using the well leg as a standard for comparison is a must.*

The position of comfort for the patient is frequently the position in which the patient is found. I prefer to begin the examination with the patient in this position. The initial examination can be particularly revealing when it occurs before the onset of effusion and muscle spasm. A single examination is not always definitive. Re-examination is essential and appropriate.

Sometimes a change in venue will help both physician and patient to relax and will result in a more productive physical examination. Ice is a useful adjunct to the physical examination as it decreases pain and promotes relaxation. The sideline is often not conducive to meticulous attention to detail required by both patient and examiner. A change of venue and circumstances may be advantageous and should be determined by the examiner.

Inspection—Look!

The injured knee must be considered in the context of the entire patient. The patient's physiologic age, body fat, and muscle mass reflect his or her previous selection of activities. I consider these to be key observations during the physical examination. The brachioradialis and gastrocsoleus are excellent muscles to observe because they are seldom developed by adult activity and thus reflect the activities of youth.

Besides the knee, the leg as a whole should be inspected. Is the skin intact? Are there abrasions, old scars, or bruising? The skin may give information about the direction, force, and mechanism of injury and the history. The alignment of the lower limb segments and any atrophy or swelling should be noted. These observations lead to the laying on of the hands—palpation.

Palpation—Feel!

The hands of the skilled examiner are a wonderful arthrometer. The palpatory examination of the knee involves a subtle gradient of force application. The initial laying on of the hands is performed on the normal side with only sufficient pressure to feel the subtleties of the knee's form. This complements the visual inspection. When the form is ascertained, more pressure is applied to distinguish induration—the firmness of the tissue planes. Induration often is the clue to the severity as well as the site of injury. Gentle flexion of the knee, where possible, is helpful during this search for induration because it may separate some of the anatomic structures and help to localize more precisely the sites of injury.

Finally, palpation is conducted with slightly more vigor to identify tenderness. This must be performed with the patient's full knowledge and cooperation, and the patient must appreciate the precision with which this portion of the examination can be conducted. Gentleness is the key to this precision.

Problems left unattended within the knee do not become easier with the passage of time. Initial subtleties become blunted by induration, edema, and effusion, which develop days after injury. One misses important details by not examining the knee-injured patient shortly after the injury occurs.

Movements—Move!

Should the examiner begin with active or passive movements? I prefer to ask the patient to move the well leg within the range of motion that is comfortable and possible. This gives a standard of comparison for the injured leg. Then I ask the patient to move the injured extremity within the bounds of comfort. This shows the range of motion available to position the leg for the ligamentous examinations.

Flexion/Extension

One of the goals of movement is to place the extremity in the optimum position for isolating and examining the different ligamentous structures. If hyperextension can be achieved, it is a good position to begin. If the knee is stable in hyperextension, the medial and lateral capsuloligamentous structures and the posterior cruciate ligament (PCL) are intact. Thus, the maximum amount of information is gained quickly. The collateral ligaments are best examined

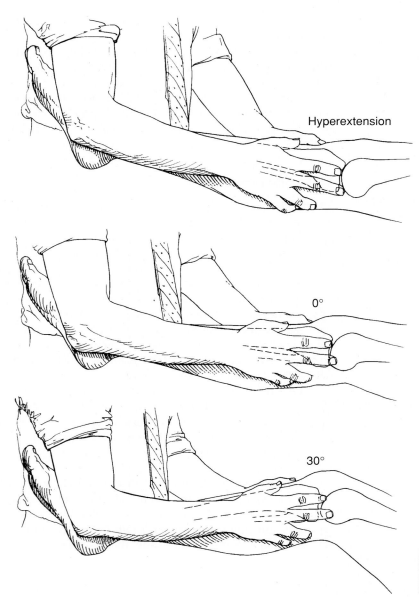

Hyperextension

0°

30°

Figure 2.1   The collateral ligaments are best examined at hyperextension, 0 degrees, and 30 degrees of knee flexion. The technique was taught to me by Smillie.

at hyperextension, neutral, and 30 degrees flexion (Fig. 2.1). The technique that Smillie (I. Smillie, Dundee, Scotland, personal communication, 1972) taught me still seems the most useful—the patient's foot is loosely constrained against the examiner's hip so both hands are free to palpate the joint lines and ligamentous structures.

Varus/Valgus Angulation

Laxity in hyperextension to varus or valgus angulation is an ominous sign that indicates disruption of key ligamentous structures. If in hyperextension the joint is lax to valgus angulation, the medial capsuloligamentous structures and the PCL are probably interrupted. If in hyperextension, the knee is lax to varus angulation, the arcuate complex and

PCL are probably disrupted. When varus and valgus are applied with the knee at 0 degrees of flexion, the ACL and PCL are slackened sufficiently that these tests are diagnostic of medial or lateral capsular injuries. At 30 degrees of flexion, the cruciate ligaments are in their most relaxed state, and pathologic laxity palpated is capsular laxity.

Anteroposterior Glide—The Lachman or Drawer Test

The essence of the physical examination is an appreciation of pathologic excursion of the tibia with respect to the femur. Anteroposterior (AP) glide is a particularly sensitive test, but may be misinterpreted if the relation of the tibia to the femur is not understood and the test is started in the wrong place.

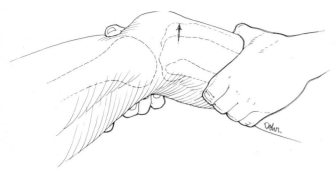

Figure 2.2   The Lachman test.

This misinterpretation most frequently occurs when the test is begun with the tibia inadvertently posteriorly subluxated on the femur. AP glide is best determined with the fingers measuring the translation of the tibia on the femur in an AP direction (Fig. 2.2). The fingers are quite accurate arthrometers, although perhaps often undertrained (see Chapter 1).

Rotation

The appreciation of increased rotatory excursion requires careful attention to detail. With the hip and knee flexed 90 degrees, internal and external rotation stress are applied first to the well and then to the injured leg (Fig. 2.3). This test can give quite meaningful information on the status of the

cruciate ligaments, as well as the complementary medial and lateral capsuloligamentous structures. I have found this test particularly useful to determine the envelope of motion.

Combined Anteroposterior Glide and Rotation

The pivot shift test is a combination of translation and rotation (Fig. 2.4). This test has been eloquently described by Losee et al.[1] and is referred to in Case Study 1 (see Chapter 3).

Patella

The patella, which after all is the second joint of the knee, is not to be underestimated or underdiagnosed. The patella should be examined for excursion, and the patient will indicate tenderness, pain, and apprehension (Figs. 2.5 and 2.6). This sometimes forgotten joint is too often the limiting factor after treatment. Thus, the initial physical examination is especially appropriate (see Case Study 3A and 3B).

PHYSICAL EXAMINATION TESTS

Lachman Test

Refinement of the physical examination has come through the work of the International Knee Documentation

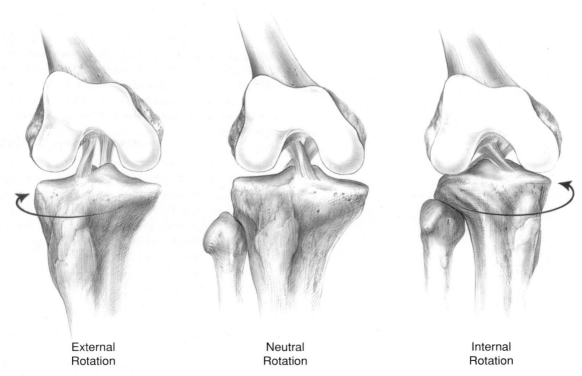

External Rotation   Neutral Rotation   Internal Rotation

Figure 2.3   Hip and knee flexed 90 degrees; tibia externally rotated, in neutral position, and internally rotated. Note the tightening of the cruciate ligaments with internal rotation.

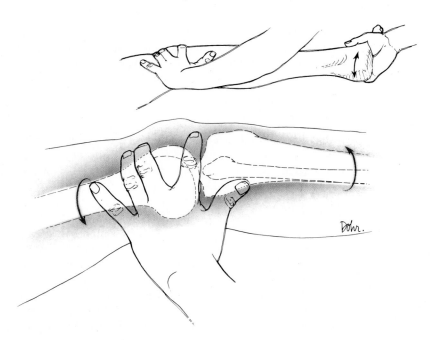

Figure 2.4 The pivot shift test as described by Losee.

Committee (IKDC). This committee, after thorough review of the anatomic and biomechanical knowledge available, proposed three key principles to physical examination:

1. The examination should define the primary restraints (ACL and PCL) and secondary restraints (MCL, posterior oblique ligament, lateral collateral ligament, and arcuate complex) so that physical examination will result in an *anatomic diagnosis.*
2. The dictum "one test—one ligament" could be accomplished (e.g., use the Lachman test with the knee at 30 degrees of flexion to evaluate the ACL as a primary restraint).
3. The pivot shift defines the three-dimensional envelope of motion. On the injured leg, the pivot shift defines the envelope of pathologic motion. The envelope of motion should be defined on every knee.

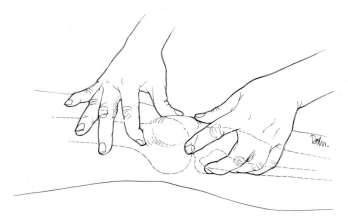

Figure 2.5 The patella is examined for excursion, pain, and apprehension.

The IKDC arrived at these principles through lengthy discussion, peer review, and consultation. These principles are the essence of the physical examination; they lead to an anatomic diagnosis and the definition of the pathologic envelope of the knee.

The Lachman and pivot shift tests are essential for every practitioner to master. The Lachman test is performed with the knee flexed at 30 degrees and the patient relaxed. The lower leg may be drawn forward on the upper leg by firmly stabilizing the femur and drawing the tibia forward on the femur (Fig. 2.2). Increased anterior excursion on this test is pathognomonic of a torn ACL. The end point should be graded as hard or soft. The end point is said to be hard when the ACL abruptly halts the forward motion of the tibia on the femur. The end point is soft when there is no ACL and the restraints are the more elastic secondary stabilizers. The Lachman test has become more refined since the work of the IKDC. Mild laxity corresponds to 0 to 5 mm pathologic laxity; moderate, 6 to 10 mm; and severe, 11 to 15 mm of excursion greater than that of the uninvolved leg. Generally, the examiner can refine the physical examination so as to expect an error of no more than ±1.5 mm on the Lachman test. The Lachman test is specific, reliable, and minimally painful to the patient. It must be mastered by those who examine the injured knee. The Lachman test can also be performed in the prone position, which is then gravity-assisted and favors small hands (Fig. 2.7).

The knee is placed in 30 degrees of flexion and the tibia is translated forward on the fixed femur. In the prone position, the knee is placed in 30 degrees of flexion and the tibia is translated forward on the flexed femur. Not only does gravity assist the examiner in this position, but the patient is usually more relaxed and the

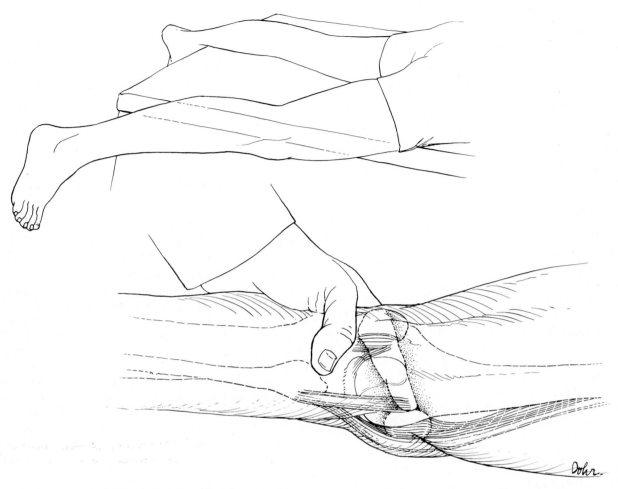

Figure 2.6 The prone position **(top)** is particularly helpful in examination of the patella. The examiner can determine the tenderness along the capsule as well as the swelling and/or tenderness of the fat pad and the inferior capsular ligaments **(bottom)**.

fingers are free to palpate the femorotibial relationship. This test gives the same information whether the patient is supine or prone.

Another test I perform in the prone position is medial-lateral translation of the lower leg on the upper leg with the knee flexed 30 degrees; a cruciate-deficient knee will manifest increased medial translation. Figure 2.8 shows how the prone medial translation test is performed. Furthermore, if the secondary lateral restraints are stretched, the medial translation becomes even more apparent and the patient can appreciate the sensation of translation. The bony anatomy, too, may come into play on this test. Those with relatively narrow femoral bicondylar distance may be inherently less stable. This may be a physical examination test that defines the "cruciate-dependent knee." In any regard, I use the medial translation test in the prone position as a *prognostic* test. When the medial translation is greatly increased in the face of cruciate deficiency, these patients seem to wear their medial compartment earlier and their natural history seems to be less satisfactory. This test has assumed great importance to me in the patient with a chronic injury when I am trying to determine how the patient will fare if he or she continues the present activity level with the specific anatomic deficit. This test is based on the work of Markolf et al.[2]

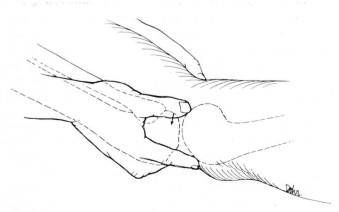

Figure 2.7 The prone Lachman test.

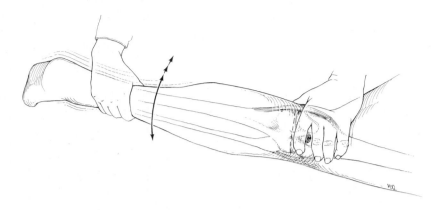

Figure 2.8   The prone medial translation test.

Pivot Shift Tests

In its various forms—for example, the Losee test (Fig.2.9),[1] the MacIntosh test,[3] the flexion-external rotation drawer test,[4] the Jakob test,[5] and the Slocum test[6]—the pivot shift test helps the examiner to determine the abnormal translation and rotation of the medial and lateral compartments of the knee. Positive results in any of these tests depend on an incompetent ACL. If the MCL is disrupted, there may not be sufficient restraining force medially for the test to be meaningful. The test may also be falsely negative because of muscle spasm. A false-positive test is quite rare and would lead one to suspect either congenital laxity or congenital absence of the ACL.

The pivot shift test, in any of its presently recognized modifications, is sufficiently useful and specific to the examiner that he or she should *master* one or more of its variants.

The IKDC recommended that the pivot shift could be graded as *negative* or *pivot glide.* A pivot glide could be either physiologic or pathologic. *Positive pivot shift is always pathologic. Gross subluxation* indicates multiple ligamentous injury. These four grades seem to capture the envelope of pathologic motion. They imply, however, that the well (noninvolved) leg has been examined first for its physiologic envelope of motion.

The form of the pivot shift test is unimportant. It can be a Losee test,[1] a MacIntosh test,[3] a Noyes test,[4] a Jakob test,[5] or a Slocum test[6]; it is the responsibility of the examiner to elicit the entire envelop of motion. Sometimes more than one of these tests is required to elicit the extent of the physiologic and pathologic motion. One cannot always do this in the office setting. Frequently, the full extent of the pathologic envelope of motion cannot be appreciated until the knee is evaluated under anesthesia with the attendant muscle relaxation.

ADJUNCT TESTS

An adjunct test is one that has become routine either because it is a specific test for a particular anatomic entity or because it has assumed significance through a clinical meaning assigned by the founder. Such adjunct tests—physical and radiographic examinations—have proven reproducible in the hands of many.

The supine or sitting position seems to be the standard for examination. Too often we forget the other side of the joint, which is brought to view when the patient is prone. I have found the prone position to be particularly helpful when performing the Lachman and medial translation tests.

The prone position is also helpful in examination of the patella. The mobility of the patella is easily ascertained, and the amount of the "capture" that may be present with injury or arthrofibrosis can be ascertained. Tenderness along the capsule can be determined, as well as the swelling and/or tenderness of the fat pad and the inferior capsular ligaments (Fig. 2.10).

Another valuable position for examination of the patellofemoral joint and the menisci has been the figure-4 position (Fig. 2.11). This position allows palpation of the retinacular ligaments of the patella, particularly the inferior medial and inferior lateral ligaments (Fig. 2.12). These ligaments are often tender and a source of symptoms. Also, the alignment of the patella with the femoral trochlea groove can be determined.

Meniscal examination in the figure-4 position is also critical in that the meniscus is retracted (Fig. 2.13), the medial collateral ligament is quite posterior, and abnormalities of the posterior horn can be appreciated through palpation as manifest by induration, tenderness, and meniscal shift. This position for physical examination of the medial meniscus complemented by magnetic resonance imaging (MRI) has led me to do many more meniscal repairs than I previously thought necessary. The patient results (to date) have been gratifying.

Besides the static examination, there is also a dynamic examination that requires assumption of different positions. Standing, walking, or running gives a keener appreciation of the limitation of function of the joint and the patient. In complex instabilities, it often is advantageous to record functional activities on videotape or film and to examine them in slow motion.

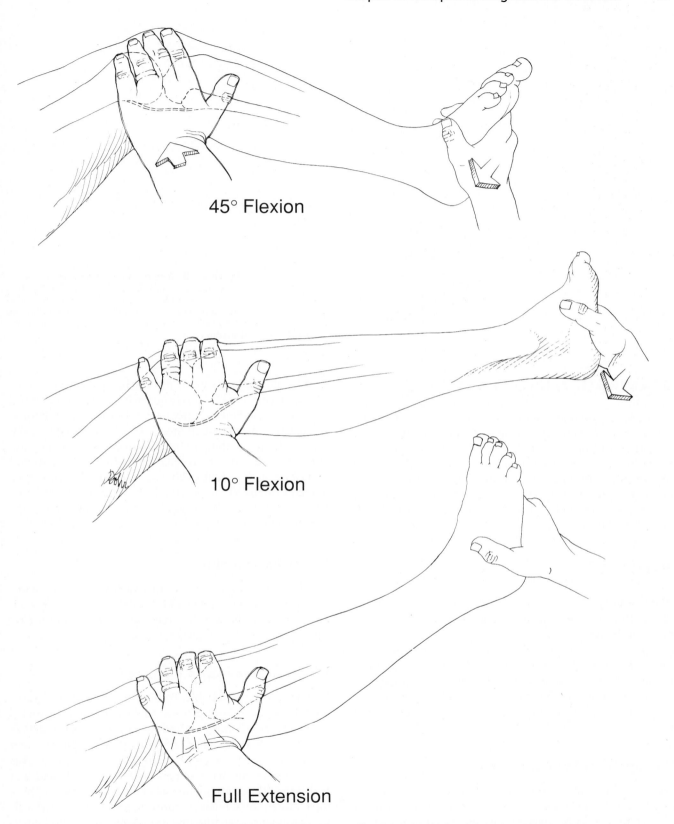

45° Flexion

10° Flexion

Full Extension

Figure 2.9   Losee's test for the pivot shift by extending the knee from a reduced to a subluxed position. **Top:** The 45 degree flexed knee is reduced with the foot and tibia twisted externally. Push the knee and pull the foot to compress the lateral joint compartment. **Middle:** Let the knee extend while maintaining strong lateral compartment compression. Let the tibia twist internally as the joint subluxes with a thud between 20 degrees and 10 degrees. **Bottom:** Complete extension quietly reduces the knee as the posterior capsule tightens.

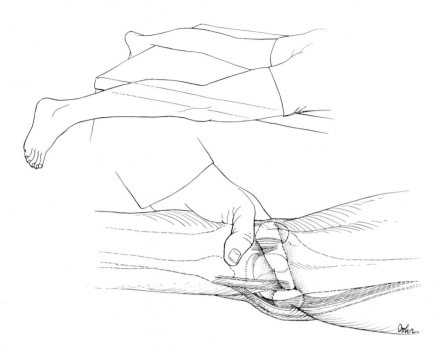

Figure 2.10   The prone position (**top**) is particularly helpful in examination of the patella. The examiner can determine the tenderness along the capsule as well as the swelling and/or tenderness of the fat pad and the inferior capsular ligaments (**bottom**).

EXAMINATION UNDER ANESTHESIA

The examination under anesthesia (EUA) should always be a concomitant of the arthroscopic examination. It is just as important during the EUA to examine the well leg first. With the muscles relaxed under anesthesia, subtle laxities may be apparent that were not fully appreciated in the office examination. It always gives a sense of satisfaction, however, when the EUA yields the same findings as the office examination.

IMAGING

What standard views and what special examinations should the examiner consider? Imaging is essential to complement the physical examination, but it is also expensive, and these resources must be taken into consideration. The role of MRI and computed tomography are ever more important. The MRI demonstrates what can be accomplished when the hardware, the software, the radiologist, the orthopaedic surgeon, and the patient cooperate to obtain the maximum information possible.

Radiographic Standard Views

What standard radiographic views should the examiner request? The lateral view is accepted as standard by most physicians. For an AP view, I prefer the weightbearing tunnel view as described by Rosenberg et al.[7] (Fig. 2.14). The knee is flexed and the beam is tangential to the tibia so that the weightbearing surfaces of the femur on the tibia and the details of the intercondylar notch are best emphasized.

Which is the best view of the patella? Many views of the patella have been described and each has its proponents. I prefer the Merchant view because it is easier to standardize. It must be realized that all these views of the patella are static, and the angles that can be measured from each are valuable but must be interpreted in light of the patient's pathology. It is doubtful that any of the views were intended to stand alone. In our clinic, we routinely obtain a lateral view of the knee, a weightbearing tunnel view, and a Merchant view of the patella.

Stress Radiographs

Stress radiographs, in both a varus/valgus and an AP plane, can be quite sophisticated and can give the physician valuable insight, although they have been used more for research than for clinical applications.

Magnetic Resonance Imaging

MRI has proven invaluable. Those who deprecate the use of the MRI have not been exposed to the good imaging that is available. Current magnets and current software can define, routinely, 1.5-mm sections of joint surface, ligament, and meniscus, as well as capsule and patellofemoral joints. This gives information that was never before available and that makes the MRI a must in the care of the complex knee. These three-dimensional images of pristine quality associated with the consultation and interpretation of the radiologist help to avoid unnecessary surgery and to plan and refine our surgical procedures. MRI can also help to determine the nature of postoperative problems such as patella capture and loss of the infrapatellar tendon interval (see Chapter 7).

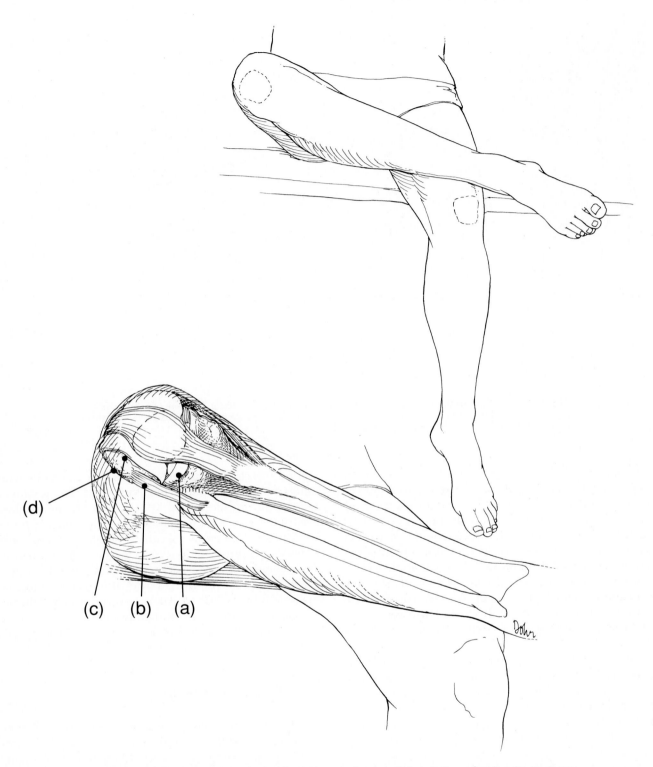

Figure 2.11 The figure-4 position **(top)**. Schematic drawing of the relations of anatomic structures **(bottom)**. Anatomic structures are: (a) medial meniscus; (b) lateral collateral ligament; (c) popliteus tendon; (d) iliotibial band.

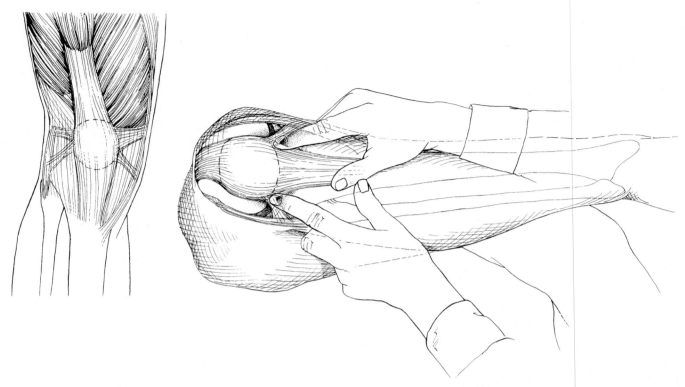

Figure 2.12   The position allows the examiner to palpate the retinacular ligaments of the patella, particularly the inferior medial and inferior lateral ligaments. The alignment of the patella with the femoral trochlear groove can also be determined.

The quality of the MRI is not only a function of the magnet, but the software, the operator, the patient's patience, and the interpretation of the radiologist. If the orthopaedic surgeon does not believe the images offered are diagnostic, then it is his or her responsibility to consult with the radiologist and seek all data available from the software and to work with the radiologists until they reach diagnostic standards expected and obtain MRIs showing the anatomy distinctly. The orthopaedic surgeon must become the patient's advocate in this matter. The work of Ho et al.,[8] Helms,[9] and Potter et al.[10] reflect the progress in MRI of the knee.

Cine-MRI gives a dimension that will help us in more effective care of patellar tracking problems and, possibly, meniscal diagnosis. The patella and its restraining ligaments, as well as adhesions and plicae, can be inspected by using motion analysis. Currently, the orthopaedist must go to the radiology suite to review these Cine studies. This is time-consuming. *Cine-MRI promises to enhance our understanding of the soft tissues and their role in knee support and function.*

ARTHROSCOPY

*The arthroscope does not replace the manual examination; rather, it augments it and provides added validity and reli-*ability. The clinician-turned-arthroscopist can focus with more certainty on the areas of pathology. Given the current state of the art, the cost of MRI must always be weighed against the cost of arthroscopy and the risks and benefits to be gained. If MRI resolves a clinical problem without need to resort to arthroscopy, it is cost-effective. If MRI enhances the accuracy and decreases the morbidity of arthroscopic surgery, it is cost-effective. Individual judgments must be made daily by the orthopaedic surgeon on behalf of the patient and in concert with third-party payers.

The arthroscope and arthroscopist have added immeasurably to the art and science of knee surgery.

DECISION-MAKING

Decision-making is often a neglected art. Decision-making is the logical conclusion of the diagnosis and selection of treatment. One of the joys of decision-making is including the informed patient and/or the family in the process. Including them implies that they are interested in, have been educated about, and understand the implications of the problem. Involving the patient (and family) is the responsibility of the treating physician. Besides being given an outline of the necessary diagnostic tests required to arrive at the point of decision-making, the patient or responsible party must understand the proposed therapy and its indi-

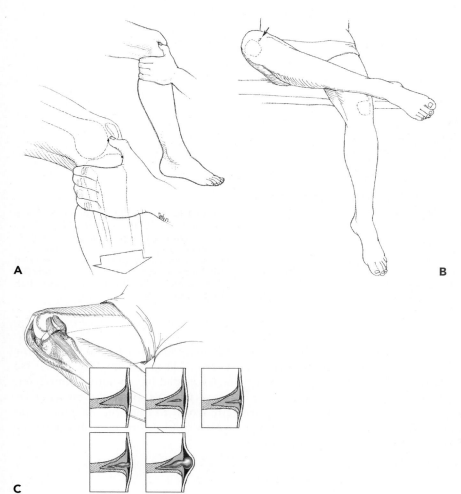

A

B

C

Figure 2.13 Examination of the meniscus. **A:** Hanging position. **B:** Figure-4 position. **C:** Cystic degeneration is the basis for radial extrusion test. (From Garrett W, Kirkendall D, Speer K, et al. *Principles and Practice of Orthopaedic Sports Medicine*, Philadelphia: Lippincott Williams & Wilkins; 2000, with permission)

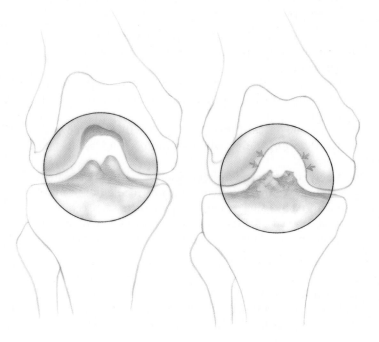

Figure 2.14 The "tunnel" view.

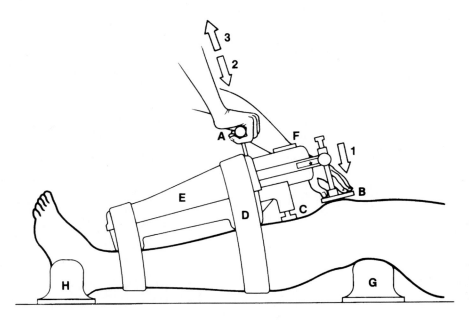

Figure 2.15 KT-1000 arthrometer. Force handle (posterior force [2] or anterior force [3]) is applied (**A**); patellar sensor pad (a constant force [1] is applied to stabilize the patellar sensor pad (**B**); tibial sensor pad (**C**); Velcro straps (**D**); arthrometer body (**E**); displacement dial (**F**); thigh support (**G**); foot support (**H**).

cations, limitations, and contraindications. These aspects are fundamental to "informed consent." The importance of rehabilitation, including its probable duration, as it relates to the proposed management must be outlined. Managing the rehabilitation of patients is a special privilege of the knee surgeon and a rightful part of our discipline. The patient must consider the necessary rehabilitation commitments before agreeing to the proposed treatment process.

REHABILITATION

I offer four principles requisite to a rehabilitation program, which are necessary to restore the knee to optimum function.

1. A close relationship among the physical therapist, patient, and surgeon is necessary for the success of all rehabilitative plans.
2. The combination of an overzealous patient and an overzealous therapist can undo even the best work of the surgeon.
3. "Life after physical therapy" (i.e., a self-motivated program) is imperative when endurance and agility are required.
4. Agility, proprioception, and balance are not adequately emphasized in our current programs. These skills can be enhanced by using existing local resources such as Pilates, yoga, martial arts, remedial dance, aerobic exercise programs, personal fitness trainers, and conditioning courses.

Objective testing should be undertaken as a reward to the patient. These tests should be performed at appropriate intervals. In addition to the muscles about the knee, hip abductors and abdominals should be tested. Simple agility drills are included to ensure that agility has not been neglected.

Use of laxity arthrometer such as KT-1000 (MEDmetric Corporation, San Diego, CA) is helpful (Fig. 2.15). We must always seek the recipe that incorporates biomechanical principles with the very best of soft tissue care. Then we must emphasize early return to function. Anaerobic and aerobic testing may be helpful for the elite athlete before full competition.

COMMENT

The total plan from examination through treatment is a subtle integration of distinct variables. Evolving the best plan is the art of medicine. This is what separates us and elevates us to our special level of service to our fellow man. The case studies (see Chapter 3) emphasize how I formulate the plan from the variables presented. Some of our colleagues, quite rightfully, would assemble the same variables and opt for a different plan. This is what makes our specialty a challenge and a responsibility.

The integration of the variables implicit in the diagnosis, treatment, and follow-up are the essence of the case studies. They will help to crystallize the principles of diagnosis and treatment. The bibliography will be a useful resource. The authors of the other chapters in Sections I and II give us their special wisdom and experience and their case studies.

Decision-making in our specialty is an art and a science. Decision-making can facilitate the treatment program because it elicits the patient's cooperation and integrates the team. Decisions are based on knowledge, technology, and experience, but nothing can replace what the dedicated knee surgeon learns daily from the physical examination and effective communication with the patient.

REFERENCES

1. Losee RE, Johnson TR, Southwick WO. Anterior subluxation of the lateral plateau. A diagnostic test and operation. *J Bone Joint Surg Am* 1978;60:1015–1030.
2. Markolf KL, Kochan A, Amstutz HC. Measurement of knee stiffness and laxity in patients with documented absence of the anterior cruciate ligament. *J Bone Joint Surg Am* 1984;66:242–252.
3. Galway HR, MacIntosh DL. The lateral pivot shift: a symptom and sign of anterior cruciate ligament insufficiency. *Clin Orthop Relat Res* 1980;147:45–50.
4. Noyes FR, Bassett RW, Grood ES, Butler DL. Arthroscopy in acute traumatic hemarthrosis of the knee. Incidence of anterior cruciate tears and other injuries. *J Bone Joint Surg Am* 1980;62: 687–695.
5. Jakob RP, Hassler H, Staeubli HU. Observations on rotatory instability of the lateral compartment of the knee. Experimental studies on the functional anatomy and the pathomechanism of the true and the reversed pivot shift sign. *Acta Orthop Scand Suppl* 1981; 191:1–32.
6. Slocum DB, James SL, Larson RL, Singer KM. Clinical test for anterolateral rotary instability of the knee. *Clin Orthop* 1976; 118:63–69.
7. Rosenberg TD, Paulos LE, Parker RD, Coward DB, Scott SM. The forty-five-degree posteroanterior flexion weight-bearing radiograph of the knee. *J Bone Joint Surg Am*. 1988;70:1479–1483.
8. Ho C, Cervilla V, Kjellin I, et al. Magnetic resonance imaging in assessing cartilage changes in experimental osteoarthrosis of the knee. *Invest Radiol* 1992;27:84–90.
9. Helms CA. The impact of MR imaging in sports medicine. *Radiology* 2002;224:631–635.
10. Potter HG, Linklater JM, Allen AA, Hannafin JA, Haas SB. Magnetic resonance imaging of articular cartilage in the knee. An evaluation with use of fast-spin-echo imaging. *J Bone Joint Surg Am* 1998;80:1276–1284.

Case Studies

3

John A. Feagin, Jr.

INTRODUCTION TO CASE STUDIES
1 AND 2 28

CASE STUDY 1: THE "ISOLATED"
ANTERIOR CRUCIATE LIGAMENT-INJURED
KNEE 29

▰▰ HISTORY 29

▰▰ COMMENTS 29
Further Comments 30
Special Considerations 31

▰▰ PLAN 31
Surgical Procedure 32

▰▰ POSTOPERATIVE CARE AND
REHABILITATION 32
Immediate 32
Long Term 32

▰▰ PROBLEMS, COMPLICATIONS, FOLLOW-UP
RESULTS 32

▰▰ SUMMARY 33

CASE STUDY 2: THE MULTILIGAMENT-INJURED
KNEE 33

▰▰ HISTORY 33

▰▰ COMMENTS 33

▰▰ COURSE OF ACTION 34
Physical Examination 34
Diagnostic Studies 34
Special Considerations 34

▰▰ PLAN 35

▰▰ SURGICAL PROCEDURE (PLAN) 35

▰▰ POSTOPERATIVE CARE AND
REHABILITATION 36

▰▰ PROBLEMS, COMPLICATIONS, FOLLOW-UP
RESULTS 37

▰▰ SUMMARY 37

INTRODUCTION TO CASE STUDIES
3A AND 3B 38

CASE STUDY 3A: SUBLUXATION
OF THE PATELLA IN THE ADOLESCENT
FEMALE ATHLETE 38

▰▰ HISTORY 39

▰▰ PHYSICAL EXAMINATION 39

▰▰ GAIT 40

▰▰ IMAGING 40

▰▰ SPECIAL CONSIDERATIONS 40

▰▰ PLAN 40

▰▰ COMMENT 41

CASE STUDY 3B: ACUTE DISLOCATION OF
THE PATELLA IN THE SKELETALLY MATURE
COMPETITIVE MALE ATHLETE 41

▰▰ HISTORY 41

■■■ COMMENTS 41

■■■ DIAGNOSTIC STUDIES 41

■■■ SPECIAL CONSIDERATIONS 42

■■■ PLAN 42

■■■ SURGERY 42

■■■ REHABILITATION 42

■■■ SUMMARY 43

INTRODUCTION TO CASE STUDIES 1 AND 2

We have come a long way in understanding the role of the anterior cruciate ligament (ACL) and the infinite pathology that can coexist or evolve. The "bone bruise," the torn meniscus, the chondral defects, concomitant injuries, the progression of laxity, functional impairment, the natural history, and degenerative arthritis are all part of the evolution of our understanding of the tear of the ACL.

Not all cruciate ligament injuries are similar; patients are dissimilar, functional demands are different, and the natural history is only vaguely known. To Dale Daniel et al.[1] and many others, we owe a huge debt for their efforts to define the natural history. To Steadman and Rodkey,[2] Sherman et al.,[3] Lubowitz and Grauer,[4] and others, we owe gratitude for their courage in revisiting primary repair. The "healing response" has been a huge step forward. Not every ACL requires reconstruction. Even prostheses are making a

reappearance for the low-demand knee. We must better identify the demands the patient expects to place on the injured knee and determine what we can and cannot do to restore the knee.

We must accept that the ACL tear occurs in a myriad of ways under a multitude of load demands and that the displacement of tibia on femur is quite variable at the instant of injury. Furthermore, compliance and expectation may determine outcome. We understand, then, that no two ACL-injured knees are the same, and the ACL-injured knee can be a complex conundrum worthy of keenest concern and attention to detail.

Dr. Jack Hughston (personal communication, 1972) challenged us vigorously on our use of "isolated" as it related to the ACL. He was correct to do so and we were naïve in our thought process. The ACL is a central pivot. The force required to disrupt the ACL and the displacement at the time of injury usually implicates other anatomic constituents—the chondral surfaces, the supporting subchondral bone, the menisci, the patella, and the secondary ligamentous restraints. All are at risk at the instant of injury.

The elucidation of the pivot shift by Losee et al.[5] has helped us to understand the complex translation and rotation, which duplicate the injury and the patient's symptoms. The magnitude and frequency of this shift is also a key to future functional impairment and the natural history. The ACL should never be addressed simplistically or naïvely as isolated. The complexity of the ACL, the biomechanical implications of the central pivot, and the frequency of injury in sport have challenged us to the limits of our scientific method. The challenge has been a worthy one. What we have learned, how we have learned, and the application of our new knowledge are not only the reasons for this book, but the rationale for Case Study 1: the "isolated" ACL-injured knee.

CASE STUDY 1

The "Isolated" Anterior Cruciate Ligament-Injured Knee

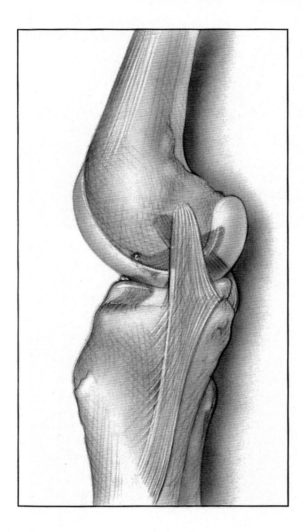

Physical Examination of 18-year-old Athlete

Diagnostic Clues	Findings
Effusion	3+ (moderate)
Tenderness	Medial and lateral joint lines
Motion	Limited: 20 to 50 degrees
Lachman test	6-mm (injured minus normal difference)
Varus/valgus laxity	Slight increase
Pivot shift test	Positive
Patella apprehension	Slightly positive
Gait	Antalgic: patient prefers crutches
Neurovascular	Intact
Radiographs	Negative except for effusion

- What do we mean by "isolated"?
- The diagnosis and care of the compromised cruciate

HISTORY

An 18-year-old secondary school athlete who has lettered in three sports sustained a noncontact injury to his right knee as he cut to the left in the second football game of his senior year. He heard a "pop" and was unable to continue play. The team physician, an orthopaedic surgeon, examined the knee on the field and felt it was "loose." Re-examination the following day in the office confirmed the on-field impressions. The following diagnostic clues and findings were recorded.

COMMENTS

The history was straightforward and suggested a tear of the ACL. The patient was a dedicated, disciplined athlete, and was determined to continue recreational sports. Physical examination with a positive Lachman test and a positive pivot shift test is indicative of a tear of the ACL. Is manual examination enough? In today's world, I prefer magnetic resonance imaging (MRI) for a more complete three-dimensional anatomic diagnosis. Although we must learn to read our own images, the presence of a radiographer schooled in joint-specific pathology is invaluable. The attending physician should settle for no less than quality imaging read by a radiographer of experience with complete diagnostic detail.

An MRI was obtained and showed a complete tear of the anterior cruciate ligament in its proximal third, a bone bruise of the lateral condyle and posterior tibia, and intact menisci. There were no obvious chondral lesions (Fig. 3.1.1).

The MRI was convincing. The patient and family wanted the knee repaired as soon as possible. They understood the implications of repair and rehabilitation.

Timing of the surgery is the next critical detail. The work of Shelbourne and Foulk[6] and others in their group has brought great attention to this variable. I concur that it is usually in the best interest of the patient to perform the surgery on an elective basis after the effusion has resolved and motion has returned. The patient described in the history attended therapy diligently and was ready for surgery 2 weeks after the injury, with the effusion resolved and a near

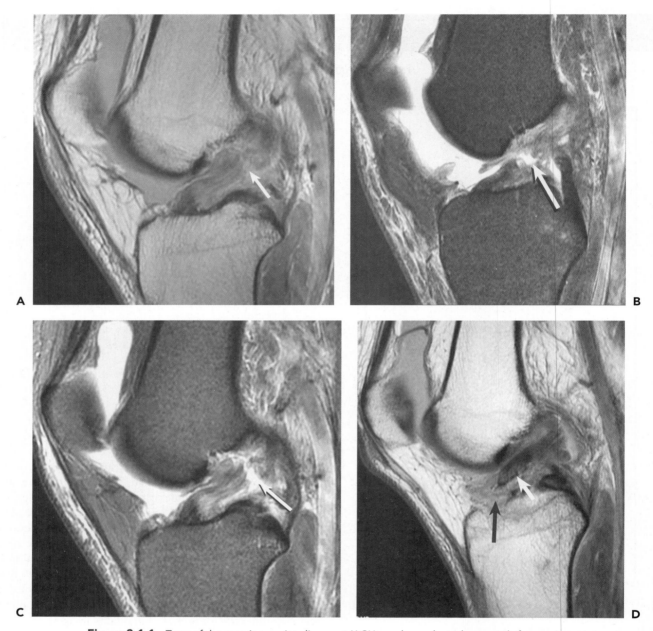

Figure 3.1.1 Tears of the anterior cruciate ligament (ACL) may be evaluated accurately for precise location and extent of the tear by magnetic resonance imaging (as shown in Figure 7.17). **A:** Sagittal proton density image shows complete disruption of the ACL *(arrow)* at the junction of middle and proximal thirds, with bowing and increased signal edema and hemorrhage within and about the proximal and distal tear ends. **B:** Sagittal fat-suppressed proton density image shows even more conspicuously the tear defect *(arrow)* and high-signal edema and hemorrhage. **C:** Sagittal fat-suppressed proton density image of a different patient reveals focal complete midsubstance tear of the ACL *(arrow)*. **D:** Sagittal proton density image of another patient shows avulsion of the distal ACL attachment, with superior and posterior retraction and posterior rotation of the avulsed fragment *(short arrow)* of the ACL insertion with defect of the anterior tibial attachment *(long arrow)*.

full range of motion. The examination before surgery confirmed a 6-mm injured-minus-noninjured knee Lachman result and a positive pivot test.

Further Comments

The philosophy and technique of the physical examination were discussed in the chapter on physical examination.

The principles I follow in the physical examination are as follows:

- Examine the patient in the position of comfort.
- Examine the well leg before the injured leg.
- Examine (feel) gently for induration and tenderness.
- Determine the status of the primary and secondary restraints.

- Make an anatomic diagnosis.
- Determine the envelope of pathologic motion through pivot shift testing and comparison with the well leg.

Examine standing alignment and evaluate gait. Be sure hip, ankle, and foot are included in the examination and that the neurovascular status is normal.

Special Considerations

The age of the patient is important, as it reflects his or her social responsibilities, lifestyle, maturation, and intended use of the limb. Adolescents and young adults rarely accept alterations in their lifestyle. Older patients will frequently adapt their lifestyle to their injury. The young adult's wishes about surgery and restoration of function must be respected. Surgeons often ask at what age ACL reconstruction surgery should not be performed. I have not found a cutoff age because I know people in their 60s who would be quite disabled by an unstable knee. Nevertheless, one must recognize that older patients are likely to suffer complications. The surgeon should be prepared to modify both the plan, the operation, and the postoperative care accordingly.

There is often pressure to do the surgery immediately, although it is "far from home." There are many considerations here, but the expertise of the surgeon, the quality of the rehabilitation, and the supervision must all be considered. Usually, surgery closer to home, where the supportive team is known, is more desirable. Continuity of care is essential and the operating surgeon is ultimately responsible for the end result.

PLAN

What makes the practice of medicine unique is the infinite variability of "the plan." We formulate the treatment plan by the subtle integration of all relevant factors—some obvious, some learned through experience, and some intuitive. The "best" treatment plan is the plan in which both the patient and surgeon have confidence. Perfecting this art of selecting the best treatment plan for each patient is an unending quest. The challenge is what keeps physicians vital through years of practice. Experience is important in formulating a treatment plan. Sometimes the surgeon is uncertain. Sometimes the patient is uncertain. Usually, I propose a tentative plan to the patient and then back off to allow response to the initial implications. *I always let patients know that their input and insight are essential in formulating a plan for their care.*

I have often found that my time is equally divided between the physical examination and formulating the plan with the patient. Ultimately, however, the physician is responsible for the contract made with the patient. If the patient finds it difficult to establish a firm contractual relationship, he or she should seek a second opinion. The surgeon should be quick to suggest further consultation when it is obvious the decision-making is difficult.

For this patient, a young dedicated athlete, the plan seemed relatively straight-forward—reconstruction of the ACL at the appropriate time with an extensive and thorough rehabilitation program to follow. Most patients wish to know which graft the surgeon is going to use. This level of sophistication is not uncommon and deserves respect. I explained to the patient that there are four choices: bone-patellar tendon-bone, hamstring grafts, allografts, and primary repair. I will usually end this brief discussion by expressing my preference for one of the four choices. This preference is not always the same. I frequently modify the choice of graft depending on the functional demands of the patient and certain anatomic features relevant to that patient. I also like to keep a window open for primary repair or "the healing response" (see Chapter 10), as I believe that sometimes this is the appropriate solution. I further explain that the final decision cannot be made until the time of surgery. Thus, I try to retain control of graft selection rather than allow the patient to pre-empt my experience on this matter.

There are cases in which the patients decline surgery. This is their right. At this juncture, I usually encourage them to seek another opinion. Sometimes it is necessary to treat a patient nonoperatively for either medical reasons or as the result of the patient's choice. For such a patient, I would consider immobilizing the knee in 20 degrees of flexion for 3 to 5 weeks. This course at least would have allowed the secondary restraints to begin healing and might have allowed the ACL to fall on the posterior cruciate ligament, and gain a secondary source of attachment and blood supply (Fig. 3.1.2). This mechanism was described by Wittek.[7] This "repair," however, is not anatomic and will not give satisfaction to a high-demand athlete.

Primary repair of the interstitially torn ACL is sometimes adequate. The work of Marshall et al.[8] and Sherman et al.[3] presents a good argument for primary repair when the repair is located proximally and the patient's demands are minimal—age is not a discriminator. The interstitial nature of the torn helicoid ACL, the scant blood supply, and the hostile nature of the intercondylar notch all make it difficult to perform a primary repair that will restore vascularity and tensile strength. Augmentation grafting has been the procedure of choice for young patients with athletic demands.

Nevertheless, with improvement in MRI diagnosis and with an understanding that proximal tears do occur, especially in skiing, there has been a re-emphasis on primary repair and "healing response." This is discussed by Dr. Steadman in detail in Chapter 8 of this book. To support the selectivity in the care of the patient, I have seen excellent results from both primary repair and the healing response. In retrospect, one third of the West Point Cadets that we reported in our original study[9] did well with primary repair. This is especially noteworthy given the activity level of this patient population. Further reflection on this early report supports the need for selectivity in patient care.

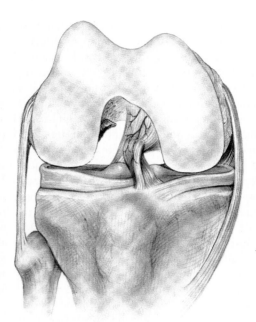

Figure 3.1.2 The torn anterior cruciate ligament falls on the posterior cruciate ligament and thus gains a secondary source of attachment and blood supply. This drawing illustrates the results of immobilization but is similar to the outcome of a surgical repair technique used by Wittek.[7]

Surgical Procedure

The procedure for the patient described in this case study was as follows:

1. The knee was re-examined under anesthesia before the tourniquet was inflated. The difference between the well leg and the injured leg served as the criteria for restoration of stability after surgery. The patient was noted to have a positive pivot shift, which further indicated augmentation grafting.
2. Arthroscopic examination showed no meniscal pathology, no chondral defects, and an interstitially torn ACL. Bone-patellar tendon-bone grafting was accomplished (see Chapter 8).
3. After graft fixation, range of motion was checked and elimination of the pivot shift was confirmed.
4. A compression wound dressing was applied.

POSTOPERATIVE CARE AND REHABILITATION

Immediate

There are three immediate postoperative goals:

- Protection of the repair
- Relief of pain
- Prevention of adhesions

Continuous passive motion (CPM) has a function in achieving all three goals and has been an effective adjunct to knee surgery. Knowing that the joint can be moved comfortably so soon after the operation gives the patient confidence toward a home mobilization program. Intra-articular anesthesia has also served to relieve some of the postoperative pain and improve function. Epidural analgesia has also proved effective in speeding return of function and rehabilitation. These practices are discussed in more detail in Chapters 8 and 13. Outpatient surgery is performed frequently, although overnight stay has its advantages. What is essential is that control is gained of the patient, the pain, and the rehabilitation process.

The postoperative dressing is important to prevent swelling and minimize pulmonary embolism. Firm compressive dressing or elastic stocking with a Cryocuff (AirCast, Summit, NJ) is applied at the end of the operation and maintained for 7 to 10 days. The thigh-length antiembolic hose has proved most satisfactory. Care is taken not to impart venous constriction through an elastic bandage about the knee.

Pulmonary embolus is a paramount consideration even in young patients. The choice of postoperative brace is again surgeon-dependent and is discussed in Chapters 6 and 8.

Long Term

Long-term rehabilitation is perhaps the most neglected portion of patient management. Return to full function is the goal of the surgical procedure, but without rehabilitation, it will not be attained. Sir John Charnley once said that a perfect operation requires little rehabilitation (personal communication, 1972). I agree, but we are far from having a perfect knee operation. As we approach perfection, we will see a decrease in the demand for rehabilitation. Indeed, we have already seen an example of this trend as arthroscopic and limited incisional surgery have replaced the open surgery of yesteryear.

Common to all long-term rehabilitation programs are the goals of strength, endurance, and agility. The SAID principle (specific adaptation to individual demands) is also applicable. These goals should be explained to the patient and objective criteria for performance established. Rehabilitation is discussed in depth in Chapter 13.

Finally, there is return to competition. It is not necessarily national or even local competition. Sometimes it is self-competition, the drive to turn the clock back and "do it again" with vigor and commitment and without pain or giving way. This is the ultimate goal. We should prepare athletic patients, such as the one described here, to work gradually toward this goal—the restoration of lifestyle for a lifetime of usage. A gratifying and unifying event for patient and surgeon is "return to competition."

PROBLEMS, COMPLICATIONS, FOLLOW-UP RESULTS

ACL surgery today is reliable to the 90th-plus percentile. Reinjury and retear do occur; they present serious problems. This is usually associated with a return to competitive sports and often reflects a reinjury of the magnitude of the original injury.

The other bedeviling complication is arthrofibrosis—limitation of motion and patellar capture. This complication has been under appreciated but is reflected in long-term morbidity. A flexed knee gait will not be accepted by the patient for long. Furthermore, capture of the patellofemoral joint through scar tissue, adhesions, and loss of the anterior interval take a toll on the patella through compression arthropathy. The physician must be alert to this complication, and be able to manage it through rehabilitation and/or arthroscopic debridement and release. I must counsel the patient both pre- and post-operatively regarding this possibility. Complications will be discussed in detail in Chapters 11 and 12.

SUMMARY

This case involved an 18-year-old outstanding athlete who sustained an "isolated ACL" during an athletic competition. The patient elected surgical repair and the central third of the patellar tendon was used for augmentation grafting. A high level of confidence in this operation by close supervision and a thorough rehabilitation program is essential to success.

The long-term results for patients treated in this manner have been excellent. The operation has proved to be reproducible. Rehabilitation, both short-term and long-term, has been stressed until strength, endurance, and agility are restored. Bracing, return to competition, and complications are discussed in Part II of this book.

CASE STUDY 2

The Multiligament-Injured Knee: Anterior Cruciate Ligament Tear, Medial Collateral Ligament Tear, Peripheral Tear of the Medial Meniscus

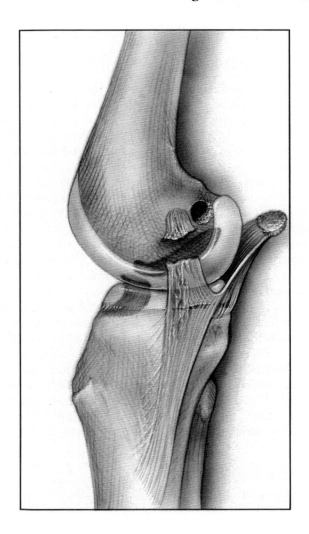

- The role of magnetic resonance imaging
- The timing of surgery
- Medial collateral ligament repair
- Meniscal repair

HISTORY

A 21-year-old college junior, a first-string running back, was struck on his planted right leg while advancing the ball. He experienced severe pain and did not attempt to rise from the turf. The examination revealed gross laxity and he was helped from the field with the leg well-splinted.

COMMENTS

This case represents the classic injury of American football as described by O'Donoghue.[10] This "triad injury" became more frequent through increased efficiency of the helmet, contact below the waist (the "crack-back block"), and enhanced fixation of the shoe-turf interface. As both the speed of the game and the force of impact increased in the late 1950s, these injuries became all too common. Game films allowed analysis of the disruptive forces that were applied to the knee through this classic mechanism. Peterson (O'Donoghue Presentation at the American Orthopaedic Society for Sports Medicine meeting, Lake Tahoe, CA, 1981), through study of game films and the injury pattern, promulgated rule changes that have been responsible for a marked decrease in this devastating injury. Regretfully, though, these devastating injuries still occur with regular frequency.

Since this patient has a chance at a professional sport future, he would be called an "elite" athlete. The next season was important to both player and coach. Because of the serious nature of the injury and the future prospects, it is important that planning proceed expeditiously and thoroughly.

COURSE OF ACTION

Physical Examination

Knee Examination of 21-year-old Collegiate Running Back

Diagnostic Clues	Findings
Effusion	Mild
Tenderness	Medially
Lachman test	8-mm (injured minus normal)
Drawer test	+3-mm positive; soft end point
Pivot shift test	Not attempted
Varus/valgus	3+ valgus opening in full extension; stable in full extension to varus testing
Patellar apprehension	Patellofemoral joint stable but apprehension with lateral displacement
Range of motion	Too painful to elicit
Gait	Unable to bear weight
Neurovascular	Intact
Imaging	Joint effusion and medial swelling

The on-field examination showed gross laxity, both to anteroposterior testing as well as medially. This indicated a multiligament-injured knee. In such cases, it is important to define the stable hinge when one exists. This allows the surgeon to plan surgery around the stable hinge.

In this case, the stable hinge appeared to be lateral. MRI is essential in cases of this magnitude to define the extent of injury and plan the surgery (Fig. 3.2.1).

Although a pivot shift may be helpful to determine the extent of injury, it would have been unnecessary to subject this patient to a subluxation test without anesthesia. *Finding the knee stable to varus testing in extension confirmed the integrity of the lateral capsular ligament and the posterior cruciate ligament.*

The patellofemoral mechanism can sometimes be disrupted in this injury. When this occurs, the lesion usually is at the origin, that is, the attachment of the superior medial patellofemoral ligament to the linea aspera and medial intermuscular septum (Fig. 3.2.2).

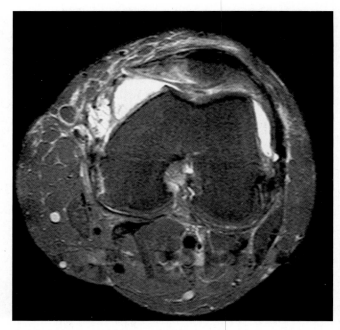

Figure 3.2.1 A magnetic resonance image illustrating the injuries to the anterior cruciate ligament, medial collateral ligament, and medial meniscus.

Diagnostic Studies

The routine radiographs were carefully studied for bony evidence of capsule or ligamentous avulsion. The MRI revealed a midsubstance interstitial tear of the ACL, an intact posterior cruciate ligament, tear of the medial collateral ligament, the posterior oblique ligament, and the medial meniscus. The lateral structures were intact. There was a bone bruise of the lateral femoral condyle (Fig. 3.2.1).

Arthroscopy must be carefully performed because of the danger of extravasation of the fluid through the disrupted medial compartment and possible compromise of the compartments of the lower leg. Arthroscopy is important, however, to prepare the medial meniscus for repair as well as to assess the damage to the medial structures and lateral compartment.

One important evaluation is the posterior horn of the lateral meniscus. The subluxation of the tibia on the femur sometimes results in a Finochietto lesion (Fig. 3.2.3).[11] This tear of the undersurface of the posterior horn, lateral meniscus, is important. At the time of arthroscopy in cases of this severity, I believe that the posterior compartment should be visualized through the intercondylar notch as further injury is often noted in this viewing, especially with a 70-degree oblique arthroscope.

Special Considerations

In injuries of this severity, I believe in early surgery. This usually occurs the morning after the game when the patient

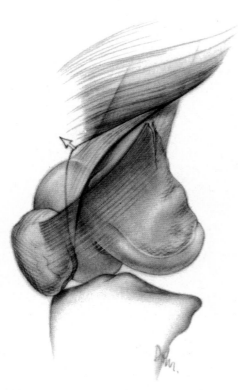

Figure 3.2.2   The lesion disrupting the patellofemoral mechanism usually occurs at the attachment of the medial patellofemoral ligament to the linea aspera and medial intermuscular septum.

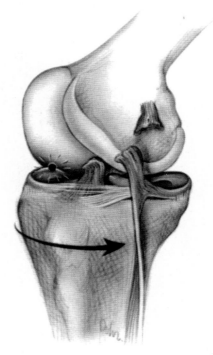

Figure 3.2.3   The markedly positive drawer test revealed that the tibia, with its conjoined menisci, could be brought quite anterior on the femur (the Finochietto sign). Both the posteromedial and posterolateral corners require careful evaluation for meniscocapsular disruption when this sign is identified.

has been hydrated, re-evaluated, and counseled. The surgical team is important in that surgery must proceed rapidly and expeditiously and tourniquet time must be limited. For an assistant, I prefer an orthopaedic surgeon or highly trained surgical assistant who has experience in knee surgery cases. Because the equipment is also highly specialized, the surgical technician and operating room nurse are critical to the case. Fortunately, specialized surgical equipment exists to affix the ACL, the meniscus, and the torn ligaments. The patient must be counseled that internal fixation devices will be used and sometimes they require removal later. The patient should further be counseled about the importance of meniscal repair, wherever and whenever possible.

PLAN

The patient was scheduled for surgery the morning after injury, and the knee had been amply iced as well as splinted immediately subsequent to the injury. The "first team" was assembled for the operative procedure. A detailed examination under anesthesia is important so that maximum use can be made of arthroscopic repair and the incisions minimized. All disrupted structures must be repaired. A diligent

intraoperative physical examination at each stage of the repair will verify the restoration of stability and ensure that a ligamentous lesion has not been overlooked.

Examination under anesthesia is a part of the operative care. It is performed immediately after induction of anesthesia, before the leg is prepared, in comparison to the well leg, and before the tourniquet is inflated. Besides the obvious laxity, the surgeon searches particularly for induration at the posterior corners of the meniscal ligamentous complexes and the limits of motion of the joint anteriorly, posteriorly, and in rotation. The stable hinge is important to define. The C-arm should be available to the operating room to verify laxities and resolution of the appropriate surgery as necessary.

SURGICAL PROCEDURE (PLAN)

Complete interstitial tear of the ACL requires augmentation grafting. Frequently, in severe cases of this nature, I use an allograft to limit surgical dissection. The patient must be thus counseled as to this preference.

The meniscal attachments are carefully defined at arthroscopy. The meniscotibial and meniscofemoral attachments are important for stability. Definition of the

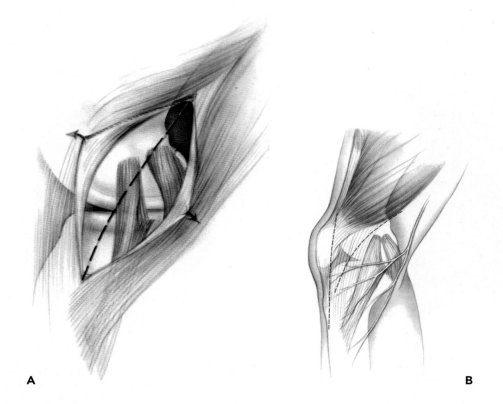

A **B**

Figure 3.2.4 A,B: The origin of the MCL in both its direct and oblique portions can be visualized by extending the medial retinacular incision obliquely along the vastus medialis obliquus muscle and reflecting the fascia or by incising the fascia along its parallel fibers overlying the tear of the deeper structures. (*Inset*) The nerve supply must be identified and preserved as well as possible. The saphenous nerve, in particular, should be protected.

posterior oblique ligament as it attaches to the meniscus must be determined and repaired. The question becomes, what is the most expeditious order to repair the components?

Furthermore, care must be taken to ensure that there are no chondral lesions, and if these are present, they should be addressed as appropriate to their extent and depth (see Chapter 9). It is obvious in this case that a limited incision will be required (Fig. 3.2.4A–B) in order to repair the medial collateral ligament and the posterior oblique ligament as well as the meniscotibial and meniscofemoral attachments. Some of this work can be done arthroscopically. This is to be encouraged wherever appropriate. Thus, the goal is an anatomic restoration of the torn structures and this usually requires some open surgery. The secret is to minimize the open surgery through preoperative planning enhanced by physical examination, MRI, and the diagnostic operative arthroscopy.

As regard to sequence of repair, I prefer to prepare the ACL tunnels for femoral and tibial insertion as a first step. Allograft will materially decrease postoperative morbidity. Then, prior to tensioning and fixation of the ACL, I address the meniscus and medial capsuloligamentous structures. Here it is important to define the posterior oblique liga-

ment, which intimately attaches to the meniscus, from the medial collateral ligament, which is not attached to the meniscus. It is also important to restore the meniscotibial ligaments and their attachments of the semimembranosus. Repair of medial structures should be accomplished according to the theoretical course of the medial collateral ligament (the line of the Burmester curve), as described by Mueller (Fig. 3.2.5).[12] Subsequent to repair of these structures, the ACL is tensioned and fixed. (For details, see Chapter 8.)

POSTOPERATIVE CARE AND REHABILITATION

Tourniquet time should be minimized. In the postoperative course, pain is decreased when tourniquet time is kept to the minimal. Also, the muscle tissues and the neurovascular structures sustain minimal damage.

Patient postoperative pain is a major concern to the surgeon. Techniques for postoperative pain are discussed in Chapters 3 (Case Study 1) and 8. Compression bandage or elastic stocking is applied firmly. Cryotherapy is a critical

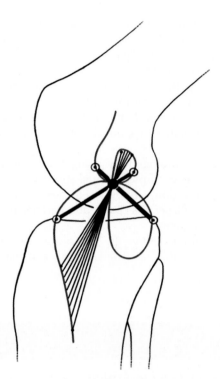

Figure 3.2.5 The repair of the medial structures must be accomplished according to the theoretical course of the medial collateral ligament and its position in relation to the Burmester curve. (Adapted from Mueller W. *The Knee. Form Function and Ligament Reconstruction.* New York: Springer-Verlag; 1983, with permission.)

component of postoperative patient care. Also, I prefer that the patient use continuous passive motion (CPM). We usually begin with 20 degrees to 70 degrees of motion. The patient is usually hospitalized for 1 or 2 days subsequent to the surgical procedure.

Even in cases of this severity much can be accomplished early. I believe in CPM, and isometric exercises, as well as toe rises and crutching walking with weightbearing to comfort. This early return of functional activities promotes a sense of well-being and ease of recovery. A detailed section on rehabilitation can be found in Chapters 8 and 13.

PROBLEMS, COMPLICATIONS, FOLLOW-UP RESULTS

The most frequent complication is stiffness. In addition to the daily use of the CPM, the therapist and patient work on flexion and extension. Also, mobility of the patellofemoral joint is a special concern. The patellofemoral joint should be mobilized daily in the superior, inferior, and mediolateral planes by both the patient and the physical therapist.

A full range of motion is desired. Surgeon, physical therapist, and patient must be alert to restrictions in motion. Early arthroscopy with lysis of adhesions and/or lateral release and restoration of the anterior interval are surgical procedures to relieve restrictions in motion (see Chapter 11).

A knee that shows increasing laxity during rehabilitation represents a serious complication. This laxity indicates that a ligamentous lesion has been overlooked or a repaired tissue has been retorn. It is best to discuss this problem with the patient as soon as it is recognized.

A third complication is sympathic dystrophy. The causes of this dystrophy are uncertain. (I have often wondered if it sometimes results from excessive compression of patellofemoral joint.) Sympathic block is sometimes appropriate to disrupt the sequence of events associated with this diagnosis. When patella compression or loss of excursion is identified, this must be corrected as soon as appropriate (see Chapter 11).

Generally, the long-term follow-up of the repaired and augmented ACL triad has been excellent. Return to function within 9 to 12 months is to be expected. Return of agility, endurance, and the cutting mechanism is usual when the principles outlined in this case study are followed. An accomplished athlete, such as the patient described here, could expect to return to football. Bracing is indicated, and a change of position for the ensuing season might be desirable. Cooperation and coordination of the team physician, trainer, coach, parent, and patient are important and must be agreed on before the patient returns to team activities.

SUMMARY

This has been the case history of an elite college football player who sustained a triad in the classic fashion. Surgical repair was elected the day after the injury, and the ACL was repaired with an allograft. The medial collateral ligament and posterior oblique ligament were anatomically repaired. The meniscotibial ligament was repaired. Early motion and early weightbearing were initiated. The patient was protected during a period of at least 6 months after his injury, until he had regained strength, endurance, and agility. Although "classic cases" such as this patient's injury are not as common as they once were, they still represent a significant portion of orthopaedic practice and are a challenge to our surgical expertise and rehabilitation skills.

INTRODUCTION TO CASE STUDIES 3A AND 3B

The patellofemoral joint is the forgotten joint of the knee. It is a "big sesamoid." The patella transmits and redirects large forces of major muscles. It is a key element of the "knee transmission."[13] Yet we have spent relatively little time understanding its complex biomechanics, developing our physical examination, or recording the natural history. The works of Trillat et al.,[14,15] Dejour et al.,[16,17] Galland et al.,[18] and the Lyon School deserve notice, as does the excellent recent text by Biedert.[19]

Magnetic resonance imaging (MRI) has helped us to understand patellar subluxation and the secondary injury that may ensue. I have come to regard and treat patella problems more critically, as I believe the natural history of the chronically subluxating patella is not good.

This case study is divided into two parts: 3A, subluxation of the patella in the adolescent female athlete, and 3B, acute dislocation of the patella in the skeletally mature competitive male athlete.

3A. Patella pathology in the active adolescent female is common. Anatomic considerations, hormonal influence, and sport all play a role. Not only is the acute injury of major concern to all involved, but also the natural history concerns me.

3B. Patella pathology in a young male athlete looking forward to a career in professional sports can signal a career-ending ambition. Not only is the acute injury a major concern to the player, his coach, and parents, but also the orthopaedic surgeon.

Both situations deserve the very best of our diagnostic and therapeutic abilities. The situation and management are dissimilar.

CASE STUDY 3A

Subluxation of the Patella in the Adolescent Female Athlete

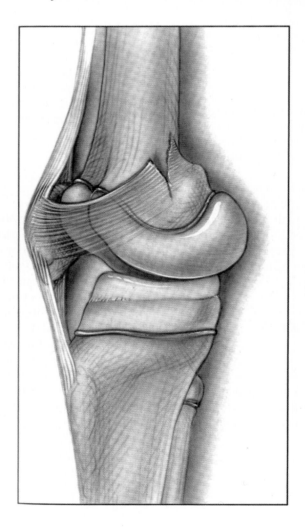

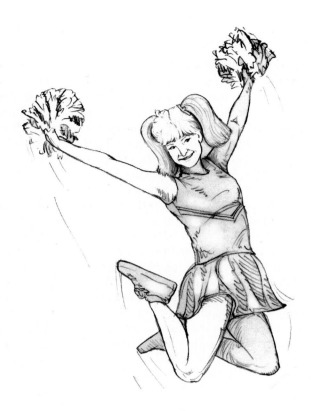

and ankle, and the rotatory component. The muscular development of the lower limb lags behind the bony development. Properly performed and explained, this part of the examination usually gets the cheerleader's attention and demonstrates your commitment, concern, and professionalism.

With the patient in the sitting position with the legs hanging off the examining table, the physician is able to examine the contours, the patella mechanism, and the tibial torsion visually. This position also allows for gentle hip rotation. The examiner can visualize the tibial tubercle alignment, the Q angle, and function of the vastus medialis oblique (VMO) muscle and can observe the patella in its most stable position, that is, seated in the trochlear groove (Fig. 3.3A.1). This position gives a further analysis of axial alignment, the muscle development, and the critical role of the superomedial patellofemoral ligament (SMPFL). In this position, I gently palpate the SMPFL for tenderness throughout its course. The origin of the ligament is just behind the medial femoral epicondyle and the junction of the VMO with the tendon of linea aspera. The SMPFL is much more visible and definable with the knee flexed at 90 degrees. During this part of the examination, the physician has control of the limb and the patient. Communication between the physician and the patient is essential during this time. The patient must be a participant throughout the examination.

HISTORY

A 15-year-old high school cheerleader felt her knee "go out" when she was jumping. A similar feeling has occurred before, but previously the symptoms never limited activity nor was there visible swelling of the knee. A few days after the injury, the cheerleader is brought to your office by her concerned parents. Her limp is prominent. The cheerleader wishes to continue being a cheerleader and wants to continue her active athletic lifestyle.

PHYSICAL EXAMINATION

This situation is one of the most challenging of all physical examinations. An accurate history is often hard to elicit because the situation is usually an acute injury superimposed on chronic symptoms. Cheerleaders wish to continue their role. Thus, the symptoms are often minimized.

The physical examination, particularly a dynamic physical examination, is critically important to decision-making. Explaining the importance of the process and eliciting cooperation and participation by the patient are critical. To instill confidence and to elicit the patient's cooperation is no easy task. Icing the knee often helps. Garbing the patient in shorts and protecting her modesty is important.

I usually begin the examination with the least-threatening component, the standing anatomic alignment. Here, I can discuss the key anatomic variables in the adolescent female—the width of the pelvis, the valgus knees, the alignment of the foot

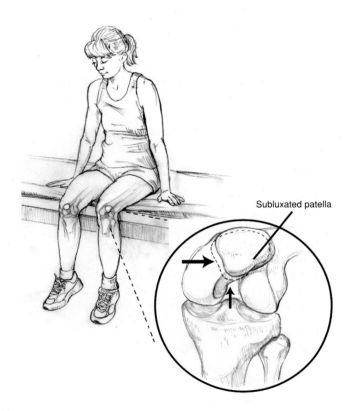

Subluxated patella

Figure 3.3A.1 The patient in the sitting position with the legs hanging off the examining table allows the physician to examine the contours, the patella mechanism, and the tibial torsion visually. This position also allows for gentle hip rotation.

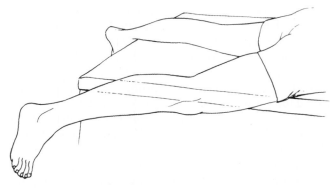

Figure 3.3A.2 In the prone examination, the hip is abducted to 45 degrees and the patient properly placed so that the edge of the table tamponades the quadriceps.

Examination of the knee in the extended position often causes pain and apprehension. Examining the patellofemoral joint with the patient in the prone position is the alternative. In the prone examination, the hip is abducted to 45 degrees and the patient properly placed so that the edge of the table tamponades the quadriceps (Fig. 3.3A.2). The examiner can examine the patella in hyperextension, with the patella disengaged from the trochlear groove. The knee is then flexed to 30 degrees and the patella can be manually contained as well as actively subluxated through a range of motion. In the prone position, a great deal of information is rapidly gained about the stability of the patellofemoral joint and the relationship between the patella and the trochlear groove.

Physical Examination of 15-year-old Cheerleader

Diagnostic Clues	Findings
Effusion	2+ the day following injury
Tenderness	Medially and laterally along the patella as well as the lateral femoral condyle
Lachman test	Negative
Drawer test	Negative
Pivot shift test	Not attempted
Varus/valgus	Stable
Patellar apprehension	Markedly positive
Range of motion	Patient will not attempt
Gait	Halting and stiff knee
Neurovascular	Intact
Other	None

GAIT

A halting gait aimed at minimizing range of motion and impact is somewhat characteristic of patellofemoral subluxation. Crutches seldom seem necessary to the patient.

IMAGING

Although there are standard patellar views, there is no standard imaging sequence. There is little agreement on the causality of patellofemoral problems. I prefer the Merchant view because it is reproducible, adequately shows engagement and alignment in the slightly flexed position, and will clearly show bone lesions if the SMPFL has pulled from the superomedial patella, either acutely or chronically. Yet the Merchant view is certainly the ultimate or necessarily the extent of our diagnostic imaging. MRI and, if possible, dynamic MRI through a range of motion has become the preferred sequence. Soft tissue injury to the SMPFL, the course of the VMO, bone bruise, and chondral damage, are all available from the MRI. The MRI complemented by a well-done physical examination offers the best diagnostic clues to an anatomically sound program.

In some instances, when the rotatory components are severe and confounding, a computed axial scan is helpful in establishing hip anteversion, and femoral and tibial torsion. Rotatory osteotomy as described by Teitge[20] is sometimes a requisite for severe cases of rotatory deformity manifested by subluxation of the patella.

The technetium (TEC) scan, although not often obtained, has helped me on several occasions in which repetitive activities caused symptoms and subluxation was suspect. Skate skiing is one such example of an activity. I believe stress fractures of the patella, although rare, are possible.

SPECIAL CONSIDERATIONS

The age and gender of the patient are important for understanding the pathologic process. Furthermore, adolescents do not tolerate alterations in their lifestyles as readily as older patients. Parental control and concern is always important. Further rehabilitation, a second opinion, and consultations are often a key to success in these difficult situations.

Because the diagnosis of patellofemoral subluxation is not universally agreed on, there is no consensus for treatment, especially the need for or efficacy of surgical treatment.

I believe integrity of the SMPFL, aided by well-developed VMO, is essential to avoid chronic subluxation, limitation of function, and degenerative arthritis in later life. This motivates my quest for an accurate anatomic diagnosis, which usually requires an MRI.

PLAN

The patient and the family understand the diagnosis, the critical features of the anatomy, and the fact that this is a chronic problem with an acute overlay. All agree that physical therapy aimed at maximizing the role of the vastus medialis obliquus (VMO) in dynamizing the superior medial patella femoral ligament (SMPFL) should be the next step.

"Cheerleading" with the patella taped or a patellar brace may be possible. No discussion about surgery should be considered until rehabilitation has rested its capacity for improvement. Patellofemoral subluxation rarely results in acute chondral damage, as distinguished from patellofemoral dislocation and spontaneous reduction, to be presented in Case Study 3B. A return to activity may be attempted as part of the rehabilitation program. Patellofemoral braces seem to assist in containment of the patella but are not 100% effective.

In the long run, to make our treatment plans, we must depend on the symptoms, the physical examination, plus an MRI coincidental with the injury. In this case the SMPFL was torn from the patella, as manifest by the tenderness and the MRI. Furthermore, the MRI showed the VMO to be stripped from the linea aspera, thus depriving this dynamizing muscle of its oblique status and its biomechanical leverage.

When surgery is accomplished, not only should the SMPFL be restored to its origin but also the obliquity of the VMO should be restored. This is a key ingredient for success. A lateral retinacular release is sometimes required to give the patella the mobility required for repair.

Surgery can be reliable and reproducible when the anatomy is restored and if there is no underlying congenital pathology, such as excessive femoral rotatory deformity or a deficient trochlea groove.

COMMENT

We hope that this in-depth discussion of a common but difficult anatomic distortion will enhance your patient care in a case such as this adolescent female cheerleader.

CASE STUDY 3B

Acute Dislocation of the Patella in the Skeletally Mature Competitive Male Athlete

HISTORY

A 21-year-old college football running back with professional football aspirations sustained a glancing blow to the knee when his foot was fixed while cutting downfield. On-field examination showed that the patella was able to be subluxated and exquisitely tender. Effusion was present immediately. The player had to be assisted off the field and he could not bear weight on the affected leg.

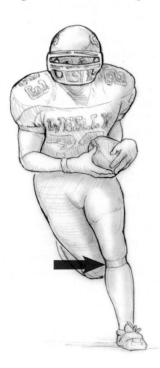

COMMENTS

The mechanism of injury is quite like that of an anterior cruciate ligament (ACL) injury. In fact, with an ACL injury, patella subluxation is not uncommon (see Case Study 2). In this case, however, the "glancing blow" dislocated the patella before the knee was flexed adequately to protect the patella in the trochlea groove. Then, because the knee was fully loaded, the quadriceps mechanism fully engaged, and flexion-extension operant, the patella relocated.

Forces three to five times the body weight are involved. An osteochondral (OC) fracture on relocation of the patella is frequent. The rapid occurrence of effusion was a reliable sign of an OC fracture. These fractures may be quite large and involve 25% to 40% of the chondral surface of the patella.

When an OC fracture is suspect, I believe in an immediate MRI and surgery as soon as possible to restore the chondral surface as best possible.

DIAGNOSTIC STUDIES

I believe immediate MRI is imperative in these cases to confirm and define the chondral damage, the damage to the SMPFL, the VMO, and the lateral femoral condyle. In addition, because the pain precludes an adequate knee examination, the MRI can rule out other injuries. The lack of an adequate preoperative knee examination does remind us to do a careful examination under anesthesia at the time of surgery, as is always done.

Physical Examination of 21-year-old Skeletally Mature Male

Diagnostic Clues	Findings
Effusion	3+ within 30 minutes of injury
Tenderness	Medially and laterally along the patella and the lateral femoral condyle
Lachman test	Negative
Drawer test	Negative
Pivot shift test	Not attempted
Varus/valgus	Stable
Patellar apprehension	Markedly positive
Range of motion	Patient will not attempt
Gait	Antalgic; stiff 30° flexed knee; prefers crutches
Neurovascular	Intact
Other	None

Figure 3.3B.1 A magnetic resonance image obtained 2 hours after injury showed evidence of patellofemoral dislocation and relocation.

SPECIAL CONSIDERATIONS

Early surgery is the major consideration. How long the cartilage retains its viability on the fracture fragments is not known, but certainly early restoration of the anatomy is the favorable choice.

Reattachment of the chondral fragments is always a challenge, but newer devices and techniques have given us great advantage in this essential technical detail.

PLAN

The MRI is obtained 2 hours after injury and shows evidence of patellofemoral dislocation and relocation (Fig. 3.3B.1). The MRI also shows disruption of the medial soft tissues—the SMPFL and VMO—a large effusion, a lateral femoral condylar bone bruise, and numerous chondral fragments in the lateral gutter.

SURGERY

Surgery is scheduled immediately. Diagnostic arthroscopy confirms the MRI and an open medial parapatellar approach is accomplished, which will allow the patellar fragments to be retrieved and replaced. The SMPFL and origin of the VMO are identified by the attendant hemorrhage and anatomically repaired. Lateral retinacular release is not necessary.

REHABILITATION

The quality of the fixation of the fragments determines the postoperative program and the rehabilitation. Hopefully, fixation is adequate to offer CPM in a limited range of motion (20 to 60 degrees). This allows the patella to remain seated in the trochlear groove and yet not be subjected to excessive shear strains. Regardless, rehabilitation will need to proceed slowly and with great specificity. Nowhere will the challenge be greater or the need for the principles (expanded in Chapter 13 on rehabilitation) be more essential.

The long-term results in these cases are uncertain. Some have been amazingly good; some have been career-ending. This unpredictability of results justifies the urgent nature of diagnosis and treatment and every attempt to restore the chondral surface.

Arthroscopic reinspection at 6 months after restorative surgery can determine the status of the healed cartilage, encourage cartilage regeneration where indicated, determine patellar tracking, release adhesions, and ensure that the patellotibial tendon interval is intact. This feature is, perhaps, the most important and underappreciated. Physical examination after relief or restoration of the patellotibial tendon interval will also confirm restoration of this key component and patellar function.[21]

Lateral retinacular release is sometimes necessary at the 6-month interval if limited mobility is apparent. Limited mobility may lead to capsuloligamentous contracture.

SUMMARY

This case study emphasizes the need for emergent care in the dislocated patella with chondral fracture. Immediate MRI is a standard, and I consider surgery emergent to restore chondral integrity as best possible.

Rehabilitation is a challenge. The shear forces on the normal patellofemoral joint are considerable as the patella engages the trochlear groove and goes into a compressive mode with the activities of daily living, such as stair climbing. The replaced chondral fragments must not be loosened through injudicious mobilization.

Arthroscopic reinspection at the appropriate interval after restorative surgery can reinforce the rehabilitation progress and fine-tune the mobilization process through elimination of adhesions and capsular contracture.

I hope this case of the football player with the traumatically dislocated patella, particularly as contrasted with the less-emergent patellar subluxation (see Case Study 3A), will give you a breadth of possibilities in how to examine and treat such injuries.

REFERENCES

1. Daniel DM, Stone ML, Dobson BE, et al. Fate of the ACL-injured patient. A prospective outcome study. *Am J Sports Med* 1994;22:632–644.
2. Steadman JR, Rodkey WG. Role of primary anterior cruciate ligament repair with or without augmentation. *Clin Sports Med* 1993;12:685–695.
3. Sherman MF, Lieber L, Bonamo JR, Podesta L, Reiter I. The long-term followup of primary anterior cruciate ligament repair. Defining a rationale for augmentation. *Am J Sports Med* 1991;19: 243–255.
4. Lubowitz JH, Grauer JD. Arthroscopic treatment of anterior cruciate ligament avulsion. *Clin Orthop* 1993;294:242–246.
5. Losee RE, Johnson TR, Southwick WO. Anterior subluxation of the lateral plateau. A diagnostic test and operation. *J Bone Joint Surg Am* 1978;60:1015–1030.
6. Shelbourne KD, Foulk DA. Timing of surgery in acute anterior cruciate ligament tears on the return of quadriceps muscle strength after reconstruction using an autogenous patellar tendon graft. *Am J Sports Med* 1995;23:686–689.
7. Wittek A. Zur Naht der Kreuzbandverletzung im Kniegelenk. *Zentralbl Chir* 1927;54:1538–1541.
8. Marshall JL, Warren RF, Wickiewicz TL, Reider B. The anterior cruciate ligament: a technique of repair and reconstruction. *Clin Orthop* 1979;143:97–106.
9. Feagin JA Jr, Curl WW. Isolated tear of the anterior cruciate ligament: 5-year followup study. *Clin Orthop* 1996;325:4–9.
10. O'Donoghue DH. Surgical treatment of fresh injuries to the major ligaments of the knee. *J Bone Joint Surg Am.* 1950;32: 721–738.
11. Finochietto B. Semilumar cartilages of the knee. The "jump sign." *J Bone Joint Surg Am.* 1935;17:916–921.
12. Mueller W. Kinematics of the cruciate ligaments. In: Feagin JA Jr, ed. *The Crucial Ligaments.* 2nd ed. New York: Churchill Livingstone; 1994;289–305.
13. Dye SF. The knee as a biologic transmission with an envelope of function. *Clin Orthop Rel Res* 1996;325:10–18.
14. Trillat A, Dejour H. Chondro-osseous fractures of the internal articular side of the patella [in French]. *Rev Chir Orthop Reparatrice Appar Mot* 1967;53:331–342.
15. Trillat A, Dejour H, Coulette A. Diagnosis and treatment of recurrent dislocations of the patella [in French]. *Rev Chir Orthop Reparatrice Appar Mot* 1964;50:813–824.
16. Dejour H, Goutallier D, Furioli J. Unbalanced patella. X: Criticism of therapeutic methods and indications [in French]. *Rev Chir Orthop Reparatrice Appar Mot* 1980;66:238–244.
17. Dejour H, Walch G, Neyret P, Adeleine P. Dysplasia of the femoral trochlea. *Rev Chir Orthop Reparatrice Appar Mot* 1990;76:45–54.
18. Galland O, Walch G, Dejour H, Carret JP. An anatomical and radiological study of the femoropatellar articulation. *Surg Radiol Anat* 1990;12:119–125.
19. Biedert R, ed. *Patellofemoral Disorders: Diagnosis and Treatment.* West Sussex, England: Wiley & Sons; 2004.
20. Teitge RA. Osteotomy in the treatment of patellofemoral instability. *Tech Knee Surg* 2006;5:2–18.
21. Feagin JA. Physical examination of the knee. In: Garrett WE, Speer KP, Kirkendall DT, eds. *Principles & Practice of Orthopaedic Sports Medicine.* Philadelphia: Lippincott, Williams & Wilkins; 2000:613–622.

SUGGESTED READINGS

Barrett DS. Proprioception and function after anterior cruciate reconstruction. *J Bone Joint Surg Br* 1991;73:833–837.
Brand RA. Knee Ligaments. A new view. *J Biomech Eng* 1986;108: 149–152.
Butler DL. Evaluation of fixation methods in cruciate ligament replacement. *Instr Course Lect* 1987;36:173–178.
Dehne E. The spinal adaptation syndrome (a theory based on the study of sprains). *Clin Orthop* 1955;5:211–219.
Fairbank TJ. Knee joint changes after meniscectomy. *J Bone Joint Surg Br* 1948;30B:664–670.
Feagin JA, Cabaud HE, Curl WW. The anterior cruciate ligament. Radiographic and clinical signs of successful and unsuccessful repairs. *Clin Orthop* 1982;164:54–58.
Feagin JA, Curl WW. Isolated tear of the anterior cruciate ligament. 5-year follow-up study. *Am J Sports Med* 1976;4:95–100.
Fithian DC, Daniel DM, Casanave A. Fixation in knee ligament repair and reconstruction. *Oper Tech Orthop* 1992;2:63–70.
Galway HR, MacIntosh DL. The lateral pivot shift. A symptom and sign of anterior cruciate ligament insufficiency. *Clin Orthop* 1980; 147:45–50.
Hunter LY, Funk FJ, eds. *Rehabilitation of the Injured Knee.* St. Louis: CV Mosby; 1984.
Merchant AC, Mercer RL, Jacobsen RH, Cool CR. Roentgenographic analysis of patellofemoral congruence. *J Bone Joint Surg Am* 1974; 56:1391–1396.
Müller W. The Knee. *Form, Function, and Ligament Reconstruction.* New York: Springer-Verlag; 1983.
Noyes FR. Flexion rotation drawer test for anterior cruciate insufficiency. In: Edmonson AS, Crenshaw AH, eds. *Campbell's Operative Orthopaedics.* 6th ed. St. Louis: CV Mosby; 1980:924.
Noyes FR, Grood ES, Torzilli PA. Current concepts review. The definitions of terms for motion and position of the knee and injuries of the ligaments. *J Bone Joint Surg Am* 1989;71:465–472.
O'Donoghue DH. The classic. Surgical treatment of fresh injuries to the major ligaments of the knee. *Clin Orthop* 1991;271:3–8. [Originally published in *J Bone J Surg Am* 1950;32:721–738.]
Pavlov H. The radiographic diagnosis of the anterior cruciate ligament deficient knee. *Clin Orthop* 1983;172:57–64.
Perkins G. Rest and movement. *J Bone Joint Surg Br* 1953;35:521–539.
Reznik AM, Daniel DM. ACL graft placement, tensioning, and fixation: part I. *Surg Rounds Orthop* 1990;August:13–15.
Reznik AM, Daniel DM. ACL graft placement, tensioning, and fixation: part II. *Surg Rounds Orthop* 1990;September:21–24.
Slocum DB, James SL, Larsen RL, Singer KM. Clinical test for anterolateral instability of the knee. *Clin Orthop* 1976;118:63–69.
Wills RP, Feagin JA, Lambert KL, et al. Intraarticular anterior cruciate ligament reconstruction without extraarticular ligament augmentation. A followup of 137 knees. Paper presented at: American Academy of Orthopaedic Surgeons; 1990; New Orleans, LA.

Classic Bibliography

John A. Feagin, Jr.

An in-depth study of any subject suggests a knowledge of the history and evolution of the subject, especially where science is concerned. I have always enjoyed the historical aspects of our care of the knee and have been privileged to know most of the major players since I entered the arena in 1967. But what of the history before my involvement? The contributions of Galen, Noulis, Battle, Hey Groves, Alwyn Smith, Campbell, Ivar Palmer, and a host of others. Their efforts, investigations, and insight must not be lost. Their contributions have helped me and often guided my thoughts. Too often we accept the limitations of a computer search for our bibliography. This "crucial" or classic bibliography is presented to stimulate the student to study in depth and learn from those who have gone before. I have immensely enjoyed preparing this bibliography and hope it will prove as valuable to you as it has for me.

Anderson AF, Federspie CF, Snyder RB. Evaluation of the knee ligament rating systems. *Am J Knee Surg* 1993;6: 67–74.

Andrews JR, Sanders R. A "mini-reconstruction" technique in treatment of anterolateral rotatory instability (ALRI). *Clin Orthop Rel Res* 1983;172:93–96.

Arnockzy SP. Anatomy of the anterior cruciate ligament. *Clin Orthop Rel Res* 1983;172:19–25.

Arnockzy SP. Blood supply to the anterior cruciate ligament and supporting structures. *Orthop Clin North Am* 1985; 16:15–28.

Arnockzy SP, Rubin RM, Marshall JL. Mircrovasculature of the cruciate ligaments and its response to injury. An experimental study in dogs. *J Bone Joint Surg Am* 1979;61: 1221–1229.

Arnoczky SP, Warren RF. Microvasculature of the human meniscus. *Am J Sports Med* 1982;10:90–95.

Battle WH. A case of suture of the crucial ligaments after open section of the knee joint. *Clinical Soc Trans* 1903;33:252.

Behr CT, Potter HG, Paletta GA Jr. The relationship of the femoral origin of the anterior cruciate ligament and the distal femoral physeal plate in the skeletally immature knee: an anatomic study. *Am J Sports Med* 2001;29: 781–787.

Berchuck M, Andriacchi TP, Bach BR Jr, Reider B. Gait adaptations by patients who have a deficient anterior cruciate ligament. *J Bone Joint Surg Am* 1990;72:871–877.

Beynnon BD, Johnson RJ, Fleming BC, et al. Anterior cruciate ligament replacement: comparison of bone-patellar tendon-bone grafts with two-strand hamstring grafts: a prospective, randomized study. *J Bone Joint Surg Am* 2002;84:1503–1513.

Beynnon BD, Uh BS, Johnson RJ, et al. Rehabilitation after anterior cruciate ligament reconstruction: a prospective, randomized, double-blind comparison of programs administered over 2 different time intervals. *Am J Sports Med* 2005;33:347–359.

Biedert RM. *Patellofemoral Disorders Diagnosis and Treatment.* Chichester, England: John Wiley & Sons Ltd, 2004.

Blankevoort L, Huiskes R, de Lange A. The envelope of passive knee joint motion. *J Biomech* 1988;21:705–720.

Blumensaat C. Die Lageabweichungen und verrenkungen der kniescheibe. *Ergeb Chir Orthop* 1938;31:149–23.

Brand RA. Knee ligaments. A new view. *J Biomech Eng* 1986;70B:149–152.

Brantigan OC, Voshell AF. The mechanics of the ligaments and the menisci of the knee joint. *J Bone Joint Surg Am* 1941;23:44–66.

Burks RT, Friederichs MG, Fink B, et al. Treatment of postoperative anterior cruciate ligament infections with graft removal and early reimplantation. *Am J Sports Med* 2003;31:414–418.

Butler DL, Noyes FR, Grood ES. Ligamentous restraints to anterior-posterior drawer in the human knee. A biomechanical study. *J Bone Joint Surg Am* 1980;62:259–270.

Cabaud HE, Rodkey WG, Feagin JA. Experimental studies of acute anterior cruciate ligament injury and repair. *Am J Sports Med* 1979;7:18–22.

Campbell WC. Reconstruction of the ligaments of the knee. *Am J Surg* 1939;43:473–480.

Cho KO. Reconstruction of the anterior cruciate ligament by semitendinosus tenodesis. *J Bone Joint Surg Am* 1975;57:608–612.

Clancy WG, Nelson DA, Reider B, Narechania RG. Anterior cruciate ligament reconstruction using one-third of the patellar ligament, augmented by extra-articular tendon transfers. *J Bone Joint Surg Am* 1982;63:352–359.

Cotton FJ, Morrison GM. Artificial ligaments at the knee. A technique. *N Engl J Med* 1934;210:1331. Reprinted as The Classic in *Clin Orthop Rel Res* 1985;196:4–6.

Coventry MB. Osteotomy of the upper portion of the tibia for degenerative arthritis of the knee: a preliminary report. *J Bone Joint Surg Am* 1973;55:23–48.

Cox JS, Cordell LD. The degenerative effects of medial meniscus tears in dog's knees. *Clin Orthop Rel Res* 1977;125:236–242.

Daniel DM. Assessing the limits of knee motion. *Am J Sports Med* 1991;19:139–146.

Daniel DM, Malcom ML, Stone ML, et al. Quantification of knee stability and function: the one-leg hop for distances. *Contemp Orthop* 1992;5:83–91.

Daniel DM, Stone ML, Riehl B, Moore MR. A measurement of lower limb function: the one-leg hop for distance. *Am J Knee Surg* 1988;1:212–214.

Daniel DM, Stone ML, Sachs R, Malcom L. Instrumented measurement of anterior knee laxity in patients with acute anterior cruciate ligament disruption. *Am J Sports Med* 1985;13:401–407.

Deehan DJ, Cawston TE. The biology of integration of the anterior cruciate ligament. *J Bone Joint Surg Br* 2005;87:889–895.

DeFrate LE, Papannagari R, Gill TJ, et al. The 6 degrees of freedom kinematics of the knee after anterior cruciate ligament deficiency: An *in vivo* imaging analysis. *Am J Sports Med* 2006;34:1240–1246.

DeHaven KE. Diagnosis of acute knee injuries with hemarthrosis. *Am J Sport Med* 1980;8:9–14.

Dye SF. Functional morphologic features of the human knee: an evolutionary perspective. *Clin Orthop Relat Res* 2003;410:19–24.

Elmqvist L-G, Johnson R. Prevention of cruciate ligament injuries. In: Feagin JA Jr, ed. *The Crucial Ligaments. Diagnosis and Treatment of Ligamentous Injuries about the Knee.* New York: Churchill Livingstone; 1994:495–505.

Elsasser JC, Reynolds DC, Omohundre JR. The nonoperative treatment of collateral ligament injuries of the knee in professional football players. *J Bone Joint Surg Am* 1974;56:1185–1190.

Fairbank TJ. Knee joint changes after meniscectomy. *J Bone Joint Surg Br* 1948;30:664–670.

Feagin JA, Cabaud HE, Curl WW. The anterior cruciate ligament. Radiographic and clinical signs of successful and unsuccessful repairs. *Clin Orthop Rel Res* 1982;164:54–58.

Feagin JA, Cooke TD. Prone examination for anterior cruciate ligament insufficiency. Brief report. *J Bone Joint Surg Br* 1989;71:863–865.

Feagin JA, Curl WW. Isolate tear of the anterior cruciate ligament: 5 year follow up study. *Am J Sports Med* 1976;4:95–100.

Feller JA, Webster KE. A randomized comparison of patellar tendon and hamstring tendon anterior cruciate ligament reconstruction. *Am J Sports Med* 2003;31:564–573.

Finochietto R. Semilumar cartilages of the knee. The "jump sign." *J Bone Joint Surg Am* 1935;17:916–921.

Fithian DC, Paxton EW, Stone ML, et al. Prospective trial of a treatment algorithm for the management of the anterior cruciate ligament-injured knee. *Am J Sports Med* 2005;33:335–346.

Fleming BC, Renstrom PA, Beynnon BD, Engstrom B, Peura G. The influence of functional knee bracing on the anterior cruciate ligament strain biomechanics in weight-bearing and nonweightbearing knees. *Am J Sports Med* 2000;28:815–824.

Friedman MJ. Prosthetic anterior cruciate ligament. *Clin Sports Med* 1991;10:499–513.

Galway RD, Beaupre A, MacIntosh DL. Pivot shift: a clinical sign of symptomatic anterior cruciate insufficiency [abstract]. *J Bone Joint Surg Br* 1972;54:763–764.

Graf B, Simon T, Jackson DW. Isometric placement of substitutes for the anterior cruciate ligament. In: Jackson DW, Drez D Jr, eds. *The Anterior Cruciate Deficient Knee.* St. Louis: CV Mosby; 1987:102–113.

Grood ES, Noyes FR. Diagnosis of knee ligament injuries. In: Feagin JA Jr, ed. *The Crucial Ligaments. Diagnosis and Treatment of Ligamentous Injuries of the Knee.* 2nd ed. New York: Churchill Livingstone; 1994:371–386.

Grood ES, Noyes FR, Butler DL, Suntay WJ. Ligamentous and capsular restraints preventing straight medial and lateral laxity in intact human knees. *J Bone Joint Surg Am* 1981;63:1257–1269.

Grood ES, Stowers SF, Noyes FR. Limits of movement in the human knee. Effect of sectioning the posterior cruciate ligament and posterolateral structures. *J Bone Joint Surg Am* 1988;70:80–87.

Griffin LY, Albohm MJ, Arendt EA, et al. Understanding and preventing noncontact anterior cruciate ligament injuries: a review of the Hunt Valley II Meeting, January 2005. *Am J Sports Med* 2006;34:1512–1532.

Groves H. The crucial ligaments. *Lancet* 1907;3:674.

Haggmark T. *A Study of Morphological and Enzymatic Properties of the Skeletal Muscles after Injuries and Immobilization in Man* [Dissertation for PhD]. Stockholm: Karolinska Institure; 1978.

Harvey A, Thomas NP, Amis AA. Fixation of the graft in reconstruction of the anterior cruciate ligament. *J Bone Joint Surg Br* 2005;87:593–603.

Hauser ED. Total tendon transplant for slipping patella. A new operation for recurrent dislocation of the patella. *Surg Gynecol Obstet* 1938;66:199–214.

Henning CE, Lynot MA, Yearout KM, et al. Arthroscopic meniscal repair using exogenous fibrin clot. *Clin Orthop Rel Res* 1990;252:64–72.

Henning CE, Yearout KM, Vequist SW, Stallbaumer RJ, Decker KA. Use of the fascia sheath coverage and exogenous fibrin clot in the treatment of complex meniscal tears. *Am J Sports Med* 1991;19:626–631.

Herzmark MH. The evolution of the knee joint. *J Bone Joint Surg* 1938;20:77–84.

Hewett TE, Myer GD, Ford KR. Anterior cruciate ligament injuries in female athletes: Part 1, mechanisms and risk factors. *Am J Sports Med* 2006;34:299–311.

Hey Groves EW. The crucial ligaments of the knee joint: their function, rupture, and the operative treatment of the same. *Br J Surg* 1920;7:505–515.

Holden DL, James SL, Larson RL, Slocum DB. Proximal tibial osteotomy in patients who are fifty years old or less. A long-term follow up study. *J Bone Joint Surg Am* 1988;70:977–982.

Houseworth SW, Mauro VJ, Mellon BA, Kieffer DA. The intercondylar notch in acute tears of the anterior cruciate ligament. A computer graphics study. *Am J Sports Med* 1980;8:106–113.

Hughston JC. *Knee Ligaments. Injury and Repair.* St Louis: Mosby Yearbook; 1993.

Hughston JC, Andrews JR, Cross MJ, Moschi A. Part I: Classification of the knee ligament instabilities. Part I: The medial compartment and cruciate ligaments. *J Bone Joint Surg Am* 1976;58:159–172.

Hughston JC, Andrews JR, Cross MJ, Moschi A. Part II: The lateral compartment. *J Bone Joint Surg Am* 1976;58:173–179.

Hughston JC, Eilers AF. The role of the posterior oblique ligament in repairs of acute medial (collateral) ligament tears of the knee. *J Bone Joint Surg Am* 1973;55:923–940.

Hughston JC, Jacobson KE. Chronic posterolateral rotatory instability of the knee. *J Bone Joint Surg Am* 1985;67:351–359.

Hughston JC, Norwoood LA. The posterolateral drawer test and external rotational recurvatum for posterolateral rotary instability of the knee. *Clin Orthop Rel Res* 1980;147:82–87.

Indelicato PA, Hermansdorfer J, Huegel M. Nonoperative management of complete tears of the medial collateral ligament of the knee in inter-collegiate football players. *Clin Orthop Rel Res* 1990; 256:174–177.

Jackson DW, Schaefer RK. Cyclops syndrome. Loss of extension following intra-articular anterior cruciate ligament reconstruction. *Arthroscopy* 1990;6:171–178.

Jackson DW, Simon TM, Kurzwell PR, Rosen MA. Survival of cells after intra-articular transplantation of fresh allografts of the patellar and anterior cruciate ligaments. DNA-probe analysis in a goat model. *J Bone Joint Surg Am* 1992;74:112–118.

Jacobson K. Osteoarthritis following insufieciency of the cruciate ligaments. *Acta Orthop Scand* 1977;48:520–526.

Jakob RP, Staubli H-U, eds. *The Knee and the Cruciate Ligaments, Anatomy, Biomechanics, Clinical Aspects, Reconstruction, Complications, Rehabilitation.* Berlin: Springer-Verlag; 1992 [Original German edition: Kniegelenk und Kreuzbander. Anatomie, Biomechanik, Klinik, Rekonstrucktion, Komplikationen, Rehabilitation. Heidelberg: Springer-Verlag; 1990.]

Jakob RP, Staulbli H-U, Deland JT. Grading the pivot shift. Objective tests with implications for treatment. *J Bone Joint Surg Br* 1987;69:294–299.

Jesse, DC. ACL insufficiency in children. In: Feagin JA Jr, ed. *The Crucial Ligaments. Diagnosis and Treatment of Ligamentous Injuries about the Knee.* New York: Churchill Livingstone; 1994:649–676.

Johnson RJ, Eriksson E, Haggmark T, Pope MH. Five-to-ten-year follow-up evaluation after reconstruction of the anterior cruciate ligament. *Clin Orthop Rel Res* 1984;183:112–140.

Johnson RJ, Ettlinger CF, Campbell RJ, Pope MH. Trends in skiing injuries. Analysis of a six-year study (1972–1978). *Am J Sports Med* 1980;8:106–113.

Jones KG. Reconstruction of the anterior cruciate ligament. A technique using the central one-third of the patellar ligament. *J Bone Joint Surg Am* 1963;45:925–932.

Jones KG. Reconstruction of the anterior cruciate ligament using the central one-third of the patellar ligaments. A follow-up report. *J Bone Joint Surg Am* 1970;52A: 1302–1308.

Kannus P, Jarvinen M, Paakkala T. A radiological scoring scale for evaluation of post-traumatic osteoarthrosis of the knee joint. *Injury* 1988;12:291–297.

Kaplan EB. The fabellofibular and short lateral ligaments of the knee join. *J Bone Joint Surg Am* 1961;43:169–179.

Kilger RH, Stehle J, Fisk JA, et al. Anatomical double-bundle anterior cruciate ligament reconstruction after valgus high tibial osteotomy: A biomechanical study. *Am J Sports Med* 2006;34:961–967.

Kim TK, Savino RM, McFarland EG, Cosgarea AJ. Neurovascular complications of knee arthroscopy. *Am J Sports Med* 2002;30:619–629.

King D. The function of the semilunar cartilages. *J Bone Joint Surg* 1936;18:1069–1076.

Kirkley A, Mohtadi N, Ogilvie R. The effect of exercise on anterior-posterior translation of the normal knee and knees with deficient or reconstructed anterior cruciate ligaments. *Am J Sports Med* 2001;29:311–314.

Kocher MS, Steadman JR, Briggs KK, Sterett WI, Hawkins RJ. Relationships between objective assessment of ligament stability and subjective assessment of symptoms and function after anterior cruciate ligament reconstruction. *Am J Sports Med* 2004;32:629–634.

Kocher MS, Steadman JR, Briggs K, et al. Determinants of patient satisfaction with outcome after anterior cruciate ligament reconstruction. *J Bone Joint Surg Am* 2002;84: 1560–1572.

Kosei, S. Allografts in knee ligament reconstruction. In: Feagin JA Jr, ed. *The Crucial Ligaments. Diagnosis and Treatment of Ligamentous Injuries about the Knee.* New York: Churchill Livingstone; 1994:623–628.

Koski JA, Ibarra C, Rodeo SA. Tissue-engineered ligament: cells, matrix, and growth factors. *Orthop Clin North Am* 2000;31:437–452.

Kurosaka M, Yashiysa S, Andrish JT. A biomechanical comparison of different surgical techniques of graft fixation in anterior cruciate ligament reconstruction. *Am J Sports Med* 1987;2:71–75.

Lambert KL. Vascularized patellar tendon graft with rigid internal fixation for anterior cruciate ligament insufficiency. *Clin Orthop Rel Res* 1989;172:85–89.

Laxdal G, Kartus J, Eriksson BI, et al. Biodegradable and metallic interference screws in anterior cruciate ligament reconstruction surgery using hamstring tendon grafts: prospective randomized study of radiographic results and clinical outcome. *Am J Sports Med* 2006;34: 1574–1580.

Lemaire M, Combelles F. Technique actuelle de plastie ligamentaire pour rupture ancienne du ligament croise anterieur [Plastic repair with the fascia lata for old tears of the anterior cruciate ligament]. *Rev Chir Orthop* 1980;66:523–525.

Liorzou G. *Le Genou Ligamentaire* [Knee Ligaments, Clinical Examination]. Heidelberg: Springer-Verlag; 1990.

Lobenhoffer P, Posel P, Witt S, Piehler J, Wirth CJ. Distal femoral fixation of the iliotibial tract. *Arch Orthop Trauma Surg* 1987;106:285–290.

Losee RE. Pivot shift. In: Feagin JA Jr, ed. *The Crucial Ligaments. Diagnosis and Treatment of Ligamentous Injuries about the Knee.* New York: Churchill Livingstone; 1994:407–422.

Losee RE, Johnson TR, Southwick WO. Anterior subluxation of the lateral tibial plateau. A diagnostic test and operative repair. *J Bone Joint Surg Am* 1978; 60:1015–1030.

Lyle MJ, Kocher MS. *The Pediatric and Adolescent Knee.* 1st ed. Philadelphia: Elsevier; 2006.

Lynch MA, Henning CE, Glick KR. Knee joint surface changes: long-term follow-up of meniscal tear treatment in stable anterior cruciate ligament reconstruction. *Clin Orthop Rel Res* 1983:172:148–153.

Lysholm J, Gillquist J. Evaluation of knee ligament surgery results with special emphasis of the use of a scoring scale. *Am J Sports Med* 1982;10:150–154.

Markolf KL, Hame SL, Hunter DM, Oakes D, Gause P. Biomechanical effects of femoral notchplasty in anterior cruciate ligament reconstruction. *Am J Sports Med* 2002; 30:83–89.

Markolf KL, Kochan A, Amstutz HC. Measurements of knee stiffness and laxity in patients with documented absence of the anterior cruciate ligament. *J Bone Joints Surg Am* 1984;66:242–243.

Marshal JL, Warren RF, Wickiewicz TL, Reider B. The anterior cruciate ligament: a technique of repair and reconstruction. *Clin Orthop Rel Res* 1979;143:97–106.

Marumo K, Saito M, Yamagishi T, Fujii K. The "ligamentization" process in human anterior cruciate ligament reconstruction with autogenous patellar and hamstring tendons: a biochemical study. *Am J Sports Med* 2005;33: 1166–1173.

McDaniel WJ Jr, Dameron TB Jr. Untreated ruptures of the anterior cruciate ligament. A follow-up study. *J Bone Joint Surg Am* 1980;62:696–705.

McDevitt ER, Taylor DC, Miller MD, et al. Functional bracing after anterior cruciate ligament reconstruction: a prospective, randomized, multicenter study. *Am J Sports Med* 2004;32:1887–1892.

McMurray TP. The operative treatment of ruptured internal lateral ligament of the knee. *Br J Surg* 1918;6:377–381.

Menschik A. The basic kinematic principle of the collateral ligaments, demonstrated on the knee joint. In: Chapchal G, ed. *Injuries of the Ligaments and Their Repair.* Stuttgart: Thieme; 1977:9–16.

Merchant AC, Mercer RL, Jacobsen RH, Cool CR. Roentgenographic analysis of patellofemoral congruence. *J Bone Joint Surg Am* 1974;56:1391–1396.

Mott HW. Semitendinosus anatomic reconstruction for cruciate ligament insufficiency. *Clin Orthop Rel Res* 1983;172:90–92.

Mueller W. *The Knee Forum, Function, and Ligament Reconstruction.* New York: Springer-Verlag; 1983.

Mueller W, Biedert R, Hefti F, et al. OAK knee evaluation. A new way to assess knee ligament injuries. *Clin Orthop Rel Res* 1988;232:37–50.

Murray MM, Martin SD, Martin TL, Spector M. Histological changes in the human anterior cruciate ligament after rupture. *J Bone Joint Surg Am* 2000;82:1387–1397.

Norwood LA Jr, Cross MJ. The intercondylar self and the anterior cruciate ligament. *Am J Sports Med* 1977;5:171–176.

Norwood LA, Cross MJ. Anterior cruciate ligaments. Functional anatomy of its bundles in rotatory instabilities. *Am J Sports Med* 1979;7:23–26.

Noyes FR. Flexion rotation drawer test. As illustrated (Fig. 9–53, p.924) In: Edmonson AS, Crenshaw AA, eds. *Campbell's Operative Orthopaedics.* 7th ed, vol 3. St. Louis: CV Mosby; 1987.

Noyes FR, Grood ES, Torzilli PA. The definitions of terms for motion and position of the knee and injuries of the ligaments. *J Bone Joint Surg Am* 1989;71:465–471.

Noyes FR, Mooar LA, Moorman CT, III, McGinniss GH. Partial tears of the anterior cruciate ligament. Progression to complete ligament deficiency. *J Bone Joint Surg Br* 1989;71:825–833.

O'Donoghue DH. Surgical treatments of fresh injuries to the major ligaments of the knee. *J Bone Joint Surg Am* 1950;32:721–738.

O'Donoghue DH. An analysis of end results of surgical treatment of major injuries to ligaments of the knee. *J Bone Joint Surg Am* 1955;37:1–13.

O'Donoghue DH. A method for replacement of the anterior cruciate ligament of the knee. *J Bone Joint Surg Am* 1963;45:905–924.

O'Donoghue DH. Facetectomy. *South Med J* 1972;65: 645–654.

O'Donoghue DH. Reconstruction for medial instability of the knee. Technique and results in sixty cases. *J Bone Joint Surg Am* 1973;55:941–955.

O'Donoghue DH. *Treatment of Injuries to Athletes.* 4th ed. Philadelphia: WB Saunders; 1984.

Paessler HH. *New Techniques in Knee Surgery.* Heidelberg, Germany: Die Deutsche Bibliothek; 2003.

Palmer I. On the injuries to the ligaments of the knee joint. A clinical study. *Acta Chir Scand* 1938;53(suppl):8–282. [Reprinted as The Classic in *Clin Orthop Rel Res* 2007; 454:17–22.]

Patel D. Proximal approaches to arthroscopic surgery of the knee. *Am J Sports Med* 1981;5:253–255.

Patel RR, Hurwitz DE, Bush-Joseph CA, Bach BR Jr, Andriacchi TP. Comparison of clinical and dynamic knee function in patients with anterior cruciate ligament deficiency. *Am J Sports Med* 2003;31:68–74.

Paulos LE, Rosenberg TD, Drawbert J, Manning J, Abbott P. Infrapatellar contracture syndrome: an unrecognized cause of knee stiffness with patella entrapment and patella infera. *Am J Sports Med* 1987;15:331–341.

Pavlov H. The radiographic diagnosis of the anterior cruciate ligament deficient knee. *Clin Orthop Rel Res* 1983;172:57–64.

Petrigliano FA, McAllister DR, Wu BM. Tissue engineering for anterior cruciate ligament reconstruction: a review of current strategies. *Arthroscopy* 2006;22:441–451.

Poehling GG, Curl WW, Lee CA, et al. Analysis of outcomes of anterior cruciate ligament repair with 5-year follow-up: allograft versus autograft. *Arthroscopy* 2005;21:774–785.

Plancher KD, Steadman JR, Briggs KK, Hutton KS. Reconstruction of the anterior cruciate ligament in patients who are at least forty years old. A long term follow-up and outcome study. *J Bone Joint Surg* 1998;80A:184–97.

Plaweski S, Cazal J, Rosell P, Merloz P. Anterior cruciate ligament reconstruction using navigation: a comparative study on 60 patients. *Am J Sports Med* 2006;34: 542–552.

Pridie KH. A method of resurfacing osteoarthritic knee joints [abstract]. *J Bone Joint Surg Br* 1959;41:618–619.

Reznik AM, Daniel DM. ACL graft placement, tensioning, and fixation: part I. *Surg Rounds Orthop* 1990;August: 13–15.

Robson M. Ruptured crucial ligaments and their repair by operation. *Ann Surg* 1903;37:716.

Rodkey WG. Laboratory studies of biodegradable materials for cruciate ligament reconstruction. In: Feagin JA Jr, ed. *The Crucial Ligaments. Diagnosis and Treatment of Ligamentous Injuries about the Knee.* New York: Churchill Livingstone; 1994:811–822.

Roe J, Pinczewski LA, Russell VJ, et al. A 7-year follow-up of patellar tendon and hamstring tendon grafts for arthroscopic anterior cruciate ligament reconstruction: differences and similarities. *Am J Sports Med* 2005;33:1337–1345.

Rosenberg TD, Paulos LE, Parker RD, Coward DB, Scott SM. The forty-five-degree posteroanterior flexion weight-bearing radiograph of the knee. *J Bone Joint Surg Am* 1988;70:1479–1483.

Salmon LJ, Refshauge KM, Russell VJ, et al. Gender differences in outcome after anterior cruciate ligament reconstruction with hamstring tendon autograft. *Am J Sports Med* 2006;34:621–629.

Salmon LJ, Russell VJ, Refshauge K, et al. Long-term outcome of endoscopic anterior cruciate ligament reconstruction with patellar tendon autograft: minimum 13-year review. *Am J Sports Med* 2006;34:721–732.

Salter RB, Simmonds DF, Malcolm BW, et al. The biological effect of continuous passive motion on the healing of full-thickness defects in articular cartilage. An experimental investigation in the rabbit. *J Bone Joint Surg Am* 1980;62:1232–1251.

Scapinelli R. Studies on the vasculature of the human knee joint. *Acta Anat* 1968;70:305–311.

Seebacher JR, Inglis AE, Marshall JL, Warren RF. The structure of the posterolateral aspect of the knee. *J Bone Joint Surg Am* 1982;64:536–541.

Segond P. Recherches clinques et experimentales sur les epanchements sanguins du genou par entorse. *Progres Med Paris* 1879;7:297–299, 320–321, 340–341, 379–381, 400–401, 419–421.

Sekiya JK, Giffin JR, Irrgang JJ, Fu FH, Harner CD. Clinical outcomes after combined meniscal allograft transplantation and anterior cruciate ligament reconstruction. *Am J Sports Med* 2003;31:896–906.

Settlage RA, Johnson DJ, Berman AB, Vireday C. ACL reconstruction with gore-tex compact diameter ligament. In: Feagin JA Jr, ed. *The Crucial Ligaments. Diagnosis and Treatment of Ligamentous Injuries about the Knee.* New York: Churchill Livingstone; 1994:797–810.

Shelbourne DK, Gray T. Results of anterior cruciate ligament reconstruction based on meniscus and articular cartilage status at the time of surgery: five- to fifteen-year evaluations. *Am J Sports Med* 2000;28:446–452.

Shelbourne KD, Nitz P. Accelerated rehabilitation after anterior cruciate ligament reconstruction. *Am J Sports Med* 1990;18:292–299.

Shelbourne KD, Wilckens JH, Mollabashy A, DeCarlo M. Arthrofibrosis in acute anterior cruciate ligament reconstruction. The effect of timing of reconstruction and rehabilitation. *Am J Sports Med* 1991;19:332–336.

Shultz RA, Miller DC, Kerr CS, Mitcheli L. Mechanoreceptors in human cruciate ligaments. A histological study. *J Bone Joint Surg Am* 1984;66:1072–1076.

Slocum DB, Larson RL. Pes anserinus transplantation. *J Bone Joint Surg Am* 1968;50:226–242.

Slocum DB, Larson RL. Rotatory instability of the knee. Its pathogenesis and a clinical test to demonstrate its presence. *J Bone Joint Surg Am* 1968;50:211–225.

Smillie IS. *Disease of the Knee Joint.* Edinburgh: Churchill Livingstone; 1980:1–27.

Smith A. The diagnosis and treatment of injuries of the crucial ligaments. *Br J Surg* 1918;6:176.

Southmayd W, Quigley TB. The forgotten popliteus muscle. Its usefulness in correction of anteromedial rotatory instability of the knee. A preliminary report. *Clin Orthop Rel Res* 1978;130:218–222.

Speer KP, Spritzer CE, Bassett FR III, Feagin JA Jr, Garrett WE Jr. Osseous injury associated with acute tears of the anterior cruciate ligament. *Am J Sports Med* 1992;20: 378–381.

Staubli H-U, Birrer S. The popliteus tendon and its fascicles at the popliteal hiatus. Gross anatomy and functional arthroscopic evaluation with and without anterior cruciate ligament deficiency. *Arthroscopy* 1990;6: 209–220.

Staubli H-U, Rauschning W. Popliteus tendon and lateral meniscus. Gross and multiplanar cryosectional anatomy of the knee. *Am J Knee Surg* 1991;4:110–121.

Steadman JR, Briggs KK, Rodrigo JJ, et al. Outcomes of patients treated arthroscopically by microfracture for traumatic chondral defects of the knee: average 11-year follow-up. *Arthroscopy* 2003;19:477–484.

Steadman JR, Cameron ML, Briggs KK, Rodkey WG. A minimally invasive technique (healing response) to treat proximal ACL injuries in skeletally immature athletes. *J Knee Surg* 2006;19:8–13.

Steadman JR, Forster RS, Silfverskiold JP. Rehabilitation of the knee. *Sports Med* 1989;8:605–627.

Sterett WI, Briggs KK, Farley T, Steadman JR. Effect of functional bracing on knee injury in skiers with anterior cruciate ligament reconstruction: a prospective cohort study. *Am J Sports Med* 2006;34:1581–1585.

Tenger Y, Lysholm J, Gillquist J. Rating systems in the evaluation of knee surgery [abstract]. *Acta Orthop Scand* 1984;55:111.

Tenger Y, Lysholm J, Gillquist J. A performance test to monitor rehabilitation and evaluate anterior cruciate ligament injuries. *Am Sports Med* 1986;14:156–159.

Terry GC. The anatomy of the extensor mechanism. *Clin Sports Med.* 1989;8:163–177.

Terry GC, Hughston JC, Norwood LA. The anatomy of the ipsiopatellar band and iliotibial track. *Am J Sports Med* 1986;14:39–45.

Torg JS, Conrad W, Kalen V. Clinical diagnosis of anterior cruciate ligament instability in the athlete. *Am J Sports Med* 1976;4:84–93.

Uhorchak JM, Scoville CR, Williams GN, et al. Risk factors associated with noncontact injury of the anterior cruciate ligament: a prospective four-year evaluation of 859 West Point cadets. *Am J Sports Med* 2003;31: 831–842.

Warren RF, Kaplan N, Bach BR. The lateral notch sign of anterior cruciate ligament insufficiency. *Am J Knee Surg* 1988;1:119–124.

Warren LF, Marshall JL. The supporting structures and layers on the medial side of the knee. An anatomical analysis. *J Bone Joint Surg Am* 1979;61:56–62.

Windsor RE, Insall JN, Warren RF, Wickiewicz TL. The hospital for special surgery knee ligament rating form. *Am J Knee Surg* 1988;1:140–145.

Wittek Von A. Kreuzbandverletzung im Kniegelenk. *Zentralbl Chir* 1935;65:103–104.

Wojtys EM, Huston LJ, Boynton MD, Spindler KP, Lindenfeld TN. The effect of the menstrual cycle on anterior cruciate ligament injuries in women as determined by hormone levels. *Am J Sports Med* 2002;30:182–188.

Yagi M, Wong EK, Kanamori A, et al. Biomechanical analysis of an anatomic anterior cruciate ligament reconstruction. *Am J Sports Med* 2002;30:660–666.

The Envelope of Function

Scott F. Dye

4

■ **INTRODUCTION 51**

■ **THE KNEE AS BIOLOGIC TRANSMISSION 52**

■ **THE ENVELOPE OF FUNCTION 52**
Factors that Determine the Envelope of Function 53
Indicators of the Envelope of Function 54
Clinical Application of the Envelope of Function 54

■ **CONCLUSIONS 55**

The primary goal of orthopaedic surgical treatment is universally considered to be "restoration of musculoskeletal function." Until now, the definition of restoration of musculoskeletal function has been conceptualized primarily in structural and biomechanical terms. It is a common belief that if one can restore normal structural and biomechanical characteristics following a joint injury such as the achievement of normal instrumented laxity in an anterior cruciate ligament (ACL)-reconstructed knee, then that joint has been "fixed" and its function restored. Further, it is thought, if function has been restored then it will be safe to return such a knee to high-demand sports like soccer and, in addition, the development of long-term arthritis will be prevented.

Recent reports have documented, however, that despite the achievement of normal structural and biomechanical indicators in knees having undergone ACL reconstruction procedures (normal laxity measurements, full range of motion, excellent muscle strength, and normal short-term x-rays), many such joints are manifesting the very disturbing development of early degenerative arthritis.[1-5] Such joints are emblematic of the failure of what can be termed the *structural and biomechanical paradigm*. This structural paradigm currently forms the conceptual foundation for most clinical orthopaedic practice (i.e., restore structural and biomechanical normalcy and function is restored). However, it is becoming increasingly apparent that restoration of normal structural and biomechanical characteristics is insufficient to prove the restoration of full physiological function of an injured musculoskeletal system. The consideration of metabolic and physiological factors—biological characteristics of *living* tissues—is essential to understand the full meaning of restoration of musculoskeletal function.

A new and alternative orthopaedic paradigm characterized by the term *tissue homeostasis* has been developed in recent years that takes into account metabolic characteristics of living musculoskeletal systems.[6,7,8] The term tissue homeostasis may be new to the reader. The word "homeostasis" is most often associated with the constant maintenance, within a certain range, of soluble factors in the blood such as levels of glucose, CO_2, or ionic calcium. The concept of *tissue* homeostasis encompasses the more complex phenomenon of normal physiologic processes of volumes of living cells within a certain range. All living musculoskeletal structures are composed of cells that, under normal circumstances, are constantly metabolically active, representing continuous molecular maintenance of these tissues. Presently, the most readily available method of manifesting tissue homeostasis is by means of technetium bone scintigraphy, which is capable of geographically revealing osseous homeostasis[9] (Fig. 4.1). The paradigm of tissue homeostasis has been formulated into a practical concept by means of the envelope of function, which represents the safe, homeostatic loading capacity of a joint or musculoskeletal system.[7] These concepts will be discussed further in this chapter.

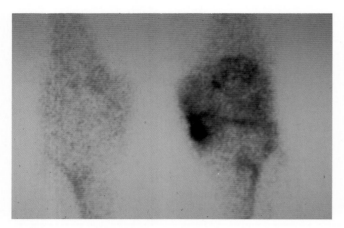

Figure 4.1 A 3-hour delayed static study anteroposterior view of the right and left knee. The study is of a 28-year-old man with symptoms of medial compartment discomfort. The magnetic resonance image (MRI) reveals a torn medial meniscus; however, radiographs of both knees were normal, as is the MRI bone signal of the left knee. One can clearly see the increased osseous metabolic activity demonstrated in the medial compartment of the left knee compared with the normal study of the right knee.

THE KNEE AS BIOLOGIC TRANSMISSION

If our task as orthopaedic surgeons is to restore musculoskeletal function, what then, is the function of a joint such as the knee? In 1988, Alfred Menschik of Vienna, Austria, in a personal communication to this author, stated that he thought the knee could be best thought of as a kind of "stepless transmission." After much consideration and discussion with many members of the international orthopaedic community, it became clear that this was an accurate and profoundly valuable insight into musculoskeletal function. The function or purpose of the knee (and by extension, all diarthrodial joints) is to accept, redirect, and dissipate a broad range of biomechanical loads without either metabolic or structural failure.

A transmission, in an automobile, for example, is a highly complex system designed to accept, redirect, and dissipate a range of mechanical loads without overheating or outright structural failure. In this analogy, the knee ligaments represent sensate, adaptive nonrigid linkages within the biologic transmission. An ACL-injured knee, for example, can thus be understood as a transmission with linkage failure that is vulnerable to symptoms of giving way, analogous to a mechanical transmission slipping out of gear. The menisci can be visualized as mobile, sensate bearings within the transmission. A knee with a torn meniscus is like a transmission with structural failure of a bearing. The patellofemoral joint functions as a large slide-bearing withstanding the highest loads within the biologic transmission. The muscles in this analogy function as living cellular engines that provide (in concentric contraction), motive forces across the knee, and (in eccentric contraction) also act as brakes and dampening systems.

THE ENVELOPE OF FUNCTION

The functional capacity of a mechanical transmission—its torque envelope—is defined as the range of loading (torque) that can be safely placed across such a system without failure (overheating or overt structural damage). One can similarly represent the safe load-transference capacity of a living human joint such as the knee, by a load/frequency distribution, which defines and delineates this safe range of load acceptance and transference in a given period of time.[7] This range of homeostatic loading is termed the *envelope of function* (Fig. 4.2). An alternative term I frequently use in communications with the lay public is the *envelope of load acceptance.*

In its simplest form, the envelope of function is a two-dimensional graph with increasing load applied across a joint on the vertical (Y) axis and increasing frequency of loading on the horizontal (X) axis. Loads applied across a living joint within the envelope of function are not only compatible with physiologic normalcy (tissue homeostasis) of all components, but are actually *inductive* of it as well. If, for example, a normal 20-year-old person is forced to decrease loading across the knees for a prolonged period of time by being kept at strict bed rest for a month, loss of tissue homeostasis manifested by muscle atrophy and calcium loss from bone will likely ensue. The pathophysiologic effects of such persistent subphysiologic underloading are often described as "disuse"[10] (Fig. 4.3).

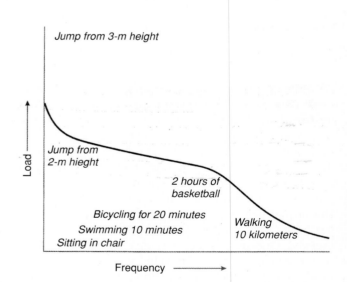

Figure 4.2 Graph representing the envelope of function for an athletically active young adult. All loading activities except jump from a 3-m height, are within this envelope of function. The shape of the envelope of function represented here is an idealized theoretical model. The actual loads transmitted across an individual knee under these different conditions are variable and are due to multiple complex factors, including the dynamic center of gravity, the rate of load application, and the angles of flexion and rotation. The limits of the envelope of function for the joint of an actual patient are probably more complex. (Reprinted from Dye SF. The knee as biologic transmission with an envelope of function. A theory. *Clin Orthop* 1996;325:12, with permission.)

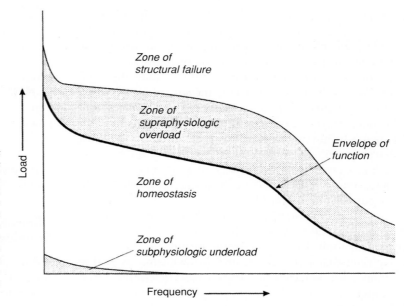

Figure 4.3 Graph showing the four different zones of loading across a joint. The area within the envelope of function is the zone of homeostasis. The region of loading greater than that within the envelope of function but insufficient to cause macrostructural damage is the zone of supraphysiologic overload. The region of loading great enough to cause macrostructural damage is the zone of structural failure. The region of decreased loading over time resulting in a loss of tissue homeostasis is the zone of subphysiologic underload. (Adapted from Dye SF. The knee as a biologic transmission with an envelope of function. *Clin Orthop Relat Res* 1996 Apr; (325):10–18, with permission.)

Most normal knees can tolerate a broad range of loading without the induction of either physiologic failure (loss of tissue homeostasis) or overt structural failure, represented by the outer edge of the envelope of function. If, however, a knee is exposed to loading beyond its physiologic load acceptance capacity, but less than that required to cause overt structural damage, then loss of tissue homeostasis will occur because of supraphysiologic overload. The term *overuse* is commonly used to describe this loss of tissue homeostasis secondary to excessive loading. A familiar clinical example would be represented by a jogger who suddenly increases his or her running distance from 5 to 15 km a day resulting in what could be termed the painful early stages of a *stress fracture* of the tibia. Such a loss of osseous tissue homeostasis is currently best manifested by a standard technetium bone scan, a metabolically oriented, rather than a structurally oriented, study. If a sufficiently great load is placed across a normal knee, an overt structural failure (e.g., ruptured ACL or fracture of a bone) can result.

Note that under normal circumstances, the outer edge of the envelope of function does not touch the horizontal x-axis (Fig. 4.2). This is because the time represented in the standard graph is during a 12-hour period. During such a short period of time, noticeable disuse will not typically ensue from too little loading. This refinement of the envelope of function concept is attributable to Dean Taylor, MD, formerly of the United States Army Medical Corps. I term this refinement, the *Taylor Gap.*

The new biologically-oriented paradigm (that of tissue homeostasis/envelope of function) thus recognizes four zones or regions of loading across a living musculoskeletal system that will (through transduction of the perceived loads at the cellular and molecular level) result in four dif-

ferent biological responses[10]: (i) *subphysiologic loading* resulting in loss of tissue homeostasis characterized as disuse, (ii) *physiologic loading* resulting in tissue/joint homeostasis, (iii) *supraphysiologic loading* resulting loss of tissue homeostasis characterized as overuse, and (iv) *loading to structural failure* of one or more components. These zones could also be simply termed *disuse, homeostasis, overuse,* and *structural failure* (Fig. 4.4).

Factors that Determine the Envelope of Function

I believe that (in addition to sex, age, and nutrition) four factors together determine the envelope of function for a

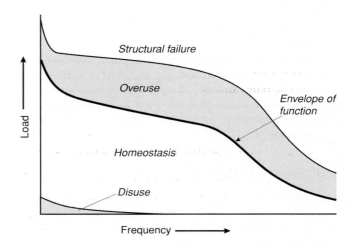

Figure 4.4 The four zones of biologic response of musculoskeletal tissues to differential loading: disuse, homeostasis, overuse, and structural failure.

specific joint or musculoskeletal system, including (i) anatomic/structural factors, (ii) kinematic/neuromuscular factors, (iii) physiologic/metabolic factors, and (iv) treatment factors (both nonoperative and operative).

Anatomic/structural factors would include the morphology (both micro and macro) and structural integrity of all components of a joint or musculoskeletal system. Also included in this category would be limb alignment and a patient's height and weight. These sets of factors are those that are manifested by structurally oriented imaging studies such as x-rays, computed tomographs, and magnetic resonance images (MRIs), and are those that most orthopaedic surgeons primarily consider.

Kinematic/neuromuscular factors are those that determine the actual motion of a joint under load with a given set of anatomic factors, and would include the proprioceptive/cerebellar muscular control mechanisms, as well as spinal reflex characteristics. These factors determine the actual temporal sequencing of motor unit contractions. Patients with excellent neuromuscular control mechanisms can adapt to the potential pathokinematic effects of many types of structural damage. For example, a patient with a damaged ACL may be able to dynamically control the knee well without any functional instability, if the patient learns to contract the musculature (cellular engines) in the proper temporal sequence. Such patients can be described as *knee copers*. This term can be interpreted as implying that there is something inherent to the knee joint itself that determines functional stability in the presence of structural failure of the ACL, whereas just the opposite is probably true. The functional stability more likely results from (anatomically) distant neuromuscular control mechanisms such as excellent cerebellar adaptive characteristics.

Physiologic factors include the effectiveness of genetically determined mechanisms of molecular and cellular homeostasis, and the ability of such systems to maintain and repair (heal) tissues. Some individuals do seem to tolerate higher degrees of loading without failure as compared with others. Also, it appears that some peoples' injured joints do heal (restoration of tissue homeostasis) quicker and better than others.

Treatment factors include nonoperative ones, such as physical therapy, bracing, and medications, as well as operative intervention. The beneficial effects of bracing in a ligamentously injured knee may arise from the enhancement of the proprioceptive neurologic output rather than from any overt biomechanical stabilization effects.

Indicators of the Envelope of Function

Clinical indicators that a joint is being loaded within its envelope of function (zone of homeostatic loading) would include the absence of pain, swelling, warmth, and instability. At present, only scintigraphic methods (e.g., positron emission tomography, technetium bone scans) are capable of geographically manifesting the presence of tissue homeostasis. These types of studies absolutely require a living, metabolically active system in order to be performed, whereas most of the other imaging modalities that are commonly used by orthopaedists, that are structural in nature, including plain radiographs (x-rays), computed tomographs, and even MRIs, do not. It may surprise the reader that, as currently configured, MRIs cannot readily distinguish between a living and cadaveric joint. In the future, it is likely that better methods of manifesting the properties of tissue homeostasis (including soft tissues) will be developed, perhaps with techniques such as functional MRI and MRI spectroscopy, among others.

Clinical Application of the Envelope of Function

The use of the envelope of function concept can be beneficial in daily orthopaedic practice. Virtually all patients with a symptomatic knee injury have been exposed to at least supraphysiologic loading conditions, if not loads sufficient to cause structural failure of one or more components. For example, anterior knee pain, often due to patellofemoral overloading (resulting in loss of tissue homeostasis, e.g., retropatellar synovitis, and increased osseous remodeling) can respond well clinically by simply decreasing the loading across this symptomatic joint to within its painless envelope of function for a sufficient period of time (along with appropriate physical therapy and an anti-inflammatory program of nonsteroidal anti-inflammatory drugs and intermittent cooling).[11,12]

I have found that the cooperation of such patients is easier to achieve by explaining the envelope of function concept, and actually drawing it out on a piece of paper. Each patient must find the limits of his or her symptomatic joint's own specific envelope by empirical means, through trial and error. Regarding physical therapy, I usually recommend an exercise day followed by a rest day for the treatment of most symptomatic joints. To be clinically within the envelope, the patient must not only be pain-free during certain activities, such as bicycling for 30 minutes, but also on the day following (because of the lag-time effect of cytokine production that can follow a supraphysiologic loading event). Mild discomfort in the muscles (cellular engines) following exercise is acceptable, whereas pain in the joint (biologic transmission) is to be avoided.

I believe that the perception of pain is the conscious aspect of a biologic negative feedback loop system, evolutionarily designed to alert the central nervous system of dangerous conditions.[13] The perception of knee pain with a certain activity is a direct indicator that it is being loaded out of its envelope. The symptoms of persistent discomfort (as well as the presence of warmth or an effusion) following maximal healing of ACL reconstructive or cartilage-oriented surgery is an indication that the knee is being persistently loaded out of its envelope of function.[10] In such cases, in addition to a Rosenberg x-ray (posteroanterior

Figure 4.5 The envelope of function 1 year after reconstruction of the anterior cruciate ligament and postoperative rehabilitation. The envelope has not been fully restored to the preinjury status. The area between the postoperative and preinjury envelopes represents a new zone of supraphysiologic overload, which potentially extends to a zone of structural failure. If a patient returns to previous high-impact loading (X), which is now outside the postoperative envelope of function, the knee will be at risk for early degenerative changes and structural failure of the graft. (A) pre-injury envelope of function; (B) envelope of function immediately after acute ACL injury; (C) envelope of function 9 months after ACL injury treated with rehabilitation alone. (Reprinted from Dye SF, Wojtys EM, Fu FH, et al. Factors contributing to function of the knee joint after injury or reconstruction of the anterior cruciate ligament. *J Bone Joint Surg Am* 1998;80:1380–1393, with permission.)

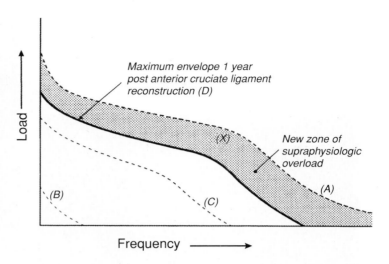

bent-knee standing x-ray of the knees), I also request a technetium bone scan. It has been demonstrated that loss of osseous homeostasis manifested by a positive bone scan precedes the development of overt radiographic degenerative changes.[14]

Posttraumatic osteoarthritis of the knee is often a phenomenon of punctuated equilibrium with periods of metabolic activation and progression of radiographically identifiable degenerative changes and periods of metabolic dormancy and nonprogression. The alarming rate of early degenerative arthrosis in knees that have had ACL reconstructions is due, in large part, to the patient believing the joints' preinjury level of function has been restored, when it has *not* been restored (Fig. 4.5). This belief then frequently results in the patient loading the knee out of its posttreatment envelope of function (which is insufficiently broad), leading initially to loss of osseous homeostasis—detectable scintigraphically, and then ultimately, structural failure—detected radiographically (Fig. 4.6A,B). If such patients are identified early (by means of a positive bone scan) at a time when the x-rays are still normal, and the patient is encouraged to decrease loading to within the current envelope, leading to restoration of osseous homeostasis, then I believe osteoarthritis can be averted.[14,15]

In my experience, patients who understand and practice the principles of restoration of tissue homeostasis by persistently loading their injured joints within their posttreatment envelopes of function rarely develop degenerative changes, barring a new injury (Fig. 4.7A,B). I never tell patients that their knee is fixed (which would imply full restoration of the preinjury envelope). Instead, in a patient with an ACL reconstruction, I say that their operated knee is like a "rebuilt transmission" rather than a factory new one, and should be protected indefinitely from excessive loading. A painless knee that functions well for decades following an injury and appropriate orthopaedic treatment is *a high-value asset,* and well worth achieving through the avoidance of certain loading activities.

An important aspect of a treatment program for a patient with a knee that is symptomatic, because it is being loaded out of its envelope, involves decreasing the loading, at least temporarily across the joint. By recommending that patients load more within their joints' own envelope of function by avoidance of certain activities, I am *not* advocating a sedentary therapeutic approach.[7,8] On the contrary, it is desirable that such a patient be as active as possible within the upper threshold limits of his or her own specific envelope. Even joints with quite restricted envelopes can often be loaded safely with an aerobic swimming or bicycling program that effectively maintains muscle strength, tone, joint flexibility, cardiovascular conditioning, and even endorphin production without supraphysiologic overload of the joint as a whole. Diminished loading across a joint identified as being at risk of developing early osteoarthritis or even one that has some overt degenerative changes along with icing, medications, and appropriate minimally invasive surgery can extend its functional capacity for years.[15]

CONCLUSIONS

I would suggest that a fundamental principle of all orthopaedic treatment is to maximize the envelope of function for a given joint or musculoskeletal system as safely and predictably as possible. A corollary principle would be: once the maximal envelope of function has been achieved, encourage the patient to continue to load within that homeostatic envelope.

With the traditional structural view of musculoskeletal injury, it is as if an astronomer were trying to understand the complexity of the universe solely with data obtained from optical telescopes that collect only visible wavelength photons. The use of metabolic imaging, such as the bone scan, can be seen as analogous to the addition of radiotelescopic data to the field of astronomy in

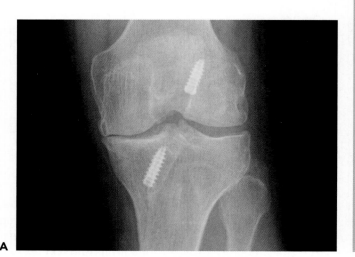

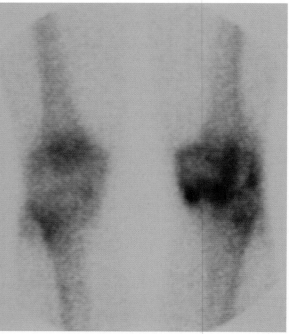

Figure 4.6   **A:** Anteroposterior standing bent-knee radiograph of a 32-year-old man showing established degenerative changes of the medial compartment of the left knee 9 years after anterior cruciate ligament (ACL) reconstruction at age 23. The patient was encouraged to pursue "accelerated rehabilitation" and was playing soccer within 6 months following surgery. This patient complained of pain in his early years, and radiographs at that time were reported as normal. One can note a near "bone-on-bone" configuration of the medial compartment as well as the retained hardware consistent with a prior ACL reconstruction. **B:** Technetium bone scan of the 32-year-old man 9 years status after ACL reconstruction showing intensely abnormal metabolic activity in the medial aspect and in general involving the entire left knee, manifesting loss of osseous homeostasis. (Adapted from Dye SF. The role of technetium bone scans in orthopaedic outcome evaluation. *Sports Med Arthroscopy Rev* 2002;10:221–228, with permission.)

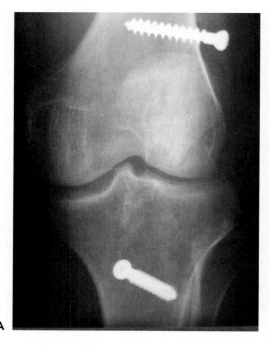

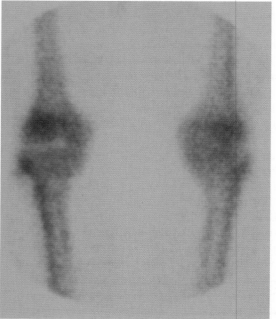

Figure 4.7   **A:** Anteroposterior radiograph of a 51-year-old man who 13 years previously (at age 38) underwent an anterior cruciate ligament reconstruction and partial medial meniscectomy showing no degenerative changes. **B:** Technetium bone scan of a 51-year-old man 13 years after anterior cruciate ligament reconstruction showing normal activity manifesting persistent maintenance of osseous homeostasis. (Adapted from Dye SF. The role of technetium bone scans in orthopaedic outcome evaluation. *Sports Med Arthroscopy Rev* 2002;10:221–228, with permission.)

the 20th century, which manifested the presence of unexpected celestial phenomenon. Based on the new information obtained from radiotelescopes (and others such as infrared and x-ray telescopes), a fundamental change in the understanding of the cosmos occurred. Similarly, the data from metabolic imaging has not only provided new insights into the dynamic pathophysiologic characteristics of symptomatic knees, but it also forces one to conceptualize joints in a fundamentally different way.[8] No longer should one view joints or musculoskeletal systems as mere assemblages of macrostructural anatomy, but as volumes of cells undergoing constant metabolic activity in an attempt to maintain tissue homeostasis under normal circumstances or restore tissue homeostasis after injury.

The tissue homeostasis paradigm and its practical application, by means of the envelope of function, provide a sufficiently broad conceptual framework to help educate patients in the subtle, but intellectually accessible principles of musculoskeletal injury and repair. This perspective has also led to therapeutic approaches that are rational, gentle, and inherently safer than those encouraged by the structural paradigm alone.

Orthopaedic surgeons with an interest in sports medicine are in an excellent clinical position to discover and document the early natural history of posttraumatic osteoarthritis of the knee. Medial compartment arthritis that develops following a medial meniscus tear can be tracked from the index injury to the possible need for joint replacement surgery. Already, there is sufficient information to indicate that loss of osseous homeostasis (manifested geographically by bone scintigraphy) precedes the development of overt radiographic degenerative changes in such patients. This phenomenon predicted by the tissue homeostasis theory thus allows for early clinical intervention that can stop the process in its earliest stages, often simply by having the patient load the knee within its envelope of function. This new pathophysiologic perspective of the development of arthritis may well have broad potential diagnostic and therapeutic implications for the early detection and prevention of arthritis of other joints.

REFERENCES

1. Daniel DM, Stone ML, Dobson BE, et al. Fate of the ACL-injured patient. A prospective outcome study. *Am J Sports Med* 1994;22: 632–644.
2. Daniel DM, Fithian DC, Stone ML, et al. A ten-year prospective study of the ACL-injured patient. *Orthop Trans* 1996–1997; 20:700–701.
3. Fithian DC. The fate of the anterior cruciate ligament injured patient: long-term follow-up: the San Diego Experience. Paper presented at: 63rd Meeting of the American Academy of Orthopaedic Surgeons; February 14, 1997; San Francisco, CA.
4. Garrick JG, Requa RK. Sports and fitness activities: the negative consequences. *J Am Acad Orthop Surg* 2003;11:439–443.
5. Salmon LJ, Russell VJ, Refshauge K, et al. Long term outcome of endoscopic anterior cruciate ligament reconstruction with patellar tendon autograft: minimum 13 year review. *Am J Sports Med* 2006;34:721–732.
6. Roe J, Pinczewski LA, Russell VJ, et al. A 7-year follow-up of patellar tendon and hamstring grafts for arthroscopic anterior cruciate ligament reconstruction: differences and similarities. *Am J Sports Med* 2005;33:1337–1345.
7. Dye SF. The knee as a biologic transmission with an envelope of function. *Clin Orthop Relat Res* 1996 Apr;(325):10–18.
8. Dye SF. The pathophysiology of patellofemoral pain: a tissue homeostasis perspective. *Clin Orthop Relat Res* 2005 Jul;(436): 100–110.
9. Dye SF, Peartree PK. Sequential radionuclide imaging of the patellofemoral joint in symptomatic young adults. *Am J Sports Med* 1989;17:727.
10. Dye SF, Wojtys EM, Fu FH, Fithian DC, Gillquist J. Factors contributing to function of the knee joint after injury or reconstruction of the anterior cruciate ligament. *J Bone Joint Surg Am* 1998;80:1380–1393.
11. Dye SF. Reflections on patellofemoral disorders. In: Biedert R, ed. *Patellofemoral Disorders: Diagnosis and Treatment.* West Sussex, England: John Wiley & Sons; 2004:1–18.
12. Dye SF, Vaupel GL. The pathophysiology of patellofemoral pain. *Sports Med Arthroscopy Rev* 1994;2:203–210.
13. Eager MR, Bader DA, Kelly JD IV, Moyer RA. Delayed fracture of the tibia following medialization osteotomy of the tibial tubercle: a report of 5 cases. *Am J Sports Med* 2004;32:1041–1048.
14. Dye SF. The role of technetium bone scans in orthopaedic outcome evaluation. *Sports Med Arthroscopy Rev* 2002;10:220–228.
15. Dye SF, Chew MH. Restoration of osseous homeostasis after anterior cruciate ligament reconstruction. *Am J Sports Med* 1993;21: 748–750.

5

Anterior Cruciate Ligament Injury Prevention: Concepts, Strategies, and Outcomes

Allston J. Stubbs   *Mininder S. Kocher*

■ **INTRODUCTION AND HISTORY 59**

■ **BIOMECHANICS AND THE FEMALE ATHLETE: THE NONCONTACT ANTERIOR CRUCIATE LIGAMENT INJURY 60**
Anterior Cruciate Ligament Injury-Prevention Studies 61

■ **BRACING THE INTACT NATIVE ANTERIOR CRUCIATE LIGAMENT 67**
The Biomechanical Experience 67
The Clinical Experience 68
Current Opinion on Prophylactic Bracing 69

■ **THE ROLE OF THE COACH AND ATHLETIC TRAINER 69**

■ **CONCLUSION 70**

INTRODUCTION AND HISTORY

A recent 10-year survey of knee injuries in 6,434 patients revealed that tears of the anterior cruciate ligament (ACL) were responsible for 20% of joint complaints.[1] It is estimated that each year between 75,000 and 250,000 individuals in the United States will suffer a new injury to the ACL. The burden of disease is particularly high in the female athlete. It is estimated that 1.4 million women and girls have torn their ACL during the last decade, and the incidence of noncontact ACL injury in female collegiate athletes is as high as 1 in 10.[2]

The epidemic of ACL injuries in both noncontact and contact athletics has resulted in a two-pronged strategy of prevention and treatment. As surgical treatment for ACL injuries carries with it morbidity, long rehabilitation and recovery, and large costs, attention has been focused on prevention of the sentinel ligament injury. During the last 35 years, orthopaedic research has contributed to a better understanding of cruciate ligament biomechanics, physiology, and failure patterns. ACL injury prevention models have been developed to address differences in cruciate injury among female athletes[3–6] and contact athletes.[7–9]

A complete tear of the ACL has been historically regarded as a significant injury. This opinion was based on the morbidity of surgical treatment, the length of time for recovery and rehabilitation, and the cost of medical treatment. The evolution of arthroscopic knee surgery, with reliable ligament reconstruction techniques, has limited the associated surgical morbidity of ACL treatment, but issues of recovery time and cost remain. Typically, ACL reconstruction requires a minimum of 6 months of functional therapy to ensure adequate muscle strength and knee joint proprioception. Additionally, the direct medical costs of a torn ACL approach $17,000 within the first year; a cumulative yearly cost of $1.5 billion in the United States.[4] This figure does not account for long-term cost of posttraumatic knee osteoarthritis or emotional cost of a major injury to active individuals.

A successful prevention strategy must address goals of efficacy, compliance, reproducibility, and cost. Several approaches to prevention have been taken, including identifying high-risk athletes, encouraging better biomechanics, and providing structural support to a healthy knee. This chapter presents current information on concepts, strategies, and outcomes related to ACL injury prevention.

BIOMECHANICS AND THE FEMALE ATHLETE: THE NONCONTACT ANTERIOR CRUCIATE LIGAMENT INJURY

The first concept of ACL injury prevention begins on the tissue level and expands to include the interaction among biologic tissues and systems. A simple hypothesis would state that achieving optimal biomechanics of a tissue system would lead to a lower chance of injury to that system. The corollary argument being that less than optimal biomechanics of a tissue system would lead to a higher chance of injury to that system. Expanding this hypothesis to the competitive athlete, one would propose that well-conditioned athletes have a lower rate of injury and that poorly conditioned athletes have a higher rate of injury. More specifically, an athlete with worse biomechanics would have a greater risk of ACL injury. A dynamic, multi-factorial model of sports injury etiology proposes that internal risk factors combine to make an athlete predisposed to injury. Exposure to external risk factors lead to a susceptible athlete who is then exposed to an inciting event, leading to injury (Fig. 5.1).[10]

What often distinguishes this injury from that of the female basketball player, however, is the presence of an external force beyond that of gravity; hence, "a contact sport." It is thus the challenge to further define the proposed hypothesis in the context of contact versus noncontact activities. The female athlete has been used as the model for the stated hypothesis in the setting of noncontact ACL injury and, thus, is the basis for this discussion.

According to Hewett et al.,[11] gender differences between male and female ACL injuries are thought to result from differences in anatomy, hormones, and neuromuscular patterns. Another study has defined these differences as nonmodifiable and modifiable.[12] Nonmodifiable differences, such as femur length,[13] femoral notch width,[14] patient height,[12] and menstrual cycle hormone levels[15-17] contribute in different capacities to ACL injury risk. Modifiable differences, such as neuromuscular patterns, appear to result from a lack of synchronization between growth and maturity of the lower extremity and appropriate neuronal control of the lower extremity in high-risk sporting movements.[18-21]

ACL injury of the female athlete has typically two defining characteristics: noncontact and deceleration. Based on these characteristics, investigators have sought to understand the implications of modifiable biomechanics on female ACL injury risk patterns and the subsequent effects of

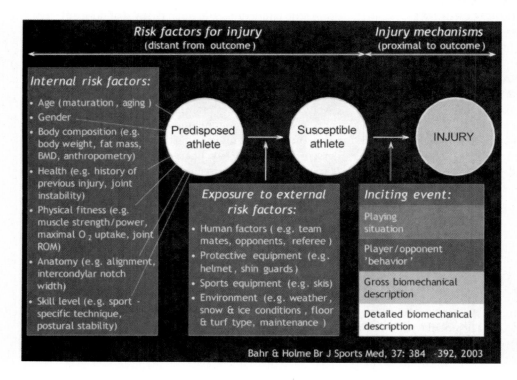

Figure 5.1 A dynamic, multifactorial model of sports injury etiology. (Adapted from Bahr R, Krosshaug T. Understanding the injury mechanisms: a key component to prevent injuries in sport. *Br J Sports Med* 2005;39:324–329.)

neuromuscular training designed to protect at-risk athletes. The female ACL injury risk pattern is best defined as a *pathokinetic chain*.[22] This chain begins as an increased adductor moment at the hip leading to lower extremity valgus and, ultimately, increased ACL strain. Hewett et al.[12] prescreened 205 female athletes for neuromuscular control using measurements of lower extremity joint angles and moments during a jump landing task. They noted that the nine athletes with subsequent ACL tears had an 8 degree greater abduction angle (knee valgus), 2.5 times greater abduction moment, and 20% higher ground reaction force as noted on the prescreening examinations. They concluded that landing task knee motion and loading are predictors of ACL injury risk in female athletes.

Other investigators have defined the at-risk position for ACL injury to be either knee varus or valgus with flexion of 10 to 30 degrees (Figs. 5.2 and 5.3).[23,24] Markolf et al.[25] were more specific in their study of ACL forces and specified that a varus force at the knee in combination with an internal rotation moment at the knee placed the ACL at greatest risk for tearing.

Encouraged by earlier investigations, Sell et al.[26] examined gender differences in planned and reactive stop-jump tasks of different directions. Comparing 18 males with 17 females of high school age, biomechanical and neuromuscular patterns were observed in the right knee. Of the three jumping directions, lateral jumping tasks to the medial aspect of the right knee demonstrated the greatest ACL risk profile by increasing ground-reactive forces, increasing

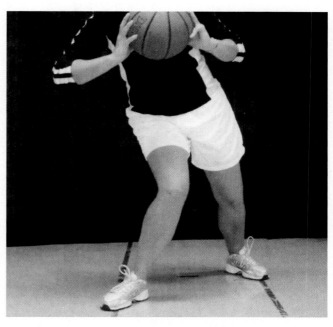

Figure 5.3   Clinical example of the valgus lower extremity at-risk alignment. (Reprinted with permission from Hewett TE, Shultz SJ, Griffin LY, eds. *Understanding and Preventing Noncontact ACL Injuries.* Champaign, IL: Human Kinetics; 2007.)

proximal tibial shear forces, increasing valgus and flexion moments, and lower flexion angles. These findings were potentiated in female athletes and by switching from a planned to a reactive task. The authors concluded that future neuromuscular and proprioceptive ACL injury prevention programs should incorporate reactive task training as well as lateral jumping strategies.

Anterior Cruciate Ligament Injury-Prevention Studies

Several ACL injury prevention studies have been performed, with many showing a reduction in the risk of noncontact ACL injury. A summary of ACL injury prevention studies is shown in Table 5.1.

Most injury-prevention schemes have focused on neuromuscular control and proprioception. Caraffa et al.[3] studied 600 soccer players in Sweden. Half (300 players) were assigned proprioceptive training and the other half no training. The players were followed for three soccer seasons. The group treated with proprioceptive training demonstrated a statistically significant decrease in the rate of ACL injury compared with the untreated group.

Hewett et al.[4] examined the effect of corrected jump and landing technique training on 11 female subjects (Figs. 5.4 and 5.5). They noted significantly reduced abduction moments at the knee. A similar study showed that phase-oriented and technique neuromuscular training in female athletes reduced the rate of ACL injuries to that seen in a male cohort.[11] A similar risk reduction was seen in elite female

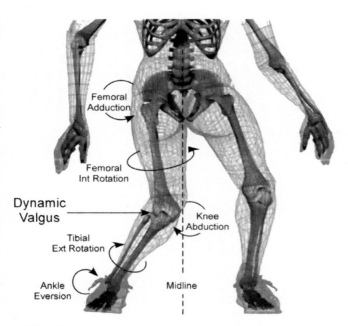

Figure 5.2   Valgus lower extremity alignment puts the anterior cruciate ligament at risk of injury. This alignment consists of hip adduction, femoral internal rotation, knee abduction, tibial external rotation, and ankle eversion. Ext, external. (Reprinted with permission from Hewett TE, Shultz SJ, Griffin LY, eds. *Understanding and Preventing Noncontact ACL Injuries.* Champaign, IL: Human Kinetics; 2007.)

TABLE 5.1
SUMMARY OF ANTERIOR CRUCIATE LIGAMENT INJURY-PREVENTION STUDIES

Study	Sport	Duration	Randomized	Equipment	Strength	Flexibility	Agility	Plyometric	Proprioception	Strengths	Weaknesses	Outcome
Caraffa et al.,[3] 1996	Soccer semi-professional and amateur; N = 600 males on 40 teams (20 intervention, 20 control)	3-season intervention (preseason)	Prospective, nonrandom	Rectangular, oblique, circular, and BAPS boards (20 min from level I to V) over 3 to 6 days a week with self-determined advancement to next level = 30 preseason days	PNF exercises	No	No	No	Balance board activities: multi-level I-V on four boards	Mechano-receptor/proprio training	Additional equipment (BAPS); not cost-effective in a large scale cohort	87% decrease in NC ACL injury: 1.15/team/season in control group compared to 0.15/team/season in intervention group (p <0.001)
Ettlinger et al.,[a] 1995	Alpine skiing; N = 4,000 ski personnel in 20 ski areas	1-year intervention (1993–94) with two previous years of historic controls (1991–93)	Prospective, nonrandom	Educational video clips of skiers sustaining ACL injuries and those that avoided injury in very similar falls; injury prevention education utilized (mechanism of injury, avoidance of high-risk behavior, fall technique)	No	No	No	No	No	Fall analysis and accident and injury analysis; cost-effective intervention and highly feasible with large skiing populations	Nonrandomized; not all potential participants trained; historic controls; exact diagnosis of serious knee sprains not always available; exact exposure to risk cannot be precisely determined	Severe knee sprains reduced by 62% among trained skiers (patrollers and instructors) compared to unperturbed group, who had no improvement during study period

Study											Outcome
Gilchrist et al.[b] 2004 (abstract only)	Soccer U-18 to U-22; N = 561 females from 61 Div I NCAA universities	1-year intervention	Yes	Educational video, cones, soccer ball	Glut med, abd, ext, HS, core training	Yes	Decel-eration, sport specific	Hip and knee position, landing technique, multiplanar	Strength on field perturbation on grass	Instructional video; Web site, compliance monitored (random site visits)	Randomized, 1-year intervention, begun at day 1 of season	Overall 72% reduction in ACL injury; 100% reduction in practice contact and NC ACLs; 100% reduction in contact and NC ACLs in last 6 weeks of season
Griffis et al.,[c] 1989	BB females	8-year intervention	Prospective, nonrandom	No	No	No	Yes	Landing technique (knee and hip flexion)	Rounded cut, deceleration patterns (3-step shuffle)	Changing cutting, deceleration, and landing techniques (encouraging knee and hip flexion)	Nonrandomized; not published (abstract only)	89% decrease in NC ACL injury in female basketball athletes
Mandelbaum et al.,[b] 2005	Soccer U-14 to U-18; N = 1041 (year 1) and 844 (year 2) females	2-year intervention	Prospective, nonrandom	Educational video, 2 in. cones, soccer ball	HS, core training	Yes	Soccer specific with decel-eration tech-niques	Hip and knee, landing technique, multiplanar	On-field program: strength, plyo, agilities on grass	Instructional video; Web site, compliance monitored (random site visits)	Nonrandomized; inherent selection (motivational) bias	Injury rates: year 1–88% reduction in NC ACL injury; year 2%–74% reduction in NC ACL injury

(continued)

TABLE 5.1
SUMMARY OF ANTERIOR CRUCIATE LIGAMENT INJURY-PREVENTION STUDIES (continued)

Study	Sport	Duration	Randomized	Equipment	Strength	Flexibility	Agility	Plyometric	Proprioception	Strengths	Weaknesses	Outcome
Myklebust et al.,[5] 2003	European team handball; N = 900 females Div I–III	3-year intervention, five-phase program	Prospective, nonrandom	Educational videotape, poster wobble board, balance foam mats	No	Yes	Planting, cutting, NM balance control activities	Landing technique (knee and hip flexion)	Balance activity on foam mats and boards	Compliance monitored by PT; instructional video poster	Nonrandomized; insufficient power	In elite division, risk of injury reduced among those who completed the program (OR: 0.06 [0.01–0.54]) compared with control; overall 53.8% and 61.5% reduction of ACL injury
Pfeiffer et al.,[d] 2004	Soccer, VB, BB HS females; N = 577 intervention, N = 862 control	2-year prospective intervention over a 9-week treatment, 15 min, two times a week	Prospective, nonrandom	No	Yes	No	No	Landing technique	No	Compliance monitored; sig. reduction in GRF and RFD in intervention	No decrease in injury in intervention group; performed posttraining; fatigue phenomenon; only 9 weeks in duration	6 NC ACL injuries: 3 intervention and 3 control = no effect
Soderman et al.,[e] 2000	Soccer females; N = 121 (control N = 100); only 62 intervention and 78 control completed study	1-season intervention (April-Oct); 10–15 min	Prospective, randomized	Balance board, 10–15 min training program in addition to regular training	No	No	No	No	Balance	Randomized clinical trail; sig. more injuries in control vs. intervention	37% dropout rate; not all subjects received same amount of training; unknown if training other than balance board was the same; numbers of ACL injuries very small	The training did not reduce the risk of primary traumatic injuries to the lower extremities; four of five ACL injuries occurred in the intervention group

Study	Sample	Design	Modality						Goals/Measures	Limitations	Results
Hewett et al.,[11] 1999	BB, VB, soccer; N = 1263: male (N = 434), female (N = 366 trained and 463 untrained)	Prospective, nonrandom	Plyometric jump box, and balance	Yes	Yes	No	Yes	Yes	Videotape, decrease peak landing forces, decrease valgus/varus perturbation, increase vertical leap, increase hamstring strength and decrease time to hamstring contraction	Nonrandomized; low VB enrollment; motivational bias; 1-on-1 program in sport facility; not feasible to implement across large cohort	14 ACLs reported: female injury rates 0.43 untrained vs. 0.12 trained vs. male control 0.9 over 6-week program; untrained group 3.6-4.8 higher injury rates of ACL injury
Heidt et al.,[f] 2000	Soccer; N = 300 females	Prospective, nonrandom	Treadmill, sports cord, plyometric box jump	Yes	Yes	Yes	Yes	Yes	Increase strength, lower overall injury rates	Not stat. sig.; 7 weeks insufficient time for NM re-education to occur at mechano-receptor level	61.2% injuries in knee/ankle; 2.4% injury rate in intervention vs. 3.1% in control
Olsen et al.,[27] 2005	European team handball (123 teams); N = 1837 players: 1586 female, 251 male	Randomized, controlled cluster trial	Wobble board (Norpro), balance foam mats (Airex)	Squats and power (bounding)	Yes	Planting, cutting, NM control	Knee over toe, proper landing technique	Balance activity on single/ double leg, mats and boards	Randomized; compliance monitored; reduction of injury; structured warm-up	Uncertain what parameter of program effective; male and female; cannot extrapolate to other sports	129 acute knee and ankle injuries overall; 81 in control (0.9 overall, 0.3 trained, 5.3 matched) vs. 48 in intervention (0.5 overall, 0.2 trained, 2.5 matched); 80% reduction of ACL injuries

6-week pre-season intervention, 1-year monitoring, 60–90 min/day for 3 days a week (Hewett et al.)

7-week pre-season intervention, 1-year monitoring, 3 days a week (one plyo and two treadmill) (Heidt et al.)

15–20 min training, 8 months (one handball season), 15 consecutive sessions and once a week thereafter (Olsen et al.)

(continued)

65

TABLE 5.1

SUMMARY OF ANTERIOR CRUCIATE LIGAMENT INJURY-PREVENTION STUDIES (continued)

Study	Sport	Duration	Randomized	Equipment	Strength	Flexibility	Agility	Plyometric	Proprioception	Strengths	Weaknesses	Outcome
Wedderkopp et al.,[g] 2003	European team handball; 236 females (17–18 years), 20 teams	10-month intervention (one season)	Randomized, controlled cluster trial	Balance board (proprioceptive) in four levels	Yes	No	No	Yes	Balance training with ankle discs	Randomized clinical trial	Specific injury types not given; description of ankle disc training not given; "warm-up" exercises also provided to trained group but not specified; compliance with all exercises not mentioned	Ankle injuries sig. greater in control group (2.4 vs. 0.2); unspecified knee injuries not sig. less in trained group (6.9 vs. 0.6); 5 knee sprains and 1 knee "luxation" in control group vs. 1 knee sprain in trained group

BAPS, biomechanical ankle platform system; PNF, proprioceptive neuromuscular facilitation; propio, proprioceptive; NC, noncontact; ACL, anterior cruciate ligament; U, under; NCAA, National Collegiate Athletic Association; Glut med, gluteus medius; abd, abduction; ext, external; HS, high school; BB, basketball; plyo, plyometric; VB, volleyball; GRF, ground-reaction force; RFD, rate of force development; sig., significantly; stat., statistically.

Adapted from: Griffin LY, Albohm MJ, Arendt EA, et al. Understanding and Preventing Noncontact Anterior Cruciate Ligament Injuries: A Review of the Hunt Valley II Meeting, January 2005. *Am J Sports Med* 2006;34:1512–1532.

[a]Ettlinger CF, Johnson RJ, Shealy JE. A method to help reduce the risk of serious knee sprains incurred in alpine skiing. *Am J Sports Med* 1995;23:531–537.

[b]Gilchrist JR, Mandelbaum BR, Melancon H. A randomized controlled trial to prevent anterior cruciate ligament injuries in female collegiate soccer players (abstract 6-7). Paper presented at: American Orthopaedic Society for Sports Medicine Specialty Day; March 13, 2004; San Francisco, CA.

[c]Griffis ND, Nequist SW, Yearout K, et al. Injury prevention of the anterior cruciate ligament. Abstracted in the American Orthopaedic Society for Sports Medicine: Meeting Abstracts, Symposia, and Instructional Courses, 15th Annual Meeting; June 19–22, 1989; Traverse City, MI.

[d]Pfeiffer RP, Shea KG, Grandstrand S, et al. Effects of a knee ligament injury prevention (KLIP) program on the incidence of noncontact ACL injury: a two-year prospective study of exercise intervention in high school female athletes. Podium presentation at American Orthopaedic Society for Sports Medicine Specialty Day; March 13, 2004; San Francisco, CA.

[e]Soderman K, Werner S, Pietila T, et al. Balance board training: prevention of traumatic injuries of the lower extremities in female soccer players? A prospective randomized intervention study. *Knee Surg Sports Traumatol Arthrosc* 2000;8:356–363.

[f]Heidt RS, Sweeterman LM, Carlonas RL, et al. Avoidance of soccer injuries with preseason conditioning. *Am J Sports Med*, 2000;28:659–662.

[g]Wedderkopp N, Kaltoft M, Holm R, et al. Comparison of two intervention programmes in young female players in European handball: with and without ankle discs. *Scand J Med Sci Sports* 2003;13:371–375.

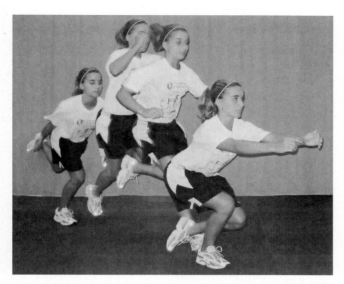

Figure 5.4 Plyometric neuromuscular training. (Reprinted with permission from Hewett TE, Shultz SJ, Griffin LY, eds. *Understanding and Preventing Noncontact ACL Injuries.* Champaign, IL: Human Kinetics; 2007.)

Norwegian handball players by Myklebust et al.[5] In the elite players, they noted that a five-phase program of neuromuscular control and planting/landing skills significantly reduced the risk of an ACL tear over the course of two seasons. This effect was not seen in a broader skill set

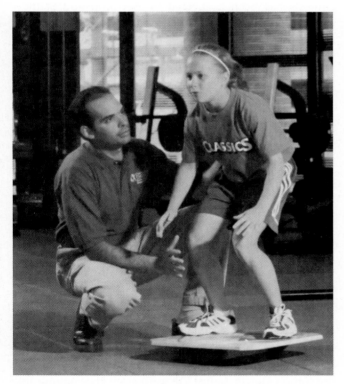

Figure 5.5 Balance board training with biofeedback. (Reprinted with permission from Hewett TE, Shultz SJ, Griffin LY, eds. *Understanding and Preventing Noncontact ACL Injuries.* Champaign, IL: Human Kinetics; 2007.)

of female players. This led the study authors to conclude that compliance and time for training likely play a role in the success of such prevention programs. Furthermore, in a randomized trial of handball clubs in Norway, Olsen et al.[27] found that a structured program of warm-up exercises to improve running, cutting, and landing technique as well as neuromuscular control, balance, and strength resulted in a reduction of knee and ankle injuries. However, a follow-up video-based intervention program studied by Arnason et al.[28] did not show a reduction in ACL injury.

More recently, Paterno et al.[29] examined the role of neuromuscular training on 41 female high school students. The intervention lasted 6 weeks and measured single-limb postural stability, anteroposterior stability, and medial-lateral stability. With focused neuromuscular training, the authors noted a significant increase in overall single-limb stability and anteroposterior stability. There was no change in medial-lateral stability. The potential for this type of neuromuscular training to reduce ACL injury in a susceptible female population will need to be determined across a larger study group.

BRACING THE INTACT NATIVE ANTERIOR CRUCIATE LIGAMENT

One of the most tangible historical and current interventions for protection against ACL injury has been knee bracing. Knee braces have been developed for prophylactic, functional, and rehabilitative purposes. Support for prophylactic knee bracing (PKB) has come from athletic trainers, coaches, physicians, and, most importantly, an athlete's family members. The effectiveness of knee bracing in protecting native ligament integrity has been studied both biomechanically and clinically.

The Biomechanical Experience

In assessing PKBs, the use of cadaveric and surrogate knee models has been viewed with skepticism. The braced knee models, while controlled, do not account for weightbearing, physiologic loads, or muscle tone. In light of these limitations, the laboratory investigations of PKBs off the playing field have provided some insight into their effectiveness in protecting against knee ligamentous injury. Further, newer laboratory methods that examine additional risk factors for noncontact injuries have led to research that accounts for the deficiencies of previous studies, including weightbearing and muscle tone.

In 1987, Paulos et al.[30] published a study of 18 cadaveric knees tested with one of two lateral stabilizing braces: Anderson Knee Stabler (Vision Quest Industries, Inc., Irvine, CA [Out of Production]) or McDavid Knee Guard (McDavid Knee-Guard, Inc. Woodridge, IL). In the presence or absence of one of the lateral braces, the application of valgus force was analyzed with respect to joint line opening and resulting ligament tensions/failure. No correlation was seen between the use of a brace and reduced joint line opening or ligament failure with application of valgus stress. The authors correlated these results to a lack of protection of the medial collateral ligament (MCL).

Also in 1987, Wojtys et al.[31] focused specifically on the influence of the Lennox Hill Brace, a functional brace, in protecting the knee from excessive anterior translation or external rotation moments. The authors used four cadaveric specimens tested at 30 degrees of knee flexion to compare nonbraced and braced ligament-intact and ligament-deficient knees. Although the sample size was too small for statistical significance, the brace was noted to decrease anterior translation in the ACL intact knee and the isolated ACL-deficient knee. No effect was noted in the braced MCL-/ACL-deficient or MCL-/lateral collateral ligament-deficient knee. With regard to rotation, the brace effectively limited external rotation in all specimens regardless of ligament condition.

The variability of cadaveric knees in biomechanics testing led some research teams to test brace wear using a surrogate knee model. These models were typically made from composite materials that could be manufactured to mimic the bulk, size, and mechanics of human tissue. Additionally, some research teams employed hybrid cadaveric-surrogate knee models to capture brace effects in a reproducible and anatomic way.

France et al.[32] introduced a human cadaver validated, free-standing, two-legged surrogate model for the assessment of lateral brace effectiveness in a contact type knee injury. Overall, six different brands of lateral prophylactic braces were tested. Brace effectiveness was based on an arbitrary standard defined as the *Impact Safety Factor* (ISF). An ISF of 1.50 or 30% load reduction across the MCL was considered adequate for protection against a lateral knee blow. The authors observed that greater brace stiffness and length were associated with a higher ISF. No brace consistently performed above the ISF rating of 1.50. This study did not examine the effect of ISF on ACL protection.

In 1990, eight PKBs were evaluated in a surrogate model by Brown et al.[33] Higher brace tension was associated with greater strain reduction across the model. All braces were noted to protect the MCL from significant strain of 20% to 30% compared with no lateral brace wear. The customized off-the-shelf braces performed better than the noncustomized braces. A year later, Paulos et al.,[34] using the model of France et al.,[32] tested the use of prophylactic bracing in a lateral knee contact to reduce MCL and ACL contact forces, contact initiation times, and ISFs. The surrogate limb in the study by Paulos et al. was rigidly fixed and the applied lateral force was increased over the 1987 model of France et al. The authors demonstrated that by increasing impact duration, a lateral brace may selectively protect the ACL over the MCL. In 1993, PKB MCL protection was seen in a surrogate knee model comparing prophylactic bracing versus no bracing.[35] Significant findings of increased valgus load to failure and MCL strain relief were noted in the models with single, upright, hinged braces. Increases in hinge length or offset, upright length, breadth, thickness, or cuff area did not lead to increased protection of the knee model.

Erickson et al.[36] published a study using a hybrid cadaveric-surrogate knee model. In eight specimens, the authors measured strain across the MCL and ACL in the setting of prophylactic bracing and lateral loading. The authors reported that the presence of a brace reduced the amount of force experienced by the knee during external contact; however, no significant change was seen in ACL strain between specimens with or without a brace. Also, there was a trend in the braced knees tested at 30 degrees for the MCL to experience less strain.

Prior criticism of the inanimate research of brace protection has led other authors to measure different clinical parameters besides load to failure, anterior joint translation, and rotation. Yu et al.[37] compared a PKB in its effect to alter landing mechanics of a stop-jump task. Using 20 human subjects with and without a specially designed knee brace, parameters of jumping performance, maximum knee flexion angle, and maximum ground-reaction force were tested. In the setting of brace wear, the authors noted a statistically significant increase of 5 degrees in maximum knee flexion angle. The other metrics of performance and ground reaction force were unchanged by brace wear. The authors concluded that special brace design may protect athletes from noncontact ACL injury through kinematic modification without compromising athletic performance.

Direct measurement techniques of ACL strain in human subjects has been pioneered by Beynnon and Slauterbeck.[38] Custom and off-the-shelf brace designs significantly reduced ACL strain values for anterior-directed loads applied to the tibia up to the maximum anterior load of 140 N. Similarly, bracing reduced ACL strain in response to internal and external rotation torques.

The Clinical Experience

The first high-profile athlete to compete with a knee brace and succeed was "Broadway" Joe Namath in the 1970s. He used the Lenox Hill Derotation Brace, a functional knee brace. Following Broadway Joe, the subsequent decade was filled with hope of a greater role for knee bracing as surgical treatment techniques for ACL-deficient knees were typically nonanatomic and rehabilitation was poorly understood. Ken Stabler, the quarterback for the 1970s Oakland Raiders, was fitted by the team's athletic trainer with a dual-hinged knee brace following an MCL injury. This experience, and that of eight other players, was detailed in the 1979 study by Anderson et al.[39] The authors speculated that braces could potentially reduce valgus loads and anteroposterior translation, and, thus, ligamentous injury to the knee. Consequently, a sports medicine movement emerged to protect the contact athlete against valgus-rotatory knee trauma and the "unhappy triad" of O'Donoghue.[40]

During the 1980s, enthusiasm for knee bracing waxed then waned. Several studies were published about knee bracing in contact athletics.[41-46] Most of these studies were inconclusive about the role of prophylactic knee bracing and some concluded that bracing could increase the rate of injuries sustained by players who wore them.[47] In response to the heightened interest within the orthopaedic community, the American Academy of Orthopaedic Surgeons (AAOS), in 1987, released a position paper entitled, "The Use of Knee Braces."[48] This manuscript stated that the AAOS remained negative to neutral at best on the role of prophylactic bracing of knees based on a lack of clear efficacy and some suggestion of potentiating injury. The orthopaedic community's response to this position paper was a retreat from recommending knee braces as a reliable way to prevent injury. Based on the expense of most knee brace systems and the purported increased risk to the player, teams across the United States avoided bracing their athletes.

Although the field of surgical treatment for ACL injury advanced with arthroscopic techniques, the concept of PKBs was not completely abandoned in the 1990s. The advances in brace technology, including polycentric hinges, lighter and stronger materials, as well as custom fitting, provided the impetus to revisit the use of knee bracing in prevention of knee injury. Further, while surgical techniques had improved to more anatomic reconstructions, the large financial cost and lengthy rehabilitation time were still substantial, leading many institutions and their teams to explore prevention alternatives. The identification of high-risk players, in conjunction with improved compliance with brace wear during at-risk activities, were fundamental to two studies published in the 1990s from West Point[7] and the Big Ten Conference.[8,9]

The West Point prospective and randomized study of 1,396 cadets during 2 years looked at the role of knee bracing in the intramural tackle football population. Outcomes of the study were measured as clinical injury of the knee preventing practice or game participation. Study subjects were controlled for shoe wear, competition exposure, brace make/model, and compliance. All of the cadets wore a noncustom brace. The study authors concluded that statistically significant reduction of injuries could be achieved with brace wear. There was also a trend toward brace wear limiting the severity of injury (e.g., MCL vs. MCL/ACL sprains) but this finding was not statistically significant. The West Point experience did not show an increased risk of injury with brace wear. A limitation of the study was the power of the study, which limited conclusions based on the severity of injury.

The Sports Medicine Committee of the Big Ten Conference commissioned a 3-year, multicenter, prospective study of MCL injuries in varsity football players. Brace wear patterns were analyzed, in conjunction with MCL injuries, across 55,722 football knee exposures. The outcome point of MCL injury was based on clinical examination. To determine the effectiveness of PKBs, players were controlled for position, string/skill level, and type of play (practice vs. game). Similar to the findings of the West Point investigation, the authors noted trends in MCL injury prevention using PKBs in the setting of practices for all players and in the setting of games for linemen, linebackers, and tight ends. During games, skill players such as cornerbacks and quarterbacks did not appear to directly benefit from protective brace wear. Once again, in contrast to the findings of Teitz et al.,[47] PKBs did not increase the quantity or quality of knee injuries sustained by National Collegiate Athletic Association varsity football players. The investigation was limited by a lack of statistical significance in all results, outcome data based on subjective assessment, and no control of brace make/model or shoe type.

Current Opinion on Prophylactic Bracing

The AAOS updated its position paper on knee bracing in 2003.[49] Based on a survey of published literature, the Academy has made the following statement regarding prophylactic knee bracing: *"American Academy of Orthopaedic Surgeons (AAOS) believes that prophylactic knee braces may provide limited protection against injuries to the medial collateral ligament in football players. Scientific studies have not consistently demonstrated similar protection by prophylactic braces to other knee ligaments, menisci, or articular cartilage."*

The orthopaedic community remains noncommittal on the use of PKBs. Global medical issues such as cost-effectiveness are a modern reality of orthopaedic sports medicine practice. Additionally, the issue of increased risk of injury with knee bracing has not been settled.[50] Despite the current era of defensive medicine, the concept of committing an athletic team financially, medically, and psychologically to prophylactic brace wear is not an accepted practice based on the available literature.

THE ROLE OF THE COACH AND ATHLETIC TRAINER

On the front lines of ACL injury prevention are the coach and athletic trainer. Both have the goal of optimizing individual and team performance. An ACL injury to any team member can be a distraction of team focus, a drain on team resources, and a detriment to a team's success. This list does not address the complex issues faced by the athlete in the setting of an ACL tear. As such, coaches and athletic trainers should have the aligned goal of ACL prevention for the benefit of the team and the health of the players.

Several strategies for ACL injury prevention have been discussed within this chapter and include identification of high-risk athletes, neuromuscular/proprioceptive training, and knee bracing. High-risk athletes include female athletes, athletes with hyperlaxity, and athletes in high-risk sports. Not all female athletes are at risk, but a majority of them require age- and skill-specific recommendations to optimize their physical condition and limit their risk of ACL injury. Hyperlaxity is a poorly defined term, but basically refers to an individual with significant ligamentous laxity. These athletes are at risk because their ligamentous restraints are compromised by disorganized collagen. Finally, high-risk sports can be noncontact or contact. Any activity, where nonlinear and pivoting motions are experienced, places the ACL at risk.

TABLE 5.2

NONCONTACT ANTERIOR CRUCIATE LIGAMENT INJURY PREVENTION TRAINING PROGRAM

Preprogram (Flexibility)
Warm-Up
   Jog line to line, shuttle run, backward running
Stretching
   Calf, quadriceps, hamstring, inner thigh, hip flexor
Neuromuscular
Strengthening
   Walking lunges, Russian hamstrings, single-toe raises
Plyometric Training
   Jump-training program → lateral hops, forward hops, single-legged hops, vertical jumps,
     scissors jumps
   Plant/landing skills
Agilities
   Shuttle run, diagonal run, bounding run
   Floor exercises: running, planting, jumping
Proprioception
   Single-leg stance
   Balance mat/wobble board: rectangular → round → multiplanar (BAPS)
   Anterior and posterior step-up
Reactive Tasks
   Sport-specific

BAPS, biomechanical ankle platform system.
Program derived from Caraffa et al.,[3] 1996; Hewett et al.,[4] 1996; Myklebust et al.,[5] 2003; and Mandelbaum et al.,[6] 2005.

Neuromuscular and proprioceptive training can be completed in the preseason conditioning phase for all athletes and continued throughout the season with higher-risk individuals as noted previously. A curriculum of correct landing and take-off, pivoting, and cutting should be introduced as an integral part of successful technique. Table 5.2 is an ACL injury prevention program modified from successful training regimens.[3-6] Endurance, conditioning, and strengthening programs should incorporate these technique recommendations. Compliance with training should be closely monitored and modified as the season progresses.

Finally, prophylactic bracing is a controversial area in ACL injury prevention. For the high-performance athlete, the effect of PKBs on speed and agility is uncertain; however, brace migration and unnatural kinematics are acknowledged nuisances.[51-53] Based on the cost, inconvenience, and lack of consistent evidence, global prophylactic knee bracing is not recommended in either the pediatric or mature athlete. In high-risk contact athletes, there may be a role for prophylactic bracing in reducing MCL sprains.

CONCLUSION

The complex challenge of ACL tear prevention lies in the variability of injury mechanisms, as well as gender-specific neuromuscular mechanics. A successful prevention program begins with identification of the high-risk athlete.

Next, a comprehensive prevention program should be developed with the athlete, the athlete's parents, trainers, and coaches. The program should incorporate a form and function approach. In regard to form, the player should be assessed for neuromuscular deficiencies that will place him or her at higher risk for an ACL tear. In regard to function, the athlete should be educated on the controversies surrounding prophylactic bracing. The use of a prophylactic brace should be based on an athlete's string, position, and game time. Additionally, the use of a brace should take into account the contact level of the sport. Based on more than 30 years of investigations into a focused ACL prevention strategy, one is left with the impression that there is not a single approach, but custom plans that must be flexible based on the needs of the athlete. Future investigations will better define prevention strategies based on an athlete's sport and position, gender, and custom biomechanical and neuromuscular profile.

REFERENCES

1. Majewski M, Susanne H, Klaus S. Epidemiology of athletic knee injuries: a 10-year study. *Knee* 2006;13:184–188.
2. Hewett TE. An introduction to understanding and preventing ACL injury. In: Hewett TE, Shultz SJ, Griffin LY, eds. *Understanding and Preventing Noncontact ACL Injuries.* Champaign, IL: Human Kinetics; 2007;xxi–xxviii.
3. Caraffa A, Cerulli G, Progetti M, et al. Prevention of anterior cruciate ligament injuries in soccer. *Knee Surg Sports Traumatol Arthroscopy* 1996;4:19–21.

4. Hewett TE, Stroupe AL, Nance TA, et al. Plyometric training in female athletes: decreased impact forces and increased hamstring torques. *Am J Sports Med* 1996;24:765–773.

5. Myklebust G, Engebretsen L, Braekken IH, et al. Prevention of anterior cruciate ligament injuries in female team handball players: a prospective intervention study over three seasons. *Clin J Sports Med* 2003;13:71–78.

6. Mandelbaum BR, Silvers HJ, Watanabe DS, et al. Effectiveness of a neuromuscular and proprioceptive training program in preventing anterior cruciate ligament injuries in female athletes. *Am J Sports Med* 2005;33:1003–1010.

7. Sitler M, Ryan J, Hopkinson W, et al. The efficacy of a prophylactic knee brace to reduce knee injuries in football. *Am J Sports Med* 1990;18:310–315.

8. Albright JP, Powell JW, Smith W, et al. Medial collateral ligament knee sprains in college football: brace wear preferences and injury risk. *Am J Sports Med* 1994;22:2–11.

9. Albright JP, Powell JW, Smith W, et al. Medial collateral ligament knee sprains in college football: effectiveness of preventative braces. *Am J Sports Med* 1994;22:12–18.

10. Engebretsen L. Discussion, summary and future research goals. In: Hewett TE, Shultz SJ, Griffin LY, eds. *Understanding and Preventing Noncontact ACL Injuries*. Champaign, IL: Human Kinetics; 2007:121–128.

11. Hewett TE, Lindenfield TN, Riccobene JV, et al. The effect of neuromuscular training on the incidence of knee injury in female athletes: a prospective study. *Am J Sports Med* 1999;27:699–706.

12. Hewett TE, Myer GD, Ford KR, et al. Biomechanical measures of neuromuscular control and valgus loading of the knee predict anterior cruciate ligament injury risk in female athletes. *Am J Sports Med* 2005;33:492–501.

13. Beynnon B, Slauterbeck J, Padua D, et al. Update on ACL risk factors and prevention strategies in the female athlete. Paper presented at: 52nd Annual Meeting and Clinical Symposia of the National Athletic Trainers' Association; June 2001; Los Angeles, CA.

14. Scoville CR, Williliams GN, Uhorchak JM, et al. Paper 62: Risk factors associated with anterior cruciate ligament injury. In: Proceedings of the 68th Annual Meeting of the American Academy of Orthopaedic Surgeons; February 28, 2001:564; San Francisco, CA.

15. Arendt EA, Bershadsky B, Agel J. Periodicity of noncontact anterior cruciate ligament injuries during the menstrual cycle. *J Gend Specif Med* 2002;5:19–26.

16. Slauterbeck JR, Hardy DM. Sex hormones and knee ligament injuries in female athletes. *Am J Med Sci* 2001;322:196–199.

17. Wojtys EM, Ashton-Miller JA, Huston LJ. A gender-related difference in the contribution of the knee musculature to sagittal-plane shear stiffness in subjects with similar knee laxity. *J Bone Joint Surg Am* 2002;84:10–16.

18. Hewett TE. Neuromuscular and hormonal factors associated with knee injuries in female athletes: strategies for intervention. *Sports Med* 2000;29:313–327.

19. Hewett TE, Paterno MV, Myer GD. Strategies for enhancing proprioception and neuromuscular control of the knee. *Clin Orthop Relat Res* 2002;402:76–94.

20. Lloyd DG. Rationale for training programs to reduce anterior cruciate ligament injuries in Australian football. *J Orthop Sports Phys Ther* 2001;31:645–654.

21. McClean SG, Lipfert S, van den Bogert AJ. Effect of gender and defensive opponent on the biomechanics of sidestep cutting. *Med Sci Sports Exerc* 2004;36:1008–1016.

22. Silvers HJ, Giza E, Mandelbaum BR. Anterior cruciate ligament tear prevention in the female athlete. *Curr Sports Med Rep* 2005; 4:341–343.

23. Delfico A, Garrett W. Mechanisms of injury of the ACL in soccer players. *Clin Sports Med* 1998;17:779–785.

24. Kirkendall DT, Garrett WE. The anterior cruciate ligament enigma: injury mechanisms and prevention. *Clin Orthop Relat Res* 2000;372:64–68.

25. Markolf KL, Burchfield DM, Shapiro MM, et al. Combined knee loading states that generate high anterior cruciate ligament forces. *J Orthop Res* 1995;12:930–935.

26. Sell TC, Ferris CM, Abt JP, et al. The effect of direction and reaction on the neuromuscular and biomechanical characteristics of the knee during tasks that simulate the noncontact anterior cruciate ligament injury mechanism. *Am J Sports Med* 2006;34:43–54.

27. Olsen OE, Myklebust G, Engebretsen L, Holme I, Bahr R. Exercises to prevent lower limb injuries in youth sports: cluster randomised controlled trial. *BMJ* 2005;26;330(7489):449–455.

28. Arnason A, Engebretsen L, Bahr R. No effect of a video-based awareness program on the rate of soccer injuries. *Am J Sports Med* 2005;33(1):77–84.

29. Paterno MV, Myer GD, Ford KR, et al. Neuromuscular training improves single-limb stability in young female athletes. *J Orthop Sports Phys Ther* 2004;34:305–316.

30. Paulos LE, France EP, Rosenburg TD, et al. The biomechanics of lateral knee bracing. Part I: response of the valgus restraints to loading. *Am J Sports Med* 1987;15:419–429.

31. Wojtys EM, Goldstein SA, Redfern M, et al. A biomechanical evaluation of the Lenox Hill knee brace. *Clin Orthop Relat Res* 1987;220:179–184.

32. France EP, Paulos LE, Jayaraman G, et al. The biomechanics of lateral knee bracing. Part II: impact response of the braced knee. *Am J Sports Med* 1987;15:430–438.

33. Brown TD, Van Hoeck JE, Brand RA. Laboratory evaluation of prophylactic knee brace performance under dynamic valgus loading using a surrogate leg model. *Clin Sports Med* 1990;9:751–762.

34. Paulos LE, Cawley PW, France EP. Impact biomechanics of lateral knee bracing: the anterior cruciate ligament. *Am J Sports Med* 1991;19:337–342.

35. Daley BJ, Ralston JL, Brown TD, et al. A parametric design evaluation of lateral prophylactic knee braces. *J Biomech Eng* 1993;115: 131–136.

36. Erickson AR, Yasuda K, Beynnon BD, et al. An in vitro dynamic evaluation of prophylactic knee braces during lateral impact loading. *Am J Sports Med* 1993;21:26–35.

37. Yu B, Herman D, Preston J, et al. Immediate effects of a knee brace with a constraint to knee extension on knee kinematics and ground reaction forces in a stop-jump task. *Am J Sports Med* 2004;32:1136–1143.

38. Beynnon BD, Slauterbeck JR. Can bracing reduce the risk of ACL injury? In: Hewett TE, Shultz SJ, Griffin LY, eds. *Understanding and Preventing Noncontact ACL Injuries*. Champaign, IL: Human Kinetics; 2007:259–264.

39. Anderson G, Zeman SC, Rosenfield RT. The Anderson knee stabler. *Phys Sportsmed* 1979;7:125–127.

40. O'Donoghue DH. Surgical treatment of fresh injuries to the major ligaments of the knee. *J Bone Joint Surg Am* 1950;32:721–738.

41. Baker BE, VanHanswyk E, Bogosian SP, et al. The effect of knee braces on lateral impact loading of the knee. *Am J Sports Med* 1989;17:182–186.

42. Garrick JG, Requa RK. Prophylactic knee bracing. *Am J Sports Med* 1987;15:471–476.

43. Grace TG, Skipper BJ, Newberry JC, et al. Prophylactic knee braces and injury to the lower extremity. *J Bone Joint Surg Am* 1988;70: 422–427.

44. Hewson GF, Mendini RA, Wang JB. Prophylactic knee bracing in college football. *Am J Sports Med* 1986;14:262–266.

45. McCarthy P. Prophylactic knee braces: where do we stand? *Phys Sportsmed* 1986;16:102–115.

46. Rovere GD, Haupt HA, Yates CS. Prophylactic knee bracing in college football. *Am J Sports Med* 1987;15:111–116.

47. Teitz CC, Hermanson BK, Kronmal RA, et al. Evaluation of the use of braces to prevent injury to the knee in collegiate football players. *J Bone Joint Surg Am* 1987;69:2–9.

48. Position Statement: *The Use of Knee Braces*. Rosemont, IL: American Academy of Orthopaedic Surgeons, October 1987.

49. Position Statement: *The Use of Knee Braces*. Rosemont, IL: American Academy of Orthopaedic Surgeons; Revised December 2003.

50. Yang J, Marshall SW, Bowling JM, et al. Use of discretionary protective equipment and rate of lower extremity injury in high school athletes. *Am J Epidemiol* 2005;161:511–519.

51. Greene DL, Hamson KR, Bay RC, et al. Effects of protective knee bracing on speed and agility. *Am J Sports Med* 2000;28: 453–459.

52. Osternig LR, Robertson RN. Effects of prophylactic knee bracing on lower extremity joint position and muscle activation during running. *Am J Sports Med* 1993;21:733–737.

53. Thomsen M, Mannel H, Spiering S, et al. Biomechanics of the tibiofemoral joint and knee braces. *Orthopade* 2002;31: 914–920.

Appendix: The Physical Examination of the Knee

John A. Feagin, Jr.

PHILOSOPHY OF PHYSICAL EXAMINATION

Physical examination of the knee is an art and a science. It serves as an introduction to the patient and a means of communication. The purpose of the physical examination is to arrive at the correct anatomic diagnosis. The examination should play a pivotal role in teaching the patient about the injury and treating the injury.

Examination of the well leg, as a standard for comparison, is a must. Function is a part of the examination. Function is the integration of all the anatomic parts as well as the symptoms that aid in diagnosis. Gait analysis is part of the functional examination for a patient with a knee injury.

The physical examination should be gentle. The patient will appreciate the art of the physician's hands-on examination and the explanations of the science involved in each part of the examination. The fact that the examination is administered so that it is nearly painless or that the patient indicates pain during certain parts of the examination is meaningful to the physician. The interaction between the patient and the examiner is the basis for a partnership during the treatment regimen.

Certain principles are essential to physical examination of the knee: (a) the unaffected side is examined first; (b) during the course of the examination, the examiner *looks* (inspection), *feels* (palpation), and *moves* both the unaffected and affected extremities; and (c) the end result is a correct anatomic diagnosis.

The physical examination will enhance the quest for truth, which is embodied in the correct and precise diagnosis. Such truth enhances and expedites patient care which is satisfying to the patient and, when combined with sound judgment, will decrease the cost of medical care to the patient.

CONDUCT OF THE PHYSICAL EXAMINATION

I attempt to examine the injured part in the position in which I find the patient. In the office situation, I presume the patient has found a comfortable position prior to my arrival. I want to observe and maintain this position as long and as possible. On the athletic field, the position in which I, as team physician, or in which the trainer finds the patient, often speaks to the forces involved, the nature of the injury, and the diagnosis and immediate care. Certainly, examining patients in the position in which they are found is most apparent in situations in which spinal injury is a suspected component of the injury.

I always examine the well leg first, and usually begin this examination gently as the patient is reciting the history. Prior to eliciting the history, I will confirm with the patient which leg is the "well" leg. Although this is an appendix on knee examination, *leg* is the proper term. We cannot isolate the examination solely to the knee because many diagnostic opportunities will be missed. Eliciting the history while examining the uninjured part is a way of communicating with the patient. In other words, I want to use the tactile sense in my hands to examine the knee, but I want to look at the patient as he or she is talking. For the chronic knee problem, a simple history can be: "Tell me all about your knee." In the acute setting, the one-question history simply may be: "*Describe* what happened to your knee." The history, elicited by a simple question, is familiar and relaxing to the patient. The examiner can examine and look at both the patient-historian, as well as the affected part. The art of eliciting the history at the same time as beginning the examination on the unaffected leg requires practice, but it is noteworthy.

I try to time the examination of the affected leg to coincide with the patient's completion of the history. Rarely will the patient talk more than a few minutes in response to a single question if he or she is not interrupted. I never interrupt patients while they are giving their history. Sometimes the history is not complete and the examiner will wish for more, but this can be mentally noted and delayed until later in the physical examination. A lack of complete history will not interrupt the flow of the physical examination. A smooth flow is important to both the examiner and the patient.

In the office situation, I usually find that the patient is sitting with the injured leg hanging over the examining table.

I know that I want to examine the knee in the flexed position, the extended position, the prone position, and in varus-valgus. Pivot shift testing is reserved until the end of the examination because frequently it is painful. Gait also must be analyzed. The anterior cruciate (ACL) and posterior cruciate ligaments (PCL), that is, the central pivot, must be defined first. The examination keys off of these two critical components, the ACL and the PCL. My first task in examining the affected leg is to compare the conformity with the unaffected leg. Conformity deals with appearance, induration, and swelling. Temperature and tenderness are also a part of the tactile examination and are elicited with the conformity. It often amazes me the sensitivity that resides in our God-given hands. In palpation of the knee, I wish to look for induration before eliciting tenderness or causing discomfort. Induration is an increase in tissue tension caused by swelling, which may be either interstitial, intracellular, or both. Fully 50% of the time, a diagnosis can be made on just this part of the examination, and the remainder of the examination is merely confirmatory. This is particularly true in meniscal lesions.

Our goal during examination is an anatomic diagnosis. Examination must be conducted in a manner that will ultimately satisfy the scientific criteria. These criteria are well outlined by the International Knee Documentation Committee, based on the work initiated by Müller et al.[1] Primary and secondary restraints, as well as the limits of motion must be defined.[2–5]

Always, as I am examining the knee, I remember the teachings of A. Graham Apley[6] on the physical examination: *Look! Feel! Move!* By thinking on these points, I will not forget anything, although I may elect to exclude some things.

Sometimes I cannot make an anatomic diagnosis on the first try with a particular patient. This usually occurs when the patient has a chronic problem or the patient is at less than their best. It also may occur when I am either hurried or tired. I will then acknowledge to the patient that I cannot arrive at the requisite anatomic diagnosis and will suggest that we do an orthopaedic examination under different conditions. Perhaps just icing the knee for 15 minutes and re-examining the knee will suffice; sometimes the patient or the examiner just needs to walk about, or break the encounter, or sometimes I ask the patient to aggravate the symptoms and return at a reappointed time. I will try to examine patients the second time at the time coincident with

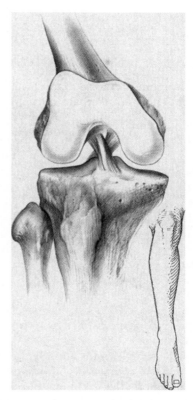

Figure A.1   The central pivot. (From Garrett W, Speer K, Kirkendall, D, eds. *Principles and Practice of Orthopaedic Sports Medicine.* Philadelphia: Lippincott Williams & Wilkins; 2000, with permission.)

their symptoms. If the problem is overuse, I may ask them to "over use" the knee by 10% to 30% for a week and then I will re-examine them in 1 week. These opportunities to repeat the physical examination have been fruitful for me and have led to more accurate anatomic diagnoses and decision-making. My judgment is usually improved by the second encounter. In the fee-for-service practice, I do not bill the patient for the second encounter.

Quite simply, *I insist on an anatomic diagnosis.* I achieve this approximately 85% of the time but must resort to re-examination and imaging for 100% diagnostic accuracy. I believe this simple criterion of an accurate anatomic diagnosis has made my life in orthopaedics a joy. Certainly, it has enhanced my ability to perform a physical examination because I have had to develop tests and techniques along the way to confirm diagnosis or diagnostic hypotheses. If physicians insist on an accurate and timely anatomic diagnosis, this will guarantee that we will never be "average" practitioners.

PRINCIPLES OF PHYSICAL EXAMINATION

Central Pivot

The ACL and the PCL form the central pivot of the knee (Fig. A.1).[7] The ACL is defined by both the Lachman and drawer tests, and the PCL is defined by the posterior drawer test.[8] The anterior and posterior drawer tests are not exactly the same.

The Lachman test is an active antigravity test that requires the patient's relaxation. In the hands of the skilled examiner, it can be quite accurate and is highly specific.[9]

The drawer test may be done with the leg hanging or with the examiner stabilizing the lower leg with the knee in 90 degrees of flexion. The former, that is, the lower leg unconstrained, is preferred because it enhances the displacements that can be appreciated while testing the ligaments. *A sound principle is to always leave one limb segment unconstrained.* This will optimize the results of the examination and is a fundamental biomechanical principle.

The posterior drawer test is a passive drop-back test with the knee in 90 degrees of flexion and depends on gravity. Patient relaxation is rarely necessary for the success of this test. Comparison with the uninvolved side is a prerequisite for the test to be a diagnostic indicator.

The Lachman Test, although it has been described by many in the past, was best described by Torg et al.[9] Torg was a resident of Lachman.

In addition to straight translation, either anterior or posterior, we are also concerned with rotation, as it may occur with translation. This combination will give some idea of the interrelationship between the central pivot, that is, the ACL and PCL, and the secondary restraints. For example, in the instance of a tear of the ACL and medial collateral ligament (MCL), one could expect a highly positive Lachman or drawer test, but one might also find a

significant degree of external rotation in addition to the anterior translation where the MCL is also incompetent. Thus, we want to elicit the entire envelope of motion,[10] be it normal or pathologic. We want to know the area under the force-displacement curve (Fig. A.2). The physical examination elicits this area under the force-displacement curve. Translational tests with the lower limb constrained do not maximize the envelope of motion for subtle pathologies. *The lower limb should be unconstrained during the ligamentous examination.*

The pivot shift test, whether it is as described by Losee et al.[11] or any of the other versions of the test,[12] is aimed at combining translation with rotation and thereby eliciting the maximum area under the force-displacement curve (Fig. A.2). Losee[13] is the master of the pivot shift (Fig. A.3). Because a positive pivot shift is diagnostic of an incompetent ACL, he uses the test to (a) verify to patients that he can reproduce the systems they have described, and (b) confirm to patients that he has corrected the problem by his operation.

Few of us use the pivot shift test in such an elegant fashion, but in his hands, it is convincing to the patient both preoperatively and postoperatively. If the pivot shift is graded as described by the International Knee Documentation Committee,[14] then the grades of negative, physiologic, or pathologic pivot glide, pivot shift, and gross subluxation are appropriate. For gross subluxation to exist, secondary restraints must also be compromised. Many adolescents and loose-jointed individuals will have a physiologic pivot glide and sometimes even a frank pivot shift, but this will

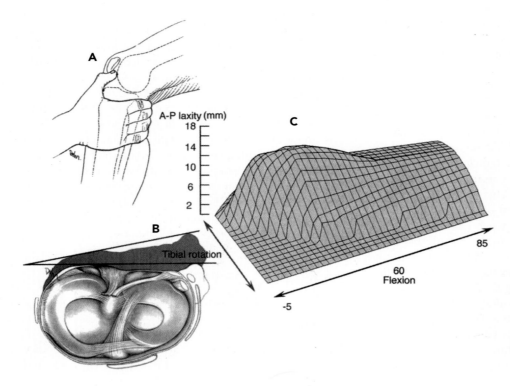

Figure A.2 The physical examination elicits the area under the force-displacement curve. A-P, anteroposterior. (From Garrett W, Speer K, Kirkendall, D, eds. *Principles and Practice of Orthopaedic Sports Medicine.* Philadelphia: Lippincott Williams & Wilkins; 2000, with permission.)

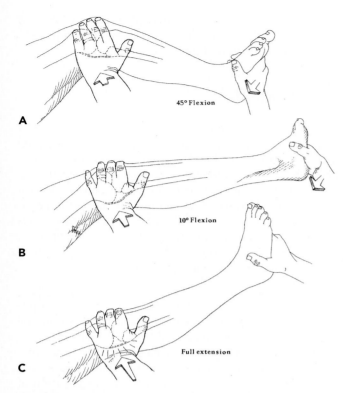

Figure A.3 The Losee pivot shift test. (From Garrett W, Speer K, Kirkendall, D, eds. *Principles and Practice of Orthopaedic Sports Medicine.* Philadelphia: Lippincott Williams & Wilkins; 2000, with permission.)

cause little concern because the unaffected leg is the basis of comparison.

After the continuity or discontinuity of the central pivot (i.e., the ACL and PCL have been determined), the secondary restraints—the MCL, lateral collateral ligament (LCL), and posterior medial and posterior lateral ligaments—are examined. The collateral ligaments are best examined at hyperextension, 0 degrees, and 30 degrees of knee flexion. If the foot is cradled loosely between the iliac crest and the examiner's elbow, then the lower limb will not be rigidly constrained and the knee can be placed in these three positions.

EXAMINATION OF THE SECONDARY RESTRAINTS

Should the examiner begin with active or passive movements? I prefer to ask the patient to move the well leg within the range of motion that is comfortable and possible. This gives a standard of comparison for the injured leg. Then I ask the patient to move the injured extremity within the bounds of comfort. This shows the range of motion available to position the leg for the ligamentous examinations.

One of the goals of movement is to place the extremity in the best position for isolating and examining the differ-

ent ligamentous structures. If hyperextension can be achieved, that is a good position in which to begin. If the knee is stable in hyperextension, the medial and lateral capsuloligamentous structures and the PCL are intact. Thus, the maximum amount of information is gained quickly. The technique that Smillie[15] taught me still seems the most useful: the patient's foot is pinioned against the examiner's hip so that both hands are free to palpate the joint lines and ligamentous structures, and the knee is then placed in hyperextension, neutral, and 30 degrees of flexion (Fig. A.4).

Varus and valgus laxity in hyperextension are ominous signs that indicate disruption of key ligamentous structures. If in hyperextension the joint is lax to valgus angulation, the medial capsuloligamentous structures and the PCL are probably interrupted. If in hyperextension the knee is lax to varus angulation, the arcuate complex, PCL, and ACL are probably disrupted. When varus

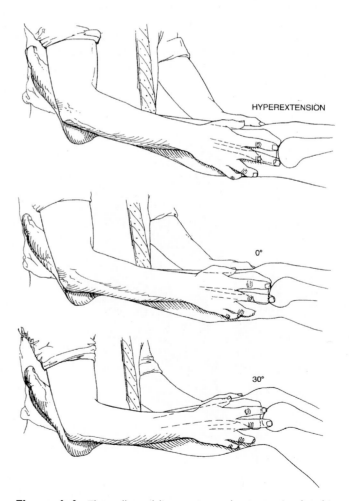

Figure A.4 The collateral ligaments are best examined at hyperextension, 0 degrees, and 30 degrees of knee flexion. The technique was taught to me by Smillie. (From Garrett W, Speer K, Kirkendall, D, eds. *Principles and Practice of Orthopaedic Sports Medicine.* Philadelphia: Lippincott Williams & Wilkins; 2000, with permission.)

angulation and valgus angulation are applied with the knee at 0 degrees of flexion, the ACL and PCL are less taut. Then these tests are diagnostic of medial or lateral posterior capsular injuries. At 30 degrees of flexion, the cruciate ligaments and posterior capsular ligaments are in their most relaxed state; then, pathologic laxity indicates MCL or LCL laxity.

I believe it is important to separate the diagnosis of the posterior medial and posterior lateral capsular complexes from the MCL and LCL because they are different layers[16] and have different functions (Fig. A.5). Posterior medial and posterior lateral capsular ligamentous are contiguous with the menisci and control meniscal motion. Thus, compromising one of these complexes will affect meniscal position and function. Further, the prognosis is not the same in that the posterior medial capsular complex retracts posteriorly with injury, and although it will heal, it does not give the same stability after healing. Also, with retraction of the posterior oblique capsular ligament there can be increased rotatory laxity, which jeopardizes the meniscus as well as function; whereas the MCL heals quite nicely *in situ* without surgery and slight laxity does not affect meniscal mechanics. In some of the literature, the MCL is not differentiated from the posterior medial

capsular complex. I believe that physical examination should make this differentiation because it is important to the future function of the knee.

THE MENISCI

Although there are traditional meniscal tests, I prefer a meniscal examination based on the pathoanatomy. The anatomy of the medial and lateral menisci is not the same. They are tethered differently through the capsular ligaments and they have different mobility. Thus, examination of the medial meniscus is not a mirror image examination of the lateral meniscus. In both menisci, the examination is based on the integrity of the radial collagen tie fibers as well as the normal mobility of the menisci under load. I examine the menisci in three positions (Fig. A.6):

1. With the knee flexed 90 degrees and the leg hanging, that is, with gravity distracting the joint. This is optimum for palpation for tenderness. In this position, the normal menisci are not palpable (Fig. A.6A).
2. The figure-4 position. In the figure-4 position, the medial meniscus is compressed and the MCL has moved further posteriorly (Fig. A.6B). This allows palpation of the injured portion of the medial meniscus as well as the MCL and posterior oblique ligament. Because the medial meniscus is most often torn in its posterior horn, this is an especially valuable position. A torn meniscus will extrude in the flexed position giving a positive "radial extrusion test" (Fig. A.6C). Cystic degeneration is the basis for the radial extrusion test.
3. If I have not found tenderness, induration, or extrusion of the meniscus in either of these positions, then I will use the third position, the McMurray[17], or other displacement tests to try to see if I can compress and displace the meniscus.

In contrast to the medial meniscus, the lateral meniscus is more likely to have pathology in the mid and anterior portion and this can be palpated better in full extension. *Thus, it is important to examine both menisci through a full range of motion.*

Magnetic resonance imaging (MRI) is highly sensitive and specific for meniscal pathology. I have gained increased confidence in the accuracy of physical examination of the menisci since I have adopted the radial extrusion test and made my palpatory examination discretely over the anterior, middle, and posterior meniscal segments. MRI has helped me to define and refine my examination of the menisci.

THE PATELLOFEMORAL JOINT

The patellofemoral joint should be examined in three positions. With the knee in extension (Fig. A.7A), with the

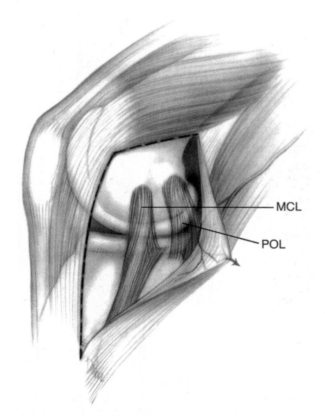

Figure A.5   The medial collateral ligament (MCL) and posterior oblique ligament (POL). (From Garrett W, Speer K, Kirkendall, D, eds. *Principles and Practice of Orthopaedic Sports Medicine.* Philadelphia: Lippincott Williams & Wilkins; 2000, with permission.)

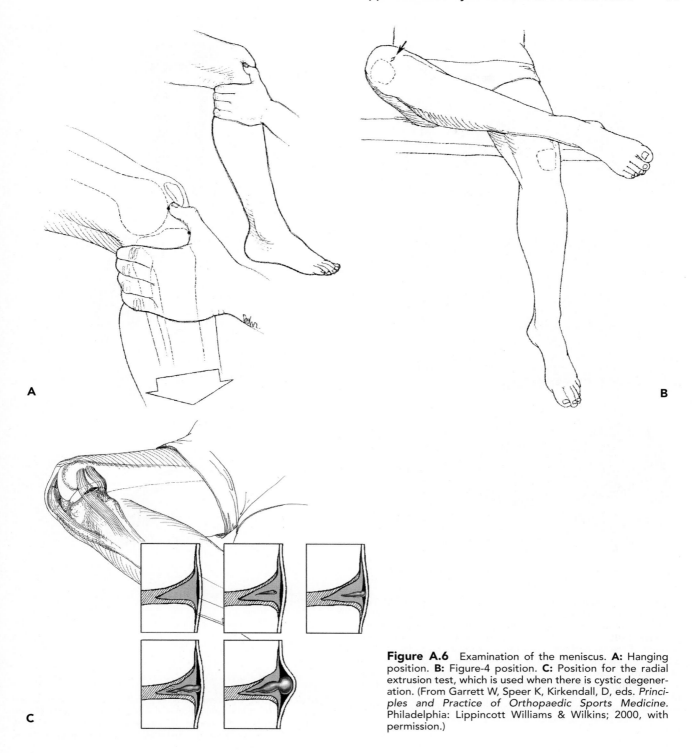

Figure A.6 Examination of the meniscus. **A:** Hanging position. **B:** Figure-4 position. **C:** Position for the radial extrusion test, which is used when there is cystic degeneration. (From Garrett W, Speer K, Kirkendall, D, eds. *Principles and Practice of Orthopaedic Sports Medicine.* Philadelphia: Lippincott Williams & Wilkins; 2000, with permission.)

knee in full flexion (Fig. A.7B), and in the prone position with the knee hyperextended (Fig. A.7C). Physical examination of the patellofemoral joint in these three positions can reveal a wealth of pathology. In addition, it is essential to examine the patellofemoral joint in a loaded condition through a range of motion as I believe that crepitus can be diagnostically revealing, and crepitus through a full range of motion is especially significant (Fig. A.8). Also, I want to know whether the crepitus occurs when the lower pole of the patella engages the trochlear groove or in extension, when the upper pole of the patella engages the trochlear groove. Furthermore, the medial and lateral alae of the fat pad can be defined by palpation; also, the size and consistency of the fat pad can be defined by palpation (Fig. A.9). In addition, using all three positions, the infrapatellar tendon can be examined in both its lax and taut positions for

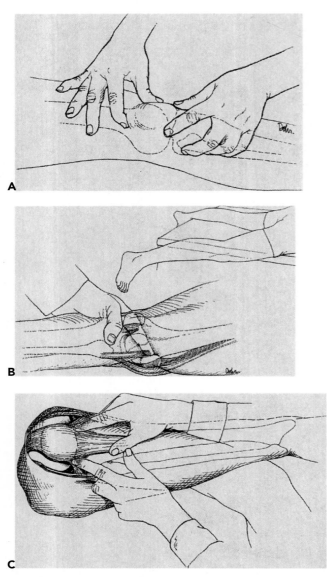

Figure A.7 Examination of the patellofemoral joint. **A:** The patella is examined for excursion, pain, and apprehension. **B:** With the patient in the prone position, the examiner can determine the tenderness along the capsule as well as the swelling and/or tenderness of the fat pad and the inferior capsular ligaments. **C:** This position allows the examiner to palpate the retinacular ligaments of the patella, particularly the inferior medial and inferior lateral ligaments. The alignment of the patella with the femoral trochlear groove can also be determined. (From Garrett W, Speer K, Kirkendall, D, eds. *Principles and Practice of Orthopaedic Sports Medicine.* Philadelphia: Lippincott Williams & Wilkins; 2000, with permission.)

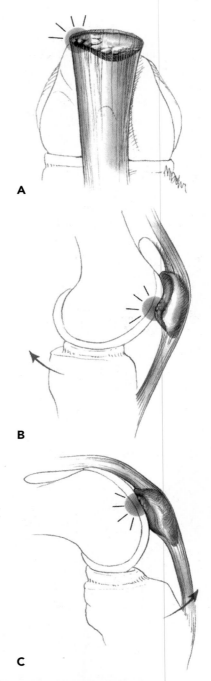

Figure A.8. A–C: Crepitus through full range of motion is especially significant in examination of the patellofemoral joint. (From Garrett W, Speer K, Kirkendall, D, eds. *Principles and Practice of Orthopaedic Sports Medicine.* Philadelphia: Lippincott Williams & Wilkins; 2000, with permission.)

pathology, such as jumper's knee and Osgood-Schlatter deformity.

In examining the patella, I believe that one should use both an apprehension test as well as a containment test (Fig. A.10). These define the medial and lateral patellar ligaments. Frequently, in the chronic ACL-deficient knee, one will appreciate lateral tilt and lateral placement of the patella as the knee assumes increasing varus deformity. The

prone position is ideal for these tests (Fig. A.10) in that one hand can be used to manipulate the knee through a range of motion, thereby changing the tension of the supporting patellar retinacular structures, while the other hand causes displacement or containment of the patella or palpates the fat pad, the patellar tendon, and inferior capsular structures for tenderness or induration.

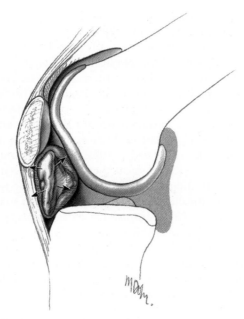

Figure A.9   The size and consistency of the fat pad can be defined by palpation. (From Garrett W, Speer K, Kirkendall, D, eds. *Principles and Practice of Orthopaedic Sports Medicine*. Philadelphia: Lippincott Williams & Wilkins; 2000, with permission.)

Another reason to examine the knee and the patellofemoral joint in the prone position is to look for masses and abnormalities of the upper or lower leg. Tumors can mimic a Baker's cyst. The knee can be flexed with the hip in extension, which checks the quadriceps for contracture and also the hips are easily checked for range of motion in this position. Sciatica can be detected as a contributing factor to knee pain or it can be ruled out. *Thus, the prone examination of the knee and patellofemoral joint is a valuable adjunct test and offers many diagnostic possibilities.*

FUNCTION

The examination of the primary and secondary ligamentous structures, the menisci, patellofemoral joint, and the enveloping capsular structures may be the first part of the examination, but these parts of the examination have not emphasized function. At some stage, I would like to determine function by moving the knee through a range of motion, comparing this to the unaffected side. In gait examination, I watch the shoulder for antalgic sway. I also use toe walking and heel walking to define pathology. Heel walking removes some of the knee shock absorbers such as the forefoot, midfoot, and subtalar joints. If the knee is arthritic, then this will accentuate an antalgic gait or sway of the shoulders. Toe walking, conversely, provides excellent shock absorption for the knee joint, but compresses the patella through quadriceps contraction. Thus, an antalgic gait in the toe-walking position indicates patellar pathology (Fig. A.11).

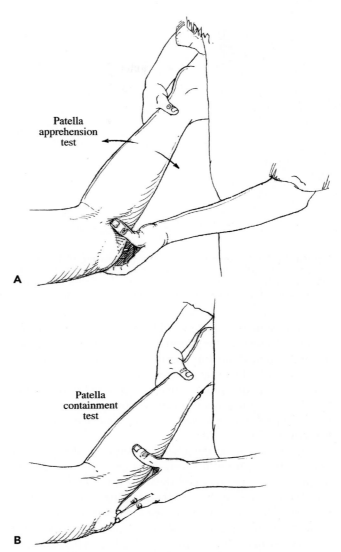

Figure A.10   One should use both an apprehension test **(A)** as well as a containment test **(B)**. (From Garrett W, Speer K, Kirkendall, D, eds. *Principles and Practice of Orthopaedic Sports Medicine*. Philadelphia: Lippincott Williams & Wilkins; 2000, with permission.)

IMAGING

I am usually able to assimilate a working diagnosis from these tests. I cannot make a definitive diagnosis, but a working diagnosis allows me to contemplate the most effective imaging and to communicate a plan of action with the patient. This is the beginning of *judgment*. Good physical examination and good judgment makes for a "good" disposition and a happy patient.

At this stage, at the very least, I order routine radiographs or review the radiographs available to me with the patient. I believe that reviewing the radiographs with the patient is an effective teaching tool and helps the patient understand the diagnosis and the decision-making process. On evaluating the radiographs, I am looking for a secondary trabecular

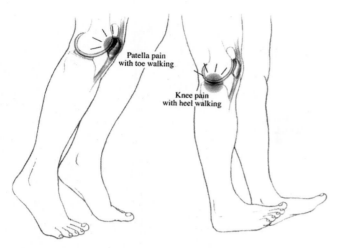

Figure A.11 An antalgic gait in the toe-walking position indicates patellar pathology. (From Garrett W, Speer K, Kirkendall, D, eds. *Principles and Practice of Orthopaedic Sports Medicine.* Philadelphia: Lippincott Williams & Wilkins; 2000, with permission.)

pattern or spurring, which would suggest overload. Because radiographs reflect a long-term history of the knee mechanics, they can be quite illuminating. I prefer to review the radiographs after I have completed the physical examination so I am not tempted to shortcut the physical examination based on the radiographic diagnosis. *Thus, imaging diagnosis should be used to complement physical examination and verify biomechanical abnormalities.*

The choice of imaging will depend on the physical examination. Our routine radiographs include an anteroposterior, lateral, weightbearing tunnel views,[18] and Merchant[19] view of the patella. Although this combination of radiographs may be seen as excessive by some, these views are helpful to make a definitive diagnosis and a plan. How often is MRI requisite? We all agree that MRI can be specific and sensitive for most structures of the knee. The cruciate ligaments, the secondary restraints, the menisci, the patellofemoral joint, the osseous structures, are all well defined by MRI. Only two disappointments with MRI remain: (a) the accuracy with regards to chondral surfaces, and (b) the ability to obtain dynamic imaging.

Both techniques are forthcoming and will greatly enhance the value of MRI to the knee surgeon. The surgeon is the patient's advocate in regards to the quality of the MRI. Less than a complete examination cannot be accepted when one is representing the patient's best interest and is involved in judgments that may lead to surgery. *The MRI as well as standard roentgenography should enhance and reinforce the physical examination.*

Adjunctive imaging such as a long film showing limb alignment, stress roentgenography, dynamic cine tomographic scan, and technetinum-99 scan are sometimes necessary, but these are highly selective and I seldom consider these early in the process.

With properly selected imaging, we should move from a working anatomic diagnosis to a definitive diagnosis. It is now time to communicate completely and effectively the diagnosis with the patient, appropriate colleagues, and write the narrative in the chart. I review the imaging and the pertinent parts of the physical examination with the patient. I want to emphasize the anatomic diagnosis so that the patient also has a working diagnosis. This leads us to decision-making. Sometimes it is appropriate to have the patient's family in attendance for the communicative portion of the diagnostic evaluation as decision-making may involve all concerned parties. Besides parents and spouses, coaches, the physical therapist, athletic trainers, and other team members may need to know the working diagnosis and the elements involved in decision-making.

The patient must be a participant in decision-making. Sometimes consultation with colleagues is necessary in decision-making. This should be used as appropriate to ensure accurate diagnosis, protect the patient, allay anxiety, and ensure successful treatment. It is important to have available colleagues who can serve as effective consultants.

DECISION-MAKING

After all the effort and expertise that is requisite to determine the patient's problem and establishing a definitive diagnosis, one certainly wants to use sound judgment and effectively articulate the best solution. The best solution is seldom apparent without the patient's participation in the decision-making process. How does the patient most effectively participate in a decision-making process in which he or she has limited experience and insight?

This is the art of our profession and can be one of the most satisfying results of a well-performed physical examination and an accurate anatomic diagnosis. The performance of the physical examination gives the patient a participatory feeling. This participatory feeling initiates the shared decision-making process. The patient will be interested in the imaging and will be interested in the review and the emphasis on the positive physical findings. Frequently, the plan will be tempered by the patient's vocational and avocational needs. Thus, these needs should be elicited prior to decision-making. I usually discuss the patient's vocational and avocational requirements during the course of the physical examination, particularly when I am in the portion of the examination that requires movement. Hopefully, the patient will focus on my query as regards to the activity status while I move the leg through the comfortable limits of motion.

SUMMARY

Physical examination, an art and science, can be mastered by almost everyone, regardless of the medical discipline. This is important because we need to communicate with the other caregivers on our team. The common denominator of communication is an anatomic diagnosis.[14,20] I expect the other caregivers on my team to be able to examine and arrive at an accurate anatomic diagnosis with the same facility and accuracy that I know. Decision-making is also an art and science. Although we know the "odds" of our surgical and nonsurgical treatments, the practice of medicine and surgery is an infinite blend of circumstances. This is why the practice of medicine can be so life-fulfilling. *Decision-making requires the integration of the science of the physical examination and anatomic diagnosis, with socioeconomic factors, as well as the patient's desires.* The patient's participation in this process should be enjoyable for patient and physician alike. The best decision and the best plan for the patient is the ultimate goal of the physical examination and the physician.

This section was copyrighted and previously published in Garrett W, Speer K, Kirkendall D, eds. *Principles and Practice of Orthopaedic Sports Medicine.* Philadelphia, Lippincott Williams and Wilkins, 2000.

REFERENCES

1. Müller W, Biedert R, Hefti F, et al. OAK knee evaluation. A new way to assess knee ligament injuries. *Clin Orthop* 1988;232:37–50.
2. Butler DL, Noyes FR, Grood ES. Ligamentous restraints to anterior-posterior drawer in the human knee. A biomechanical study. *J Bone Joint Surg Am* 1980;62:259–270.
3. Fukubayashi Y, Torzilli PA, Sherman MF, Warren RF. An in vitro biomechanical evaluation of anterior-posterior motion in the knee. *J Bone Joint Surg Am* 1982;64:258–264.
4. Grood ES, Noyes FR, Butler DL, Suntay WJ. Ligamentous and capsular restraints preventing straight medial and lateral laxity in intact human knees. *J Bone Joint Surg Am* 1981;63:1257–1269.
5. Grood ES, Stowers SF, Noyes FR. Limits of movement in the human knee. Effect of sectioning the posterior cruciate ligament and posterolateral structures. *J Bone Joint Surg Am* 1988;70:80–97.
6. Apley AG. *A System of Orthopaedics and Fractures* 4th ed. London: Butterworth Publishers, Ltd.; 1973:1.
7. Grood ES, Noyes FR. Diagnosis of knee ligament injuries. In: Feagin JA Jr, ed. *The Crucial Ligaments. Diagnosis and Treatment of Ligamentous Injuries of the Knee.* 2nd ed. New York: Churchill Livingstone; 1994:371–386.
8. Noyes FR, Grood ES, Butler DL, Paulos L. Clinical biomechanics of the knee ligament restraints and functional stability. In: Funk FJ, ed. *Symposium on the Athlete's Knee. Surgical Repair and Reconstruction.* St. Louis: CV Mosby; 1980.
9. Torg JS, Conrad W, Kalen V. Clinical diagnosis of anterior cruciate ligament instability of the athlete. *Am J Sports Med* 1976;4:84–93.
10. Blankevoort L, Huiskes R, deLang A. The envelope of passive knee joint motion. *J Biomech* 1988;21:705–720.
11. Losee RR, Johnson TR, Southwick WO. Anterior subluxation of the lateral tibial plateau: A diagnostic test and operative repair. *J Bone Joint Surg Am* 1978;60:1015–1030.
12. Galway HR, MacIntosh DL. The lateral pivot shift. A symptom and sign of anterior cruciate ligament insufficiency. *Clin Orthop* 1980;147:45–50.
13. Losee RE. Pivot shift. In: Feagin JA Jr, ed. *The Crucial Ligaments. Diagnosis and Treatment of Ligamentous Injuries about the Knee.* New York: Churchill Livingstone; 1994:407–422.
14. Daniel MD. Assessing the limits of knee motion. *Am J Sports Med* 1991;19:139–147.
15. Smillie IS. *Diseases of the Knee.* Edinburgh: Churchill Livingstone; 1980:1–27.
16. Warren LF, Marshall JL. The supporting structures and layers of the medial side of the knee. An anatomical analysis. *J Bone Joint Surg Am* 1979;61:56–62.
17. McMurray TP. The operative treatment of ruptured internal lateral ligament of the knee. *Br J Surg* 1918;6:377–381.
18. Rosenberg TD, Paulos L, Parker RD, Coward DB, Scott SM. The forty-five-degree posteroanterior flexion weight-bearing radiograph of the knee. *J Bone Joint Surg Am* 1988;70:1479–1483.
19. Merchant AC, Mercer RL, Jacobson RH, Vool CR. Roentgenographic analysis of patellofemoral congruence. *J Bone Joint Surg Am* 1974;56:1391–1396.
20. Noyes FR, Grood ES, Torzilli PA. The definitions of terms for motion and position of the knee and injuries of the ligaments. *J Bone Joint Surg Am* 1989; 71:465–471.

II

Applied Surgical Care: Microfracture, Healing Response, and "The Package"

Philosophy of Knee Care

J. Richard Steadman

6

The evolution of my philosophy of knee care began to take shape during my residency, when I was exposed to the ideas of Dr. Ernst Dehne, a surgeon whose work I greatly respected. Dr. Dehne's radical (at that time) proposal advocated that treatment of tibial fractures with a cast combined with early ambulation and weightbearing not only resulted in a healed tibia, but produced well-nourished and healthy joints above and below the fracture when the cast came off. Encouraged by the improvement I had seen in the joints that had been treated that way, I decided to treat tibial fractures with motion and early weightbearing whenever possible. This prevented the permanent adverse changes in joints that occur with prolonged immobilization and no weightbearing.

When I first started practicing orthopaedics, these as well as other techniques helped to shape the development of my treatment protocol. The AO group provided me with another revolutionary concept that I took to heart. Their idea was that if a fractured extremity was mobilized after rigid fixation, the joints above and below the fracture could tolerate later immobilization with no ill effects.

It was obvious that cast immobilization without weightbearing created problems. Sometimes there was no other choice, but by 1973–1974, I was convinced that the injury site itself was only one component of the treatment protocol, and consequently I developed a strategy to include joint mobilization whenever possible.

At the same time, I noticed that if the injured area could be protected, aerobic exercise could be done safely, and that this not only affected the fitness level, it gave a psychological boost to the injured patient's attitude. As time went on, I came to realize that exercising the injured limb (as long as there was no deformation) actually enhanced healing. The additional discovery that exercising the *uninjured* extremity resulted in strength gains on the injured side also became part of my rehabilitation philosophy. This was first employed in the medial collateral ligament, and then later applied to the anterior cruciate ligament and the ankle.

I began my orthopaedics practice in a small resort town in the mountains of California, treating injured skiers from surrounding ski areas, as well as victims of various other kinds of accidents. My office was so small that there was only room for one guest chair, but I was very busy from the beginning, and thoroughly enjoyed my work. At that time, my philosophy was simple but straightforward: I was determined to give my best to my patients.

In the mid to late 1970s and early 1980s, although surgical techniques were quickly improving, they did not yet address the anatomy as we know it to be today. With this in mind, I focused not only on producing the best surgical results I could, but realized over time that appropriate rehabilitation could transform a good surgical result into a great clinical outcome.

Another thing that I noticed during the same period was how beneficial it was for the patient to have a positive state of mind. I observed that active rehabilitation had a significantly good effect on the patient's attitude, as well as on the rate of recovery. The perfectly conditioned athlete who is seriously injured and in a hospital bed has also suffered a devastating psychological blow. I concluded that if there was no contraindication, the uninjured extremities should begin protected exercises right away, so that an active aerobic workout could be achieved, releasing the endorphins that would improve the patient's outlook on life. As I put this idea into practice, I became more and more convinced of its positive effects, not only from a physiological standpoint, but from a psychological one as well.

In the mid 1980s, I realized that developing and implementing surgical techniques and designing rehabilitation protocols was not all I wanted to do. Becoming directly involved in basic science research was a logical next step, and with this in mind, I started to collaborate with others in basic science research projects, looking at surgical procedures and their effectiveness and how they meshed with rehabilitation to produce outcomes. The research not only allowed us to prove that the rehabilitation programs we had designed were appropriate, it also led to improvements in, and validation of, surgical techniques.

The Steadman Sports Medicine Foundation was formed in 1988, allowing me to expand on my research ideas. Over time it grew and evolved into the Steadman Hawkins Research Foundation, a well-known and very productive research entity. The Foundation started on a small scale, but had great aspirations. From its inception, the plan included a basic science arm, a biomechanics arm, and data collection to assess the results of procedures. Many talented and hard-working people at the Steadman Hawkins Research Foundation are responsible for the development of the database and its contribution to the field of sports medicine.

In conclusion, many of my colleagues have contributed to the evolution of my philosophy of the knee. As a team, we have set high goals, and we are all working to provide our patients with the best possible care. All treatments, rehabilitation, understanding of the healing mechanism, and our analyses of results can be improved. To accomplish this, we need to be humble, intuitive, hard-working, knowledgeable, and always looking for ways to achieve better outcomes. If follow-up does not validate the effectiveness of a procedure, then that procedure either needs to be improved, or we should be looking for a new one to take its place.

Imaging of the Knee

Charles P. Ho

7

▰ **INTRODUCTION 87**

▰ **RADIOGRAPHIC IMAGING 87**

▰ **MAGNETIC RESONANCE IMAGING 87**
Meniscus Imaging 89
Articular Cartilage and Bone Imaging 89
  Chondral Imaging Technique 90
  Clinical Practice of Chondral and Bone Imaging 91
Ligament Imaging 96
  Cruciate Ligaments 98
  Collateral Ligaments 103
  Posterolateral Corner and Other Secondary Restraints 105
Tendon and Muscle Imaging 107

▰ **CURRENT EXPECTATIONS AND FUTURE DEVELOPMENTS 112**

Comprehensive examination of the symptomatic knee frequently may require diagnostic imaging to complement and supplement the physical examination for full diagnosis and prognosis of injury. The many derangements may present as overlapping pain syndromes, for which imaging information may provide clarification. Even with specific known injury, detailed imaging may be invaluable for treatment planning and monitoring. The many imaging techniques now available may be selected to address bone and soft tissue injury, for screening and for more specific evaluation.

RADIOGRAPHIC IMAGING

Conventional radiography is the most widely available and used imaging modality for the orthopaedic patient. Based on the tissue properties for attenuation of x-ray beams projected through the patient's knee and then sensed by appropriate film or other detectors for display, radiographs reveal details and contrast for high-attenuation materials such as bone, calcification, and metallic foreign bodies or hardware. Soft tissues have much lower and less variable attenuation properties and therefore much less radiographic contrast for delineation and evaluation of their structures.

Thus, radiographs are excellent for evaluation of the symptomatic knee for osseous fracture and reaction and for metallic implants. Radiographs assist in evaluation of the mechanical axis and alignment of bone and joints, including in the weightbearing stance. The screening radiograph also aids in finding the unexpected underlying process, such as tumor and other destructive lesions, or for metallic foreign bodies.

However, radiographs have limited value when soft tissue injury is the concern of the patient and treating physician. The utility of radiographs for evaluation of internal derangement of the knee is limited beyond screening for large effusions and for nonspecific soft tissue swelling. Purely soft tissue damage to menisci, chondral surfaces, ligaments, and tendons may not be apparent on radiographs. Milder osseous injury from contusion to impaction or avulsion fractures with little or no displacement may be difficult to see on radiographs. Radiographic findings of joint-space narrowing, sclerosis, osseous remodeling, marginal and central osteophytes, subchondral and subcortical cysts, and heterotopic bone formation are all late reactive changes, sequelae to severe chronic joint internal derangement, and soft tissue injury.

MAGNETIC RESONANCE IMAGING

The advent of magnetic resonance imaging (MRI) has been truly revolutionary for diagnostic imaging, including orthopaedic imaging. By using radiofrequency waves to stimulate mobile protons, specifically hydrogen nuclei, in body tissues and then detecting the signals given off by those protons when they return to the nonexcited state, all under the influence of a high magnetic field to increase the strength of weak signals, MRI systems can then construct high-resolution images of those tissues and structures being imaged.

The overwhelming strengths of MRI lie in the areas that are limitations that we find in radiographic imaging. The abundant hydrogen nuclei in the varying tissue environments of the musculoskeletal system provide excellent signal and contrast for superb imaging of the soft tissues as well as the osseous structures about the knee. MRI also has volume and multiplanar tomographic capability that can be optimized for imaging, as various portions of complex three-dimensional structures (including those of the knee) are best evaluated in each of the three standard orthogonal planes. Customized planes of imaging, although not generally needed, can also be tailored to specific structures when warranted.

These structures have specific normal morphologic and signal characteristics and can be evaluated for derangement of both. In more acute injuries, edema, inflammation, and hemorrhage disturb the tissue's normal signal and present as increased signal within and about the injured structures on fluid-sensitive T2-weighted MRI sequences. These are particularly conspicuous when the background high signal of marrow fat and soft tissue fat planes are eliminated by fat-suppression MRI techniques. With chronic injuries, the benefit of an increased signal indicating edema or inflammation may no longer be present, but disturbances of morphology generally are still present to be evaluated. Thus, meniscal tears, chondral defects, and ligament and tendon tears that are not apparent on radiographs are accurately evaluated by MRI.[1-7] Bone contusions and stress reactions and even fractures,[8] particularly when incomplete or with little or no displacement, may not be visible on radiographs, but are also sensitively apparent on MRIs as in-

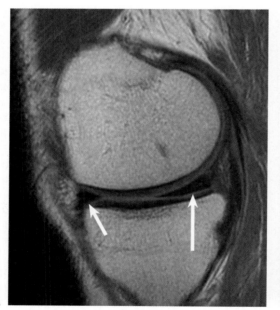

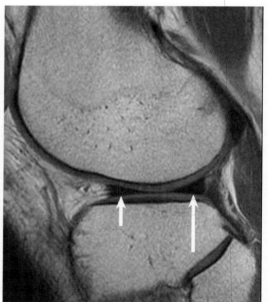

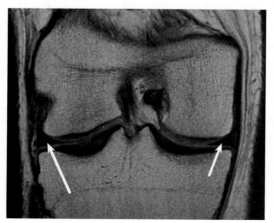

Figure 7.1 Normal magnetic resonance imaging appearance of medial and lateral menisci. Menisci should have low signal with smooth margins and a triangular cross section on sagittal and coronal images. **A:** Sagittal proton density image through the medial compartment shows normal smaller anterior *(short arrow)* and larger posterior *(long arrow)* horns of medial meniscus. **B:** Sagittal proton density image through lateral compartment demonstrates normal anterior *(short arrow)* and posterior *(long arrow)* horns, of nearly equal size, of the lateral meniscus. **C:** Coronal proton density image shows normal medial *(short arrow)* and lateral *(long arrow)* menisci at the mid meniscal body portions.

creased signal edema and hemorrhage within the bone and the surrounding soft tissues. The accurate evaluation by MRI of soft tissue and bone injury can assist the treating physician in planning management.

Limitations of current MRI techniques must also be considered. MRI may not be able to resolve small fracture lines or fragments or small areas of calcification, which are often still better detected and evaluated by radiologists or other examiners on conventional radiographs and particularly on computed tomography (CT) scans. Also, while MRI is sensitive and excellent for detecting and staging unexpected, as well as clinically apparent osseous and soft tissue masses, the MRI characteristics of such masses may not be specific. Evaluation and correlation for such masses can be much more specific on radiographs. Often radiographs may be needed in addition to the MRI.

Meniscus Imaging

One of the initial applications of MRI to the musculoskeletal system was in evaluation of the knee meniscus.[9] Both medial and lateral menisci are best evaluated using both sagittal and coronal plane images, such that the various portions of the menisci can be studied in cross section from the central free edge to the peripheral margins and synovial junction. The normal meniscus has well-defined smooth margins and, with few mobile protons in the fibrocartilage to generate signal, low or no signal on all MRI sequences (Fig. 7.1).

With repetitive stress and aging contributing to degeneration of the meniscus, the margins may become irregular, with roughening and fraying. Intrasubstance degeneration manifests as an increased signal within the meniscus.[9] It may begin as a poorly defined increased signal within the more peripheral meniscal tissue, possibly extending to the meniscosynovial junction. The degeneration may progress to coalesce as intrasubstance cleavage planes or "closed tears," presenting as more prominent and discrete, usually horizontal, longitudinal linear increased intrameniscal signals. When these cleavage planes and the corresponding MRI high signal reach and disrupt the meniscal articular margins, the characteristic degenerative horizontal longitudinal cleavage tear may be seen.

With traumatic meniscal injury, tears of even otherwise normal low-signal meniscal tissue are seen as disruptions of the normal margins and position, with possible displacement of the meniscus tissue in other more discrete tear patterns such as focal free-edge tears to radial tears, vertical-to-oblique longitudinal flap tears, and bucket-handle tears (Figs. 7.2 to 7.4). The meniscosynovial junction may also be disrupted with separation and displacement of the detached or stripped meniscus. The tear location and morphology as well as displaced fragments or flaps can be accurately evaluated by a radiologist on the sagittal and coronal MR images,[10,11] often usefully supplemented by the axial images particularly for displaced fragments or flaps. The accurate MRI evaluation and report can be extremely helpful to the treating physician for prognosis and treatment plan-

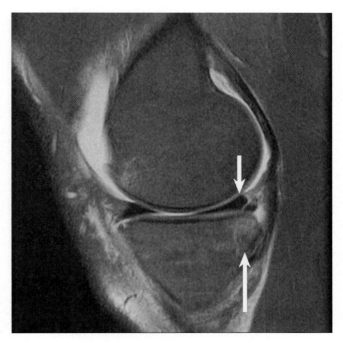

Figure 7.2 Vertical longitudinal tear demonstrated as a high signal line disrupting peripheral superior and inferior margins of the medial meniscus posterior horn (*short arrow*) on a sagittal fat-suppressed proton density image through the medial compartment. Note the geographic bone edema and contusion of the underlying posterior medial tibial plateau (*long arrow*) shown as abnormal high bone signal on fat-suppression image.

ning, assisting in finding potentially unstable meniscal lesions, and can serve as an intraoperative roadmap to detect displaced fragments that may be trapped and not readily visible by standard arthroscopic views.

Understanding the injury mechanism and pattern can be helpful in accurate evaluation of the imaging examination, as well as in the clinical examination. Characteristic mensical tear patterns may be seen in specific injury patterns. For example, with tears of the anterior cruciate ligament (ACL) involving internal rotation valgus forces and corresponding pivot-shift, oblique longitudinal tears and flap tears of the lateral meniscus posterior horn extending toward the notch as well as often oblique radial tears of the lateral meniscus at junction of body and anterior horn portions are commonly seen, likely corresponding to the areas of impaction force of the anterior lateral femoral condyle against the posterior lateral tibial plateau in the forced pivot-shift and rebound (Fig. 7.4). Peripheral vertical longitudinal and meniscosynovial junction tears of the medial meniscus posterior horn to body are also commonly encountered. These tears are likely associated with the contusion and impaction injury of the posterior medial tibial plateau often associated with ACL tears (Fig. 7.2).

Articular Cartilage and Bone Imaging

MRI has enabled accurate imaging evaluation of articular cartilage damage that could previously only be inferred in

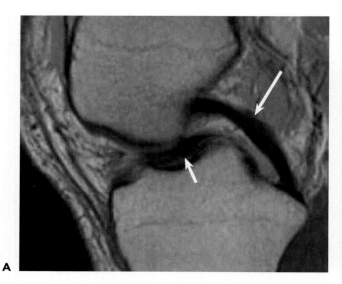
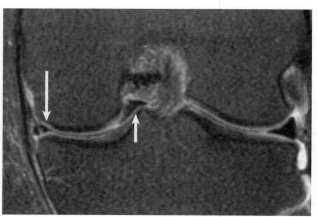

Figure 7.3   Bucket-handle tear of medial meniscus displaced into intercondylar notch. **A:** Sagittal proton density image through the notch shows displaced bucket-handle meniscal tissue (*short arrow*) within notch anterior and inferior to the posterior cruciate ligament (*long arrow*). **B:** Coronal fat-suppressed proton density image confirms the meniscal bucket-handle (*short arrow*) displaced into notch away from the peripheral remnant of the medial meniscus body (*long arrow*).

severe chronic settings by late radiographic osseous and joint-space changes. Soft tissue contrast and multiplanar imaging strengths of MRI are particularly well suited for assessment of the complex curved articular surfaces of the knee, including such areas as the femoral trochlea that can be treacherous to both clinical and imaging diagnosis. Detection of earlier stages of degenerative as well as traumatic changes, is now feasible, and may enable earlier treatment that could potentially slow or even arrest progression to late or end-stage sequelae.

MRI enables noninvasive direct imaging of morphologic changes such as chondral fibrillation, fissuring, focal defects and corresponding fragments, and more diffuse thinning and wear, all manifesting as changes of the chondral thickness and surface at the cartilage interface to joint fluid and synovium. Earlier chondral degenerative changes, such as softening or blistering, to later fibrotic change can also be visible as intrasubstance areas of MRI signal change and inhomogeneity, although such evaluation is still qualitative in standard clinical practice.

Chondral Imaging Technique

As with other applications in clinical musculoskeletal MRI, numerous types of MRI sequences are available for and have been applied to chondral imaging.[12–18] The clinical results and experience have been quite varied, and the choice of imaging protocol may be particularly important for evaluation of articular cartilage. The MRI appearance of articular cartilage varies considerably with the type of sequence applied. Specialized "cartilage-specific" sequences have been used, generally based on various gradient echo techniques that usually result in chondral signal that is relatively high

or bright compared with subchondral bone and overlying joint fluid and synovium. The high contrast between the bright cartilage and dark underlying bone delineates well the cartilage-to-bone interface, but the lower contrast with the overlying higher signal fluid and synovium demonstrates more poorly the cartilage surface and interface to the fluid. Small, more focal chondral fissures or flaps may be difficult to appreciate as small areas of lower signal in a background of bright cartilage. Sensitivity to partial or even full-thickness chondral thinning to focal defects may also be poor. Also, the gradient echo techniques tend to have poor contrast differentiation and resulting limited sensitivity for evaluation of the subchondral bone as well as the remainder of the soft tissues about the knee.

Spin echo or turbo/fast spin echo sequences have also been used, generally producing a cartilage signal that is low compared with the overlying fluid and synovium. The high contrast demonstrates the chondral surface interface well. Fibrillation, fissures, flaps, and defects are easily seen as focal high-signal and high-contrast changes in a low-signal chondral background. The low cartilage signal on spin echo sequences provides less contrast for evaluation of the cartilage interface to the low or absent signal of the underlying bone plate. This interface is also further obscured by a chemical shift artifact between the fat signal of the underlying bone marrow and the water signal of cartilage. However, fat-suppression techniques may be added to eliminate the chemical shift artifact, as well as to suppress the image high background signal of marrow fat and soft tissue fat planes. This suppression of fat signal expands and magnifies the dynamic range of display of the remaining chondral and other soft tissue and bone signals for better sensitivity

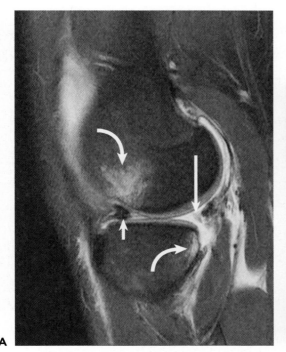

A

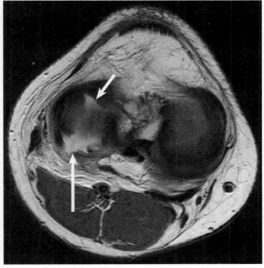

B

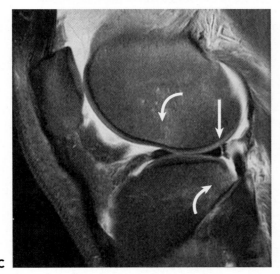

C

Figure 7.4 Lateral meniscus anterior and posterior horn tears. **A:** Sagittal fat-suppressed proton density image reveals radial tear of the meniscus at junction of anterior horn and body portions *(short arrow)*, and segmental defect tear of the posterior horn along and posterior to the popliteus hiatus *(long arrow)*. Note the associated bone high-signal edema of contusion and mild impaction injuries of the anterior lateral femoral condyle and posterior lateral tibial condyle/plateau *(curved arrows)* in this patient with acute tear of the anterior cruciate ligament (not shown on these images). **B:** Axial proton density image further confirms the extent of the radial *(short arrow)* and segmental defect *(long arrow)* tears of the lateral meniscus of the same patient as in Figure 7.4A. **C:** Sagittal fat-suppressed proton density image of a different patient with acute tear of the anterior cruciate ligament identifies peripheral vertical longitudinal tear of the lateral meniscus posterior horn *(straight arrow)* along the popliteus hiatus. Note also the bone high-signal edema and contusions of the anterior lateral femoral condyle and posterior lateral tibial condyle/plateau *(curved arrows)*.

and visibility of the cartilage-to-bone interface, as well as the cartilage substance and surface/interface to overlying fluid and synovium. Injury and resulting signal changes of bone and of soft tissue structures about the knee may also be better demonstrated.

Clinical Practice of Chondral and Bone Imaging

Spin echo and turbo/fast spin echo techniques, without and with fat suppression, remain the mainstay of MRI, and have proven accurate in evaluation of chondral as well as other soft tissue and bone derangement. A standard imaging protocol employing these sequences can then provide a comprehensive knee examination for essentially all clinical indications. Images should be obtained in all three orthogonal

planes about the knee, as the planes are all complementary and each plane is best suited for evaluation of specific portions of the complex three-dimensional structures including chondral surfaces of the knee.

Articular cartilage is often and easily overlooked in imaging examinations. Perhaps more than for any other part of the knee, the chondral surfaces should be evaluated consciously and specifically in each imaging sequence and examination. The tibial plateaus and femoral condyles are well delineated on sagittal and coronal images. The patella and particularly the complex curved trochlea surfaces should be evaluated fully by combining sagittal and axial images.

Chondral fibrillation, fissures, and flaps should be evaluated and described precisely (Figs. 7.5 and 7.6). Acute

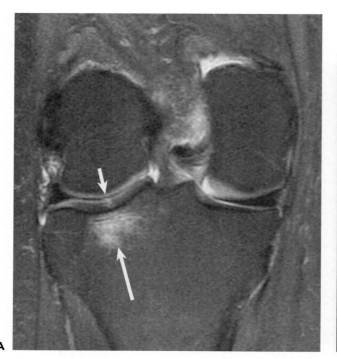

A

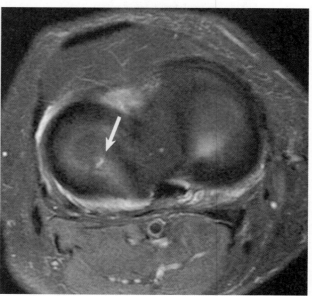

B

Figure 7.5 Focal chondral fracture of the lateral tibial plateau. **A:** Coronal fat-suppressed proton density image demonstrates bone high signal edema of contusion/impaction injury of the lateral tibal plateau *(long arrow)* with high-signal fluid in the focal fracture *(short arrow)* of the overlying articular cartilage. **B:** Axial fat-suppressed proton density image confirms the high signal focal chondral fracture *(arrow)* of the lateral tibial plateau.

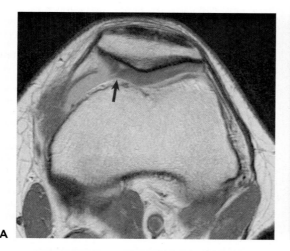

A

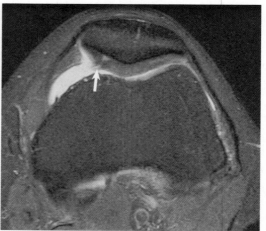

B

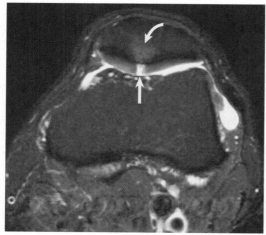

C

Figure 7.6 Patellar chondral focal fissuring and fracture to bone. **A:** Axial proton density image shows the chondral fraying and more focal high signal fissure *(arrow)* to bone over the medial facet of the patella. **B:** Axial fat-suppressed proton density image at the same level shows more conspicuously the high-signal focal fissure *(arrow)* to bone over the medial facet. **C:** Axial fat-suppressed proton density image of a different patient reveals high signal fluid in a focal sharply marginated chondral fracture *(straight arrow)* to bone on the patella median ridge with poorly defined high signal edema of contusion of the underlying bone *(curved arrow)*.

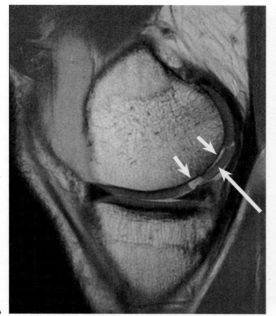

A

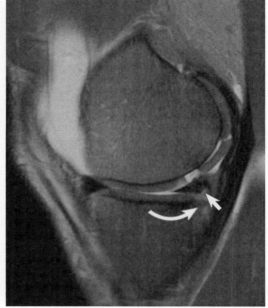

B

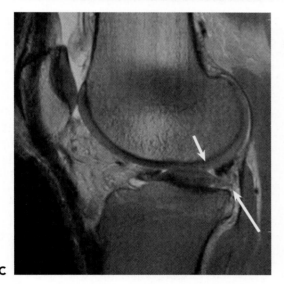

C

Figure 7.7 Chondral defect and fragment of medial femoral condyle, and chondral flap of lateral tibial plateau. **A:** Sagittal proton density image reveals focal chondral defect *(short arrows)* of posterior weightbearing aspect of medial femoral condyle, with corresponding crescentic chondral fragment *(long arrow)* partially displaced within the defect. The sharp margins of defect and fragment indicate an acute injury. **B:** Sagittal fat-suppressed proton density image at the same level demonstrates more conspicuously the high-signal fluid within the defect and outlining the fragment, as well as the peripheral inferior surface tear of the medial meniscus posterior horn *(straight arrow)* and the underlying chondral fissuring and bone edema *(curved arrow)* of the posterior margin of the medial tibial plateau. **C:** Sagittal fat-suppressed proton density image of the lateral compartment shows chondral undermining and flap *(long arrow)*. Note also the corresponding small radial free edge tear of the overlying lateral meniscus posterior horn *(short arrow)*. The posterior lateral injury forces have damaged both of these soft tissue structures.

chondral defects should be differentiated from chronic grade 4 chondral loss, as treatment and prognosis may be quite different. More focal sharply marginated defects may indicate more acute injury and the corresponding fragments should be found and reported (Fig. 7.7). The subchondral bone should also be evaluated for more acute contusion or impaction injury with resulting high-signal edema, best seen on fat-suppressed images and often seen in conjunction with the more acute chondral injury. More diffuse chondral thinning may indicate chronic degenerative wear, possibly from remote trauma,[19] which should be evaluated and reported (Fig. 7.8). More chronic reactive osteitis of the subchondral bone may be seen as relatively increased signal, typically in combination with other chronic osseous changes of sclerosis, remodeling, cystic change,

and osteophyte formation. In practice, the subchondral bone changes when identified in both acute and chronic settings are important and extremely helpful indicators of likely overlying chondral changes. For example, the forces producing acute contusion or an impaction fracture injury of the subchondral bone must be transmitted through and also will likely cause injury to the overlying articular cartilage.[20] The cartilage should then be specifically examined to find or exclude the anticipated corresponding chondral derangement (Fig. 7.5).

With acute bone injury, the high-signal intraosseous edema and hemorrhage are conspicuously seen on fat-suppressed images. MRI is exceedingly sensitive for identifying acute bone injury[21] (Fig. 7.9). However, fracture lines or avulsion fragments may be difficult to identify, particularly

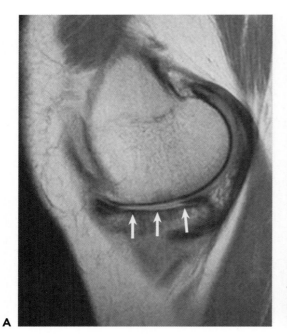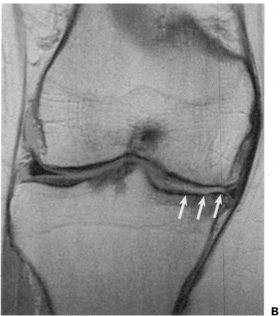

A   **B**

Figure 7.8 Grade 4 chondral thinning to bone of the medial tibial plateau *(arrows)* greater than to adjacent medial femoral condyle. The diffuse extensive chondral absence with subchondral bone low-signal sclerosis and flattening and remodeling correspond with more chronic degenerative chondral loss. **A:** Sagittal proton density image. **B:** Coronal proton density image.

when they are incomplete or when little or no displacement is present. Correlation with radiographic imaging may assist in evaluation. CT examinations particularly can assist in detecting more discrete fracture lines, fragments, and alignment, and should be considered when such additional information may influence treatment. MRI is also sensitive for repetitive stress or overuse injuries of bone in athletes,[8] from stress reactions with poorly defined bone edema to more discrete stress or insufficiency trabecular fracture lines (Fig. 7.10). However, again, the more focal cortical fracture lines may be difficult to see on MRI. CT correlation may be helpful when warranted for treatment decisions.

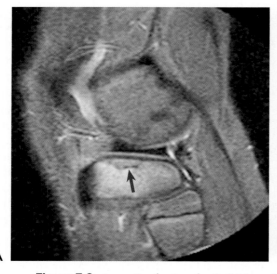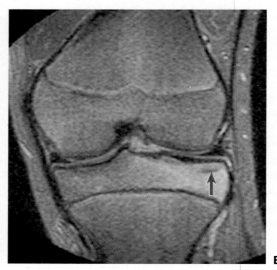

A   **B**

Figure 7.9 Impaction fracture football injury of the lateral tibial plateau with little or no displacement in 11-year-old boy. The high-signal, poorly defined bone edema of the contusion/impaction injury outlines conspicuously the more focal linear low-signal fracture line *(arrow)*. **A:** Sagittal fat-suppressed proton density image. **B:** Coronal fat-suppressed proton density image.

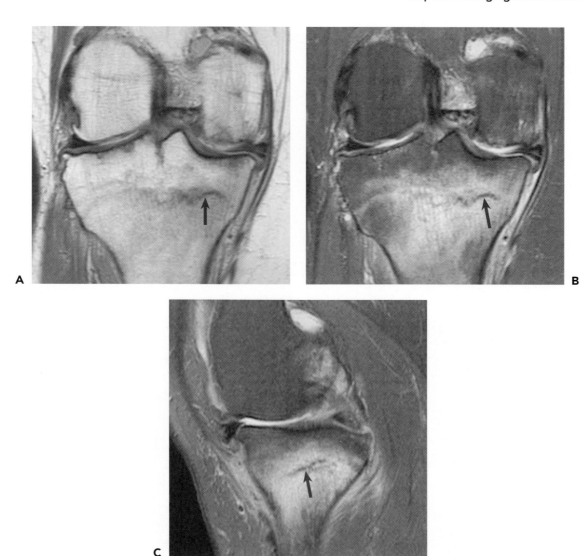

Figure 7.10 Insufficiency stress fracture of proximal medial tibia in a 57-year-old woman. The incomplete low-signal fracture line *(arrow)* is outlined by prominent, poorly defined bone edema that has intermediate signal on the proton density image and a more conspicuous high signal on fat-suppressed proton density image in which the previously high background signal of fatty marrow has been suppressed, leaving the now more conspicuous high signal of bone edema. **A:** Coronal proton density image. **B:** Coronal fat-suppressed proton density image at the same level. **C:** Sagittal fat-suppressed proton density image.

MRI may assist in selecting chondral resurfacing treatment and evaluating response to treatment and evolution of chondral resurfacing.[22–27] More focal and likely acute chondral defects may be better candidates with better prognosis for resurfacing (Fig. 7.7). A patient with more chronic diffuse chondral thinning to bone with chronic subchondral sclerosis or eburnation and cystic change may be a less likely candidate with poorer prognosis (Fig. 7.8). With microfracture or autologous chondrocyte implantation,[28–35] the filling and maturation of new cartilaginous material in treated chondral defects can be monitored (Figs. 7.11 to

7.13). Perhaps more importantly, when clinical course is not meeting expectations, poor filling or early and abortive breakdown of new material in the treated defect can be identified by reading the MRI examination. With osteochondral autograft or allograft treatment,[36] the incorporation and healing of the graft to surrounding native bone and cartilage may be evaluated (Fig. 7.14). Graft alignment, including potential problems of angulation or step-off of the graft from depression or elevation relative to the surrounding native articular surface, may be evaluated on the MRI (Fig 7.15).

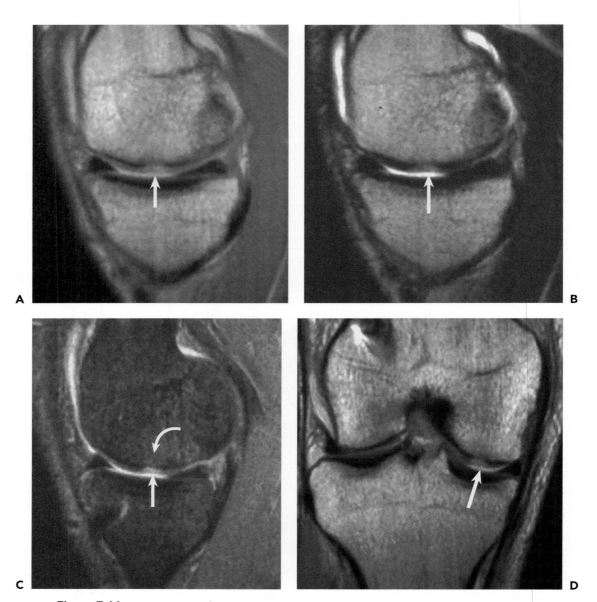

Figure 7.11   Immature microfracture of medial femoral condyle shows filling of previous chondral defect with hybrid cartilaginous material 2 months after the procedure in a football player. There is good filling with still immature-appearing material that is still slightly thinner with higher signal and indistinct margins *(arrow)* compared with the surrounding native hyaline cartilage. The subchondral bone shows mild increased signal edema *(curved arrow)* on fat suppression, indicating ongoing bone reaction and healing. **A:** Sagittal proton density image. **B:** Sagittal T2-weighted image. **C:** Sagittal fat-suppressed (STIR [short tau inversion recovery]) image. **D:** Coronal proton density image.

Ligament Imaging

Injuries to the major ligaments as well as secondary capsular and ligamentous restraints about the knee may also be accurately assessed by MRI.[3,37–39] The normal ligament collagen tissue has little or no MRI signal and the normal ligament should appear as a dark, smoothly marginated, and well-defined continuous structure coursing between the osseous attachments. The acutely injured ligament typically demonstrates an increased high signal indicating edema and hemorrhage within and about the ligament margins in sprain injury and may appear elongated and stretched from interstitial tearing. More severe injury and more discrete tears may be identified by discrete defects and retraction of the torn ligament ends. With more chronic injury, edema and hemorrhage may no longer be present to yield high signals. Chronic scar has little if no signal, but may be differentiated from normal ligament by morphologic changes such as irregular and thickened margins. A chronically torn ligament may also resorb and retract, with resulting attenuated or even

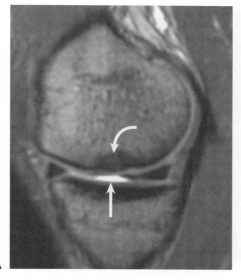

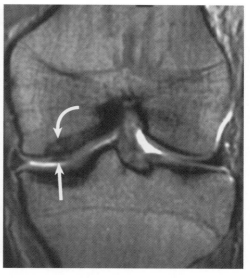

Figure 7.12 Mature microfracture of medial femoral condyle shows good smooth filling of previous chondral defect with mature-appearing hybrid cartilaginous material *(arrow)* 3 years after the procedure in a football player. The hybrid cartilaginous material has relatively lower signal and smooth well-defined surface margin congruent with the surrounding native hyaline cartilage. The subchondral bone shows low signal indicating mature bone healing with relative sclerosis *(curved arrow)*. **A:** Sagittal gradient echo image with T2* (Effective T2 on gradient echo sequence)-weighting and magnetization transfer contrast. **B:** Coronal T2* gradient echo image with magnetization transfer contrast.

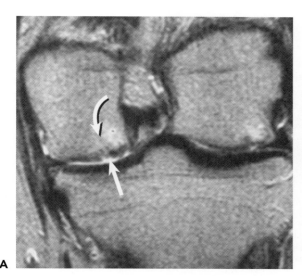

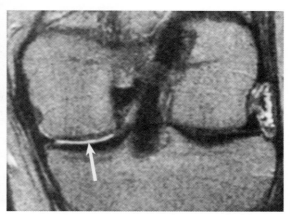

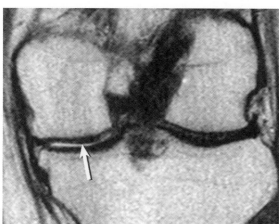

Figure 7.13 Evolution and maturation of microfracture filling in of chondral defect in patient with chronic anterior cruciate ligament (ACL) tear from basketball injury. Coronal T2-weighted images. **A:** Focal chondral defect *(straight arrow)* of medial femoral condyle with subchondral cortical irregularity and pitting and underlying bone edema *(curved arrow)* is present. ACL is chronically torn with residual scarring. **B:** After 7 months from ACL reconstruction and microfracture of the chondral defect, there is good fill of the previous defect with hybrid chondral material *(arrow)* that is smoothly marginated, nearly congruent, and similar in signal to the surrounding native hyaline cartilage. **C:** After 15 months, the microfracture material shows smooth congruent complete fill. The hybrid cartilaginous material is more mature with somewhat lower signal compared with the surrounding hyaline cartilage.

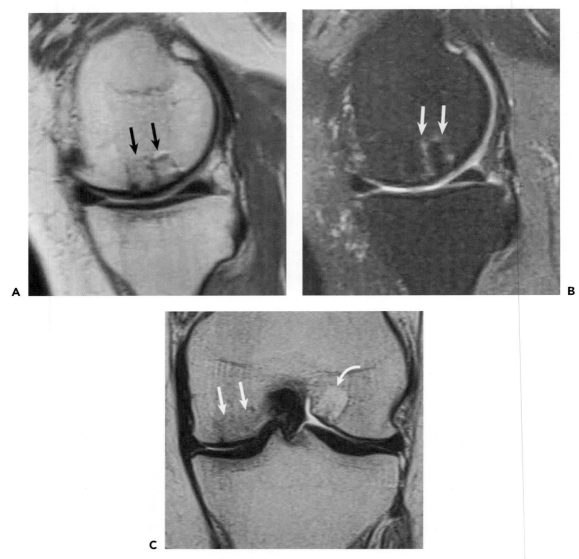

Figure 7.14 Osteochondral graft of previous defect of medial femoral condyle after 12 months with good congruency and healing. **A:** Sagittal proton density image shows grafts in place *(arrows)* with good match and congruency of the cortical and chondral margins with the surrounding condyle. **B:** Sagittal fat suppressed proton density image shows near-complete healing and incorporation of the bone graft with slight residual bone edema *(arrows)* about the remaining areas of the previous interface with the surrounding condyle cancellous bone. **C:** Coronal T2-weighted image shows the good congruency and healing of the graft *(straight arrows)* with the surrounding medial femoral condyle. Note the good healing and filling in of graft harvest site *(curved arrow)*, which had been packed with bone graft material along the lateral aspect of the notch.

absent ligament tissue or ends. Chronic degeneration may also be present, and may produce poorly defined increased intrasubstance signal, possibly progress into more focal and discrete areas of high-signal myxoid change to chronic intrasubstance ganglion cysts. All the ligaments of the knee should each be evaluated in imaging in all three orthogonal planes.

Cruciate Ligaments
The ACL along its length to the tibial attachment is well seen on sagittal images. However, the femoral attachment is poorly demonstrated on sagittal images and much better evaluated on coronal and axial images. The individual posterolateral and anteromedial bundles of the ACL are also poorly differentiated along their length on sagittal images, but routinely and accurately evaluated in cross section on the coronal and axial images, with the normal low-signal bundles separated by relatively high-signal synovial and fat tissue on the images (Fig. 7.16). This evaluation of the ligament cross section is particularly helpful and important for the physician treating patients with partial tears or sprains that may preferentially injure one of the ACL bundles.

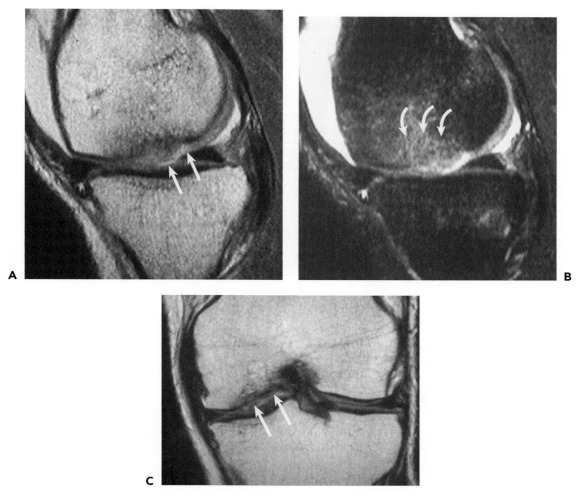

Figure 7.15 Osteochondral graft of previous defect of medial femoral condyle after 8 months with incongruency offset and angulation relative to the surrounding condyle and incomplete healing with prominent ongoing reactive surrounding bone edema. **A:** Sagittal proton density image. Note the incongruency of the graft with offset and focal chondral thinning and fissuring at the interface with surrounding condyle *(arrows)*. **B:** Sagittal fat-suppressed proton density image shows also the very prominent ongoing bone edema *(curved arrows)* and incomplete incorporation and healing of the graft to the surrounding cancellous bone of the condyle. **C:** Coronal proton density image confirms the incongruity offset and angulation of the graft with focal chondral fissuring and thinning at the interface with surrounding condyle *(arrows)*.

Complete ACL tears can be and should be differentiated from a partial tear and sprain, and the location and severity of ACL tears should be evaluated and described precisely, as the treatment options may vary. Proximal tears may be suitable for the healing response primary repair. Midsubstance tears, generally not amenable to primary repair and with poor prognosis with nonoperative management for the active patient, may require ACL reconstruction. The typical distal ACL bone avulsion can be identified and the size, angulation, and displacement of the avulsed tibial eminence fragment with the distal ACL insertion can be accurately evaluated for feasibility and planning of operative reattachment fixation (Figs. 7.17 and 7.18).

The posterior cruciate ligament (PCL) along its length to both femoral and tibial attachments is well seen on sagittal images (Fig. 7.19). However, the ligament cross section is best seen proximally on the coronal images and distally on the axial images, which can be extremely helpful for partial-thickness injuries. Although the normal individual anterolateral and posteromedial bundles of the PCL are not routinely differentiated and separated on MR images, the preferentially injured bundle in sprain or partial tears can be identified by thickening, irregularity, and increased signal edema and hemorrhage on the ligament cross section. Complete ligament tear can be differentiated from distal bone avulsion with the PCL tibial insertion. The distal PCL bone avulsion fragment can then also

(*text continues on p. 103*)

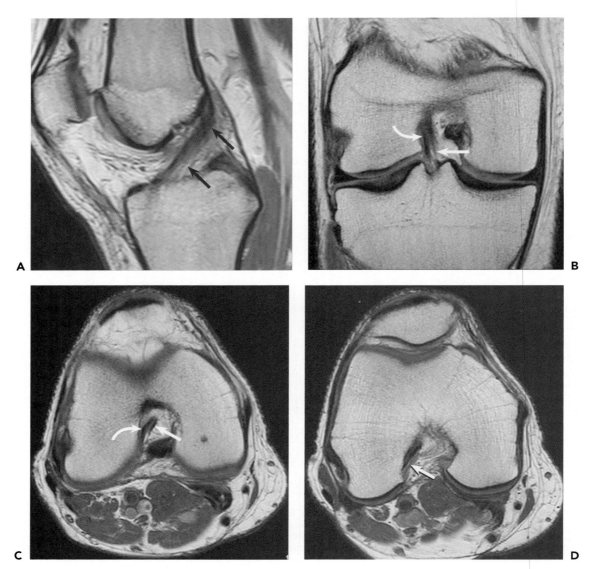

Figure 7.16 Normal anterior cruciate ligament (ACL) imaging appearance. The normal ACL shows well-defined low-signal anteromedial and posterolateral bundles with intervening higher-signal synovial and fat tissue. Proton density images. **A:** Sagittal image through the intercondylar notch demonstrates the straight appearance of a normal ACL from posterior superior femoral to anterior inferior tibial eminence attachments *(arrows)*. **B:** Coronal image through the intercondylar notch shows the normal ACL straight course from superior lateral femoral to inferior medial tibial eminence attachments. The anteromedial *(straight arrow)* and posterolateral *(curved arrow)* bundles can be appreciated and differentiated as separate distinct low-signal bands. **C:** Axial image shows the posterolateral bundle *(curved arrow)* beginning to attach to the superior lateral margin of the intercondylar notch. The anteromedial bundle *(straight arrow)* has not yet reached its origin. **D:** Axial image more proximally identifies the attachment of the anteromedial bundle *(arrow)* more posterior and superior to that of the posterolateral bundle as shown in Figure 7.16C.

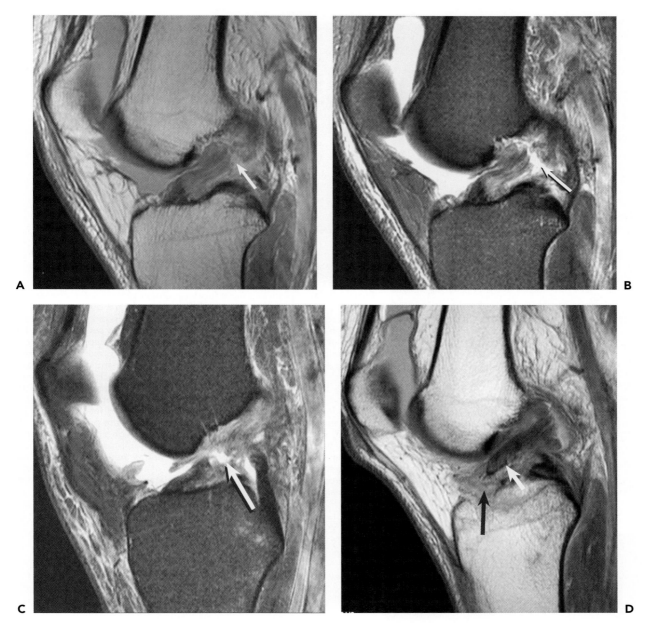

Figure 7.17   Tears of the anterior cruciate ligament (ACL) may be evaluated accurately for precise location and extent of the tear by magnetic resonance imaging. **A:** Sagittal proton density image shows complete disruption of the ACL *(arrow)* at the junction of middle and proximal thirds, with bowing and increased signal edema and hemorrhage within and about the proximal and distal tear ends. **B:** Sagittal fat-suppressed proton density image at same level as shown in **A** shows even more conspicuously the tear defect *(arrow)* and high-signal edema and hemorrhage. **C:** Sagittal fat-suppressed proton density image of a different patient reveals focal complete mid-substance tear of the ACL *(arrow)*. **D:** Sagittal proton density image of another patient shows avulsion of the distal ACL attachment, with superior and posterior retraction and posterior rotation of the avulsed fragment *(short arrow)* of the ACL insertion with defect of the anterior tibial attachment *(long arrow)*.

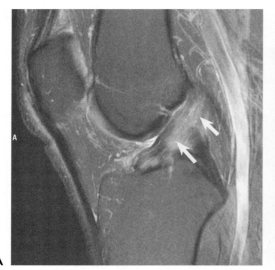

A

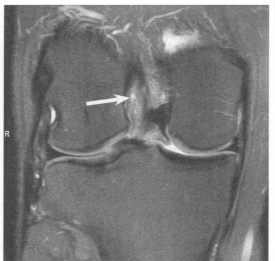

B

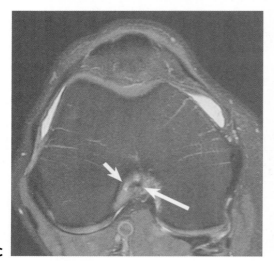

C

Figure 7.18 Sprain and more focal partial tear of the proximal anterior cruciate ligament (ACL) involving primarily the posterolateral bundle. **A:** Sagittal fat-suppressed proton density image shows an irregular, proximally thickened ACL with high-signal edema and hemorrhage *(arrows)*. The severity and extent of tearing of the proximal ligament diameter is difficult to appreciate in the sagittal plane because of partial volume averaging of the proximal ACL substance with the adjacent posterior cruciate ligament medially and the lateral margin of the notch laterally. Evaluation is possible and more precise in the other planes in which the short-diameter cross section of the proximal ligament is better seen and separated from the posterior collateral ligament and lateral notch margin, in the coronal and the axial planes. **B:** Coronal fat-suppressed proton density image shows the focal partial tear defect of the proximal third of ACL involving primarily the posterolateral band, with high-signal fluid and hemorrhage within the tear defect *(arrow)*. **C:** Axial fat-suppressed proton density image at level of the proximal third of ACL confirms the focal high signal hemorrhage in the partial tear defect *(short arrow)* of the posterolateral bundle, while the adjacent anteromedial bundle is still relatively well-defined with more normal low signal intact fibers *(long arrow)*.

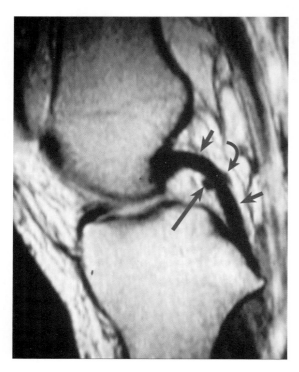

Figure 7.19 Normal posterior cruciate ligament (PCL). Sagittal proton density image through the intercondylar notch demonstrates the normal contour and bowing and low/dark or no signal of the well-defined intact PCL *(short arrows)*. Note the normal meniscofemoral ligaments of Humphrey *(long arrow)* and Wrisberg *(curved arrow)* coursing across the anterior and posterior aspects of the PCL.

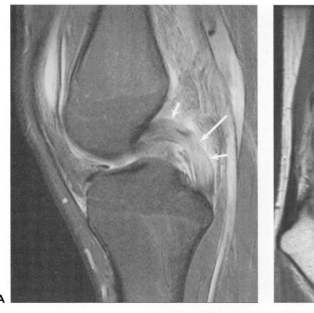
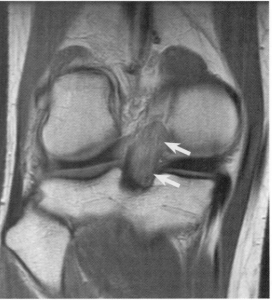
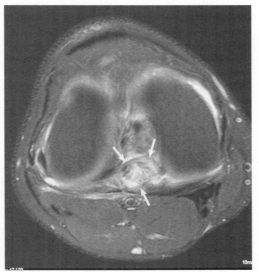

Figure 7.20 Midsubstance tear of the posterior cruciate ligament (PCL). **A:** Sagittal fat-suppressed proton density image shows diffuse thickening of the ligament with increased signal edema and hemorrhage within and about the entire PCL *(short arrows)*, with more focal mid substance tear *(long arrow).* **B:** Coronal proton density image through the posterior aspect of the notch shows the distal portion to tibial attachment of the PCL, with diffuse thickening and increased signal edema and hemorrhage *(arrows)*, unlike the normal well-defined low/dark signal of the normal PCL as shown in Figure 7.19. **C:** Axial fat-suppressed proton density image through the inferior portion of the notch shows the grossly abnormal thickening and increased/high-signal edema and hemorrhage within and about the transverse cross section of the distal PCL *(arrows)* just above its tibial attachment.

be evaluated for planning of operative fixation (Figs. 7.20 and 7.21).

Collateral Ligaments

The medial collateral ligament (MCL) is well seen along its length from femoral proximal attachment to tibial distal attachment on coronal images. Its cross section is best seen on axial images for most accurate assessment of

extent of ligament diameter damage (Fig. 7.22). Combined assessment of the MCL in both planes allows evaluation of precise location and extent of sprain or a more focal tear injury.

Although most MCL sprains and tears respond well to nonoperative management, select tears may require operative treatment, for which precise evaluation and description may be invaluable (Fig. 7.23). Identifying tears with

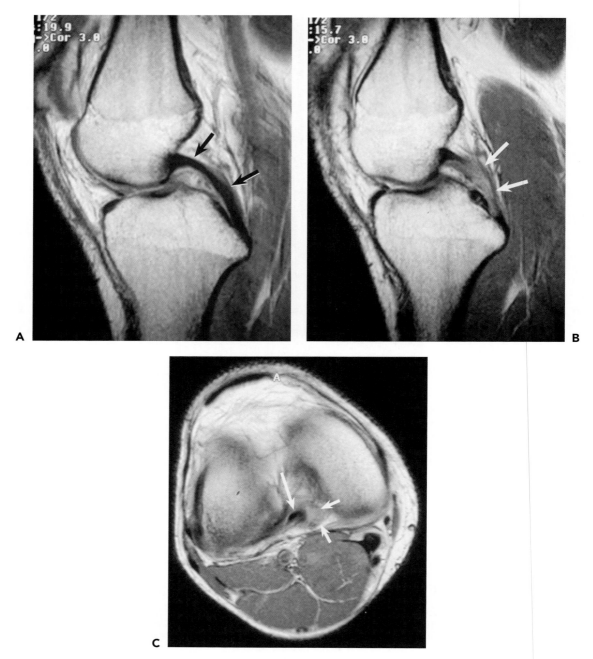

Figure 7.21   Sprain and more focal partial tearing of the posteromedial bundle of the posterior cruciate ligament (PCL). **A:** Sagittal proton density image through the notch shows a normal-appearing well-defined and low-signal PCL (arrows). **B:** However, the next more medial image of the sagittal proton density image series shows a very abnormal appearance with thickening, irregular and indistinct margins, and high signal of the mid-to-distal PCL (arrows), strongly indicative of injury. **C:** Axial proton density image through the inferior portion of the notch evaluates more reliably the mid-to-distal PCL in short-diameter transverse cross section (compared to evaluation in longitudinal appearance in the sagittal images in **A** and **B**), and confirms accurately the focal partial tearing of the PCL involving the posteromedial bundle, which is markedly thickened and irregular with high-signal edema and hemorrhage (short arrows), while the intact anterolateral bundle (long arrow) still shows more normal low-signal and well-defined margins.

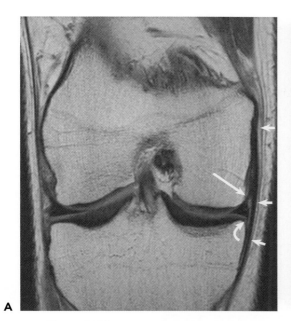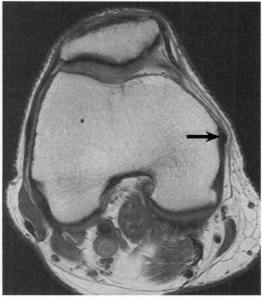

A   B

Figure 7.22 Normal medial collateral ligament (MCL). **A:** Coronal proton density images shows the smooth margins, low signal, and relatively uniform thickness of the superficial MCL *(short arrows)* extending from superior femoral attachment inferiorly. Note the deep component coronary ligaments: the meniscofemoral *(long arrow)* and meniscotibial *(curved arrows)* ligaments and underlying recesses extending above and below the medial joint line. **B:** Axial proton density image at the level of superior portion of the notch and the femoral condyles demonstrates the smooth low-signal transverse cross section of the normal proximal MCL *(arrow)* toward the femoral attachment.

widely separated and displaced ligament ends may prompt repair. Tears at the medial joint line with disruption of the deep meniscofemoral or meniscotibial ligaments and meniscocapsular junction and with trapping of torn superficial MCL end in the medial joint compartment may not heal adequately and functionally. These tears require repair. A distal tear or stripping of the MCL with prominent proximal retraction of the ligament end may also require repair, particularly as the ligament end may be trapped superficially with the distal pes tendons extending to pes anserinum interposed between the MCL end and its proper tibial insertion, thus preventing healing of the MCL in the appropriate functional state and position (Fig. 7.24). This may be a concern when a distal MCL injury is present. However, when high-resolution imaging of the knee is performed with a small field of view for optimal evaluation of internal derangement, the distal tibial attachment of the MCL may at times extend below the edge of the image field of view. When distal clinical and/or imaging findings suggest MCL distal injury at the tibial insertion, including distal edema and hemorrhage, and elongation and retraction of the visualized distal portion of MCL at the inferior margin of the images, additional supplemental axial and coronal images obtained more inferiorly are warranted. Precise and complete imaging assessments and descriptions are required.

The lateral collateral ligament (LCL), because of its more oblique course from more anterior superior at its femoral attachment to more posterior inferior at its primary insertion at fibular head, may require evaluation on sequential coronal images along its length, rather than a single coronal image. It may be followed more reliably in cross section on sequential axial images from proximal to distal attachments (Fig. 7.25). Although sprains may respond to nonoperative management, more discrete tears, including distal avulsions of the fibular head, may require repair, particularly when wide displacement and retraction of tear ends and avulsed fragments are present (Fig. 7.26). Again, accurate imaging evaluation and reporting is necessary, reasonable, and required to plan treatment.

Posterolateral Corner and Other Secondary Restraints

Assessment of secondary supporting structures[3,5,40] may be vital when evaluating knee ligamentous injury for treatment planning and prognosis. MRI can provide vital information for the accuracy of the total clinical evaluation. The posterolateral corner, because of complexity and three-dimensional course of its many component structures, including posterolateral capsule and arcuate ligament, popliteus, popliteofibular ligament, and component bands from the lateral collateral ligament and iliotibial band, should

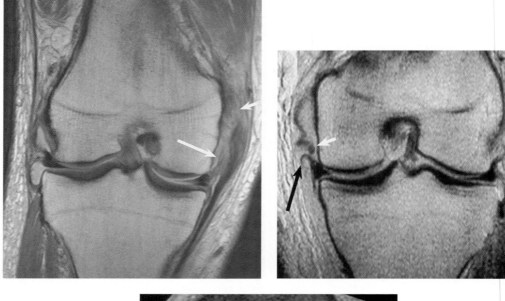

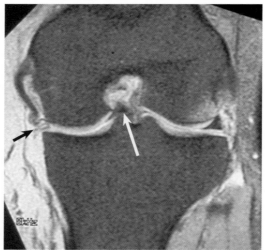

Figure 7.23   Medial collateral ligament (MCL) tears can be evaluated precisely and accurately for location and extent of tears by magnetic resonance imaging. This information may be valuable for management decisions because some MCL tears may require operative repair. **A:** Complete tear of the proximal MCL *(short arrow)* at and just below the femoral attachment. The underlying meniscofemoral coronary ligament *(long arrow)* has also been torn and stripped from the femoral attachment. The tear ends are mildly displaced, but with no intervening tissue to block scarring and healing to their anatomic origins. This type of MCL tear will generally respond well and heal/scar with nonoperative management. **B:** Coronal proton density image. Midsubstance complete disruption of the MCL at the level of the medial joint line. The underlying coronary ligaments have also been torn. The proximal end of the torn MCL *(short arrow)* is trapped, interposed between the medial femoral condyle and the displaced torn end of the meniscofemoral ligament *(long arrow)*. This tear is unlikely to heal functionally without operative repair. **C:** Coronal fat-suppressed proton density image. Another midsubstance complete tear of the MCL in a different patient with disruption of the coronary ligaments and the menicosynovial/capsular junction of the body portion of the medial meniscus, which is displaced entirely into the intercondylar notch *(long arrow)*. The torn ends and remnants of the coronary ligaments and the proximal end of the MCL *(short arrow)* extend along and into the medial joint line and may be trapped. Again, this MCL tear will not heal functionally and requires operative repair.

be assessed in images in all three orthogonal planes of the knee (Fig. 7.27). Sprain or strain injury to more discrete tears can all be demonstrated as changes in the normal smooth margins and low or absent signal of the capsule, ligament, and tendon component structures (Figs. 7.28 and 7.29). The Segond avulsion fracture of the proximal lateral tibial margin is one such secondary support injury that has been found in high association with ACL tears, and that involves avulsion of the tibial insertion of likely a coalescence of bands from the lateral collateral ligament

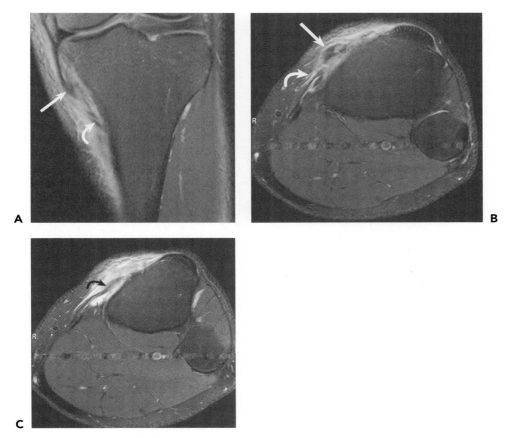

Figure 7.24 Complete distal tear and stripping of medial collateral ligament (MCL). The torn ligament end is retracted proximally superficial to the distal pes tendons and pes anserinum. The normal distal MCL and attachment is underneath, deep to the distal pes tendons and pes anserinum. This patient's torn MCL end is trapped away from its anatomic insertion by the intervening pes tendons. It is unlikely to heal functionally to its anatomic insertion without operative repair. **A:** Coronal fat-suppressed proton density image delineates the retraction of the distally torn MCL *(arrow),* proximal and superficial to the distal pes tendons *(curved arrow).* **B:** Axial fat-suppressed proton density image of the proximally retracted torn end of the MCL *(arrow).* At this level the pes tendons *(curved arrow)* are still posterior but already appear somewhat deep compared with the MCL end. **C:** Axial fat-suppressed proton density image more inferior to **B.** The MCL is no longer seen, as it is retracted above the level of this image. The pes tendons *(curved arrow)* are seen coursing more inferiorly and anteriorly compared with the more proximal image, deep to the proximally retracted MCL end, and show strain irregularity with extensive surrounding high-signal edema and hemorrhage associated with the pes strain as well as the complete tear and stripping of the distal MCL.

and the iliotibial band.[41] The small avulsion fragment from the lateral tibial margin may be difficult to appreciate on cursory inspection of the MR images, but the total injury is well delineated on the coronal and axial images, with the fibrous and ligamentous bands inserting on the avulsed fragment with associated surrounding bone and soft tissue edema and hemorrhage (Fig. 7.30).

More severe partial-to-complete tears, particularly when widely separated and retracted, may require operative treatment, because long-term insufficiency or deficiency of the secondary supporting structures may otherwise result with associated instability that may adversely contribute to outcome. Precise imaging evaluation and description contribute immensely to treatment planning.

The posteromedial corner and other secondary supports, including tendons and muscles about the knee, should be evaluated on the comprehensive knee MRI examination.

Tendon and Muscle Imaging

Normal tendons, as with ligaments, contain no MRI signal and should be smoothly marginated and dark, with little or no signal on all sequences and images. Typically, they are uniform in thickness along their length from myotendinous junction to insertion. Muscles also should be smoothly marginated, with low-to-intermediate signal on all sequences. When injured, distortion of image signal and morphology are found, with high signal of edema and hemorrhage within and

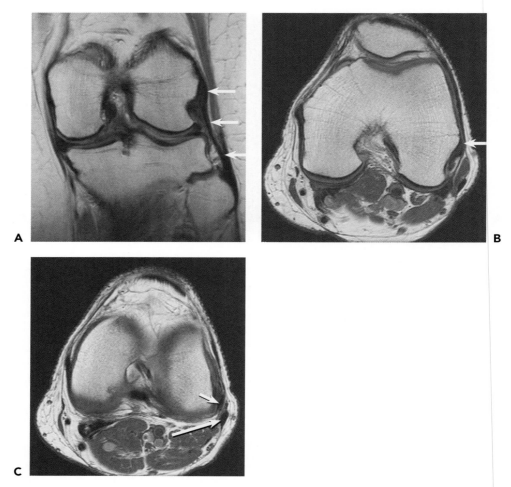

Figure 7.25 Normal lateral collateral ligament (LCL). The LCL should be smoothly marginated with low signal and intact surrounding fat planes from the proximal femoral attachment to the distal conjoined attachment with the biceps femoris at the fibular head. **A:** Coronal proton density image. The entire length of the LCL *(arrows)* is demonstrated on this image. However, because of the oblique course of the LCL from anterior superior to posterior inferior, the proximal-to-distal portions of the ligament are more frequently seen on sequential more anterior to more posterior coronal images. The LCL is evaluated more reliably in a short-diameter transverse cross section on sequential axial images, as delineated later. **B:** Axial proton density image at the level of proximal portions of the femoral condyles shows the well-defined low-signal cross section and clean intact surrounding fat planes of the proximal LCL *(arrow)* at and just below its femoral attachment. **C:** Axial proton density image more inferiorly, now at the level of the inferior notch, shows the well-defined intact LCL *(short arrow)* coursing more posteriorly and inferiorly toward the biceps femoris tendon *(long arrow).* The ligament and tendon can be followed for any evidence of injury on sequential more inferior axial images to join at the fibular head insertion.

about the tendon and muscle and with irregularity to discrete tear defects and retraction of the muscle and tendon margins.

The extensor tendons and mechanism, from distal quadriceps tendon to the patella to the patellar tendon to the tibial tubercle insertion should be evaluated along their length on sagittal images and in cross section on axial images (Fig. 7.31). The normal quadriceps tendon, in a slight departure from other tendons, typically has a relatively discrete trilaminar appearance, with superficial rectus femoris, middle vastus medialis and lateralis, and deep vastus intermedius components, which are seen as low-signal bands separated by intermediate-to-higher signal fibrofatty tissue.

Quadriceps injury can be evaluated for location and severity from strains to partial tears to complete rupture and retraction using the sagittal and axial images in combination. When complete rupture and substantial retraction are present, the proximal tendon end may be above the superior margin of the image field of view on a high-resolution knee MRI. To assist in operative planning, supplemental, more proximal sagittal and axial images may be warranted for complete evaluation and reporting of the tear defect and location of retracted tear ends.

The patellar tendon should be evaluated along its length on sagittal images and in cross section on axial images for

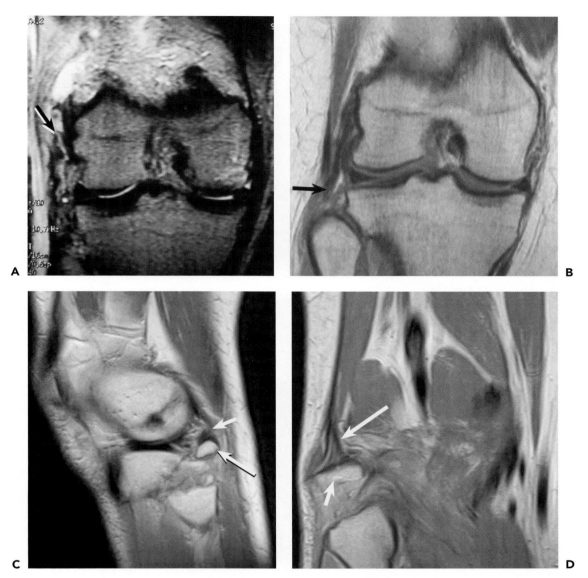

Figure 7.26   Tears of the lateral collateral ligament (LCL) also should be evaluated and reported accurately for severity and location of tear. **A:** Coronal T2-weighted image shows complete proximal tear and stripping of the LCL *(arrow)* with mild distal retraction, with associated high-signal hemorrhage extending proximally. **B:** Coronal proton density image reveals high-grade tear and stripping of the distal LCL *(arrow)* and biceps femoris, with poorly defined elongated higher signal tissue remaining distally to the fibular head representing residual fibers that have stretched with interstitial tearing. **C:** Sagittal proton density image shows avulsion of the distal LCL *(short arrow)* with a triangular to crescentic avulsion fragment *(long arrow)* of the fibular head styloid retracted proximally with the LCL to the level of the posterolateral joint line. The retracted avulsion fragment has been described on conventional radiographs as the arcuate sign of posterior lateral ligamentous disruption. **D:** Coronal proton density image in a different patient shows a larger avulsion fragment *(short arrow)* of the fibular head with proximal retraction with the conjoined distal biceps femoris and LCL attachment *(long arrow)*.

location and severity of strain to a tear injury. More chronic scarring and tendinosis are seen as irregular thickening and poorly defined low-to-intermediate increased intrasubstance signal of the tendon. More focal severe myxoid-to-cystic change, such as typically found proximally at the patellar attachment in clinical "jumper's knee," is seen as focal globular areas of high signal similar to fluid, often with

associated more poorly defined increased signal of edema and inflammation in the bone of the lower patella margin at the tendon attachment and in the underlying infrapatellar fat pad. Both areas are more conspicuously seen on fat-suppressed images (Fig. 7.32). More chronic stress-related or posttraumatic patellar tendinosis and scarring and associated osseous remodeling and heterotopic ossification

(*text continues on p. 112*)

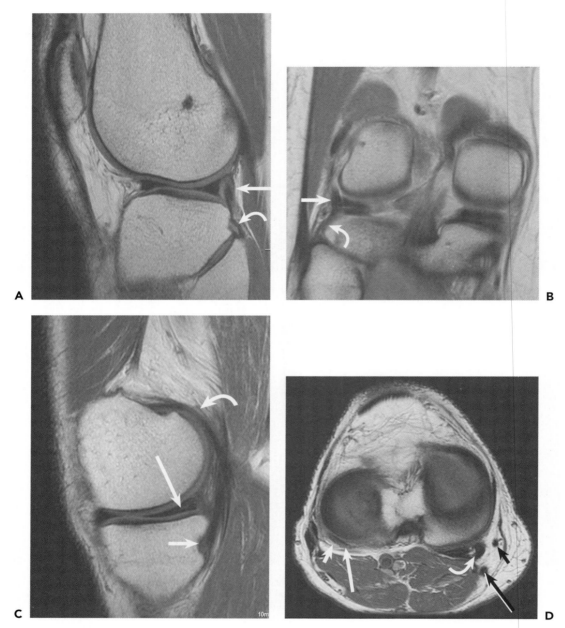

Figure 7.27   Normal posterolateral and posteromedial corners. These secondary restraint structures can be evaluated accurately by magnetic resonance imaging for evidence of injury. The capsular, ligamentous, and tendinous structures should all be well defined, with smooth margins and low signal. **A:** Sagittal proton density image of popliteus hiatus of lateral meniscus posterior horn and the posterolateral corner. The intact popliteus *(short arrow)* and lateral gastrocnemius tendons, the meniscopopliteal fascicles, and the popliteofibular ligament *(curved arrow)* are all well delineated. **B:** Coronal proton density image through the popliteus hiatus and posterolateral corner. The popliteus tendon *(short arrow)* and popliteofibular ligament *(curved arrow)* are intact with normal low-signal and well-defined margins. **C:** Sagittal proton density image through the normal posteromedial corner demonstrates the intact distal semimembranosus *(short arrow)* and proximal medial gastrocnemius *(curved arrow)* tendons to their respective tibial and femoral attachments, as well as the posteromedial capsule and meniscocapsular junction of the medial meniscus posterior horn *(long arrow)*. **D:** Axial proton density image at the level of the menisci and femoral-tibial joint line shows the normal well-defined low-signal structures of posterolateral and posteromedial corners, with intact surrounding synovial tissues and fat planes. Note the posterolateral capsule *(short arrow)* and popliteus tendon *(long arrow)* laterally, and the semimembranosus *(curved arrow)*, gracilus *(short black arrow)*, and semitendinosus *(long black arrows)* tendons medially.

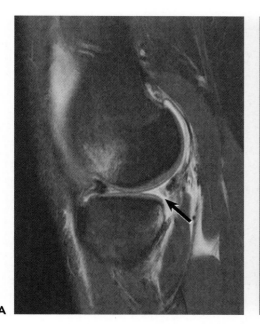
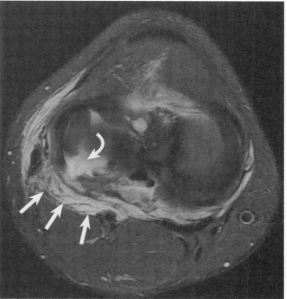

Figure 7.28 Posterolateral corner disruption in a patient with anterior cruciate ligament tear and lateral meniscus tear, discussed previously in Figure 7.4. **A:** Sagittal fat-suppressed proton density image shows tearing of the posterolateral capsule and popliteus hiatus, with disruption of the lateral meniscus posterior horn and the meniscopopliteal fascicles *(arrow)*, and high-signal fluid and hemorrhage about the strain of the popliteus and lateral gastrocnemius muscles. **B:** Axial fat-suppressed proton density image confirms in another plane the high-signal edema and hemorrhage about the posterolateral corner including within and about the popliteus muscle and tendon and posterolateral capsule *(short arrows)*, as well as the segmental tear defect of the lateral meniscus posterior horn and popliteus hiatus *(curved arrow)*.

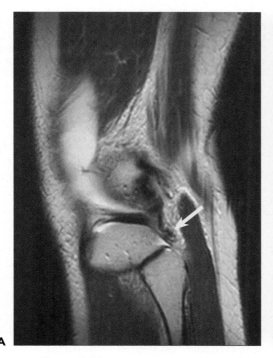
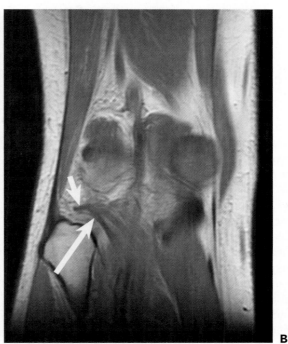

Figure 7.29 Popliteofibular ligament distal tear, stripping in patient with posterolateral corner injury. **A:** Sagittal T2-weighted image shows the torn and proximally retracted remnant of the ligament *(arrow)*, stripped from its distal fibular attachment, with surrounding high-signal edema. **B:** Coronal proton density image confirms the tear in the ligament *(short arrow)* with distal stripping and retraction from the fibula and the proximal fusion of the ligament with the popliteus *(long arrow)*.

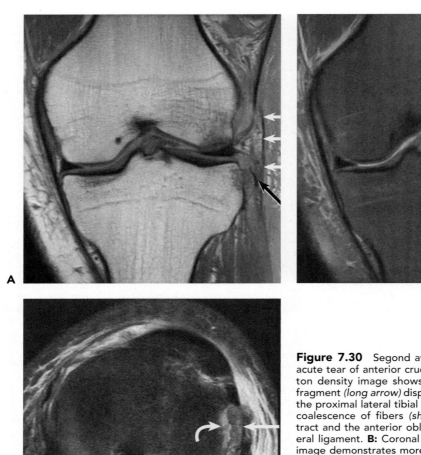

Figure 7.30 Segond avulsion fracture in patient with acute tear of anterior cruciate ligament. **A:** Coronal proton density image shows the small crescentic avulsion fragment *(long arrow)* displaced laterally from its origin at the proximal lateral tibial margin with the avulsed lateral coalescence of fibers *(short arrows)* from the iliotibial tract and the anterior oblique band of the lateral collateral ligament. **B:** Coronal fat-suppressed proton density image demonstrates more conspicuously the high signal of underlying bone edema *(curved arrow)* of lateral tibial margin and the soft tissue edema and hemorrhage surrounding the avulsed fragment *(short arrow)* and attached lateral ligament and iliotibial tract fibers. **C:** Axial fat-suppressed proton density image shows conspicuously in another plane the bone *(curved arrow)* and soft tissue high-signal edema about the Segond avulsion fragment *(long arrow).*

(possibly with bone increased signal edema) may also be seen at proximal and distal patellar tendon attachments at the lower patellar margin, as in Sinding-Larsen-Johansson syndrome, or the tibial tubercle as in Osgood-Schlatter disease. Discrete rupture tears or avulsions of the patellar tendon are well delineated with the associated retinacular tears and avulsions (Fig. 7.33). Precise imaging evaluation of the severity of injury, tear ends, and retraction by MRI can assist greatly in operative planning.

The hamstring and pes tendons and posterior muscles should also be evaluated.[42] Because of their more oblique course, they should be studied along their length on both sagittal and coronal images and in cross section on axial images. Strains or more discrete tears should be identified and described precisely for planning management, which may include operative repair when needed, such as complete tendon tears or avulsions when widely separated and retracted (Fig. 7.34).

In the comprehensive MRI examination of the knee, the tendons should also be evaluated and described, even when they are not symptomatic, because they may be potential autograft harvest sites for reconstruction, such as for tears of the ACL.

CURRENT EXPECTATIONS AND FUTURE DEVELOPMENTS

The value of the contribution that diagnostic imaging can make to the clinical assessment of the symptomatic knee has continued to grow with the development and continued evolution of MRI in orthopaedic applications. The clinically valuable information that can and should be found and reported from the comprehensive knee MRI examination has grown as the imaging technology has continued to improve. Advances include higher resolution,

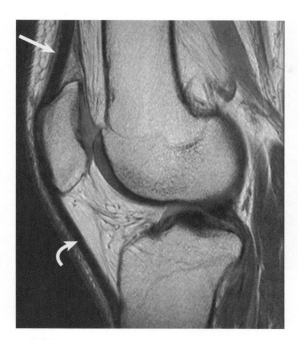

Figure 7.31 Normal knee extensor mechanism with normal distal quadriceps tendon *(arrow)*, extensor tendon/retinaculum along the anterior patella, and patellar tendon *(curved arrow)* inserting distally at the tibial tubercle. The quadriceps tendon may show normal trilaminar longitudinal structure normally, but otherwise these extensor tendons should be smoothly marginated with uniform thickness and low signal.

greater speed, improved tissue contrast capability, improved magnet design with increased magnet field strength and gradient strength, improved coil design (including knee coil and other orthopaedic application coils), and improved imaging sequence design and development of new sequences.

Similarly, the clinical experience and expectations of MRI have grown, both for the imaging radiologist and the treating physician and surgeon. One of the earliest orthopaedic MRI applications was in the knee, specifically for diagnosing the presence of meniscal tears. Little was expected or found for the remainder of the knee in symptomatic derangement. The capability and expectation for the comprehensive "standard" knee MRI examination and report have increased tremendously—far beyond simply the presence or absence of meniscal tear. Menisci, chondral surfaces, bone, ligaments, tendons, and muscles about the knee now can and should be evaluated accurately, not only for the presence of injury, but also for specific details of location and severity of injury, including size and location of tear defects, displaced meniscal or chondral fragments, and ligament and tendon tear ends.

It is incumbent on the treating physician or surgeon to communicate with the radiologist about all clinically important information that the treating doctor needs and hopes to obtain from the imaging examination for assessment of the

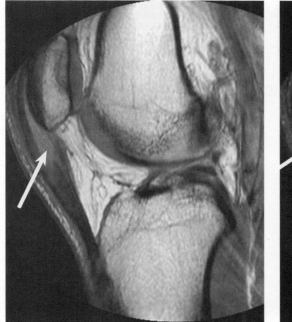 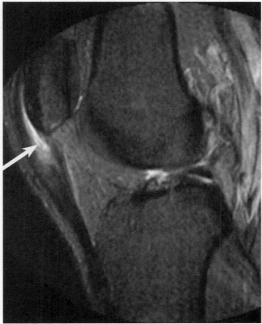

A **B**

Figure 7.32 Severe proximal patellar tendinosus with severe myxoid change and high-grade partial tearing at the patellar attachment extending more proximally along the deep portion of the extensor tendon/retinaculum along the superficial patellar margin in 23-year-old football player. Sagittal proton density **(A)** and fat-suppressed proton density **(B)** images reveal prominent thickening of the proximal patellar tendon with more focal globular to longitudinal area of high-signal myxoid change and hemorrhage of partial tear defect *(arrow)*.

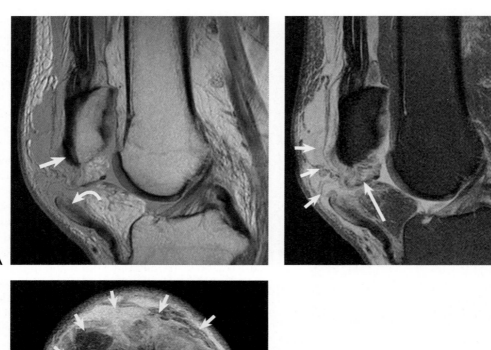

Figure 7.33 Proximal patellar tendon rupture and sleeve avulsion. **A:** Sagittal proton density image shows the proximally retracted patella *(short arrow)* and distally retracted avulsed tendon end *(curved arrow).* **B:** Sagittal fat-suppressed proton density images demonstrates more conspicuously the associated extensive surrounding high-signal fluid and hemorrhage and the tearing of the underlying infrapatellar fat pad *(long arrow)* and the overlying subcutaneous fat, with extravasation of fluid and hemorrhage dissecting superficially *(short arrows).* **C:** Axial fat-suppressed proton density image at the level of the tear defect confirms the associated tearing and avulsion of the medial and lateral retinacula *(arrows)* as well as the absence of the torn and retracted patellar tendon.

patient's knee when planning treatment. The imaging doctor must learn about the clinically important questions and should continue to improve and optimize the knee MRI examination to obtain answers that are clinically relevant. As experience and expectations have grown, sports medicine musculoskeletal imaging has developed as a specialty focus within radiology, just as orthopaedic sports medicine has developed within orthopaedics.

The collaboration between physicians in musculoskeletal imaging and orthopaedics has also benefited from the growth of teleradiology technology and practice models. Imaging has become largely digital information, with digital radiography as well as CT and MRI. With the evolution of data transmission technology and security and of digital image workstations, the knee MRI and other orthopaedic imaging examinations can be moved quickly and routinely to radiologists experienced in and focusing on orthopaedic and sports medicine imaging when the local medical community does not have that experience or focus. The teleradiology practice model includes appropriate and necessary professional services contract agreements, transmission speed and

security, medical licensing, and medical insurance and malpractice policies. Patient medical records including the MRI examination report can be securely transmitted at high speed. The patient may benefit in this manner from having the experienced and focused radiologist evaluating his knee MRI examination for all the clinically important information that may be found, regardless of where the MRI examination is obtained, just as the patient benefits from having the experienced sports medicine orthopaedist examining and treating his or her knee clinically.

The potential of MRI, including for musculoskeletal applications, is greater and is by no means exhausted. MRI technology and techniques continue to improve and evolve. Resolution, speed, and contrast continue to improve. Higher-field strength systems continue to be developed and are becoming more feasible in cost for standard clinical use. With higher field strength comes greater signal-to-noise ratios for imaging, which may be exploited for higher resolution and speed, such as required for chondral imaging. Greater speed also is promising for true dynamic MRI, which may enable virtually real-time study of joint

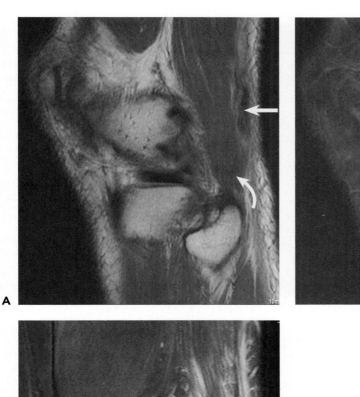

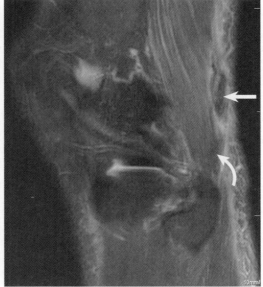

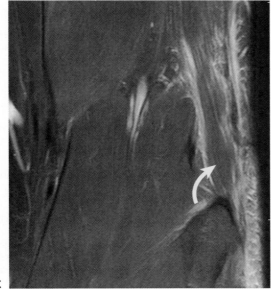

Figure 7.34 Distal biceps femoris tendon tear. The torn, stripped tendon end *(short arrow)* is retracted proximally from the fibular head, with surrounding high-signal edema and hemorrhage. This patient has a prominent distal muscular extension and insertion of the biceps *(curved arrow)* on the fibular head, deep to the tendon, that is still in continuity but strained with intramuscular also abnormal high-signal edema and hemorrhage. **A:** Sagittal proton density image. **B:** Sagittal fat-suppressed proton density image. **C:** Coronal fat-suppressed proton density image.

motion[43] with physiologic muscle, tendon, and ligament forces all in play.

Newer imaging techniques continue to be conceived and developed. For example, potentially powerful new sequences such as ultra short echo time projection reconstruction techniques, contrast-enhanced imaging, including delayed (after administration of intravenous gadolinium contrast agent) contrast-enhanced chondral imaging, diffusion-weighted imaging, and sodium MRI, are being investigated. They show great potential for assessment of even early degenerative changes of articular cartilage including derangement of chondrocytes and extracellular matrix, such as loss of glycosaminoglycans concentration and disorder of collagen structure.[44-46] These techniques are still largely investigational, time-consuming, and not yet clinically vali-

dated or widely available. They have yet to affect standard clinical imaging practice, but the potential of these (and invariably of other techniques still to come) is great.

REFERENCES

1. Bikkina RS, Tujo CA, Schraner AB, et al. The "floating" meniscus: MRI in knee trauma and implications for surgery. *AJR Am J Roentgenol* 2005;184:200–204.
2. Costa CR, Morrison WB, Carrino JA. Medial meniscus extrusion on knee MRI: is extent associated with severity of degeneration or type of tear? *AJR Am J Roentgenol* 2004;183:17–23.
3. Ho CP, Marks PH, Steadman JR. MR imaging of knee anterior cruciate ligament and associated injuries in skiers. *Magn Reson Imaging Clin North Am* 1999;7:117–130.
4. Irie K, Yamada T, Inoue K. A comparison of magnetic resonance imaging and arthroscopic evaluation of chondral lesions of the knee. *Orthopedics* 2000;23:561–564.

5. Juhng SK, Lee JK, Choi SS, et al. MR evaluation of the "arcuate" sign of posterolateral knee instability. *AJR Am J Roentgenol* 2002; 178:583–588.

6. Nakamura N, Horibe S, Toritsuka Y, et al. Acute grade III medial collateral ligament injury of the knee associated with anterior cruciate ligament tear: the usefulness of magnetic resonance imaging in determining a treatment regimen. *Am J Sports Med* 2003;31:261–267.

7. Oeppen RS, Connolly SA, Bencardino JT, et al. Acute injury of the articular cartilage and subchondral bone: a common but unrecognized lesion in the immature knee. *AJR Am J Roentgenol* 2004; 182:111–117.

8. Gaeta M, Minutoli F, Scribano E, et al. CT and MR imaging findings in athletes with early tibial stress injuries: comparison with bone scintigraphy findings and emphasis on cortical abnormalities. *Radiology* 2005;235:553–561.

9. Stoller DW, Martin C, Crues JV, et al. Meniscal tears: pathologic correlation with MR imaging. *Radiology* 1987;163:731–735.

10. Jee WH, McCauley TR, Kim JM, et al. Meniscal tear configurations: categorization with MR imaging. *AJR Am J Roentgenol* 2003;180: 93–97.

11. Vande Berg BC, Malghem J, Poilvache P, et al. Meniscal tears with fragments displaced in notch and recesses of knee: MR imaging with arthroscopic comparison. *Radiology* 2005;234:842–850.

12. Bredella MA, Tirman PF, Peterfy CG, et al. Accuracy of T2-weighted fast spin-echo MR imaging with fat saturation in detecting cartilage defects in the knee: comparison with arthroscopy in 130 patients. *AJR Am J Roentgenol* 1999;172:1073–1080.

13. Disler DG. Fat-suppressed three-dimensional spoiled gradient-recalled MR imaging: assessment of articular and physeal hyaline cartilage. *AJR Am J Roentgenol* 1997;169:1117–1123.

14. Friemert B, Oberlander Y, Schwarz W, et al. Diagnosis of chondral lesions of the knee joint: can MRI replace arthroscopy? A prospective study. *Knee Surg Sports Traumatol Arthroscopy* 2004;12:58–64.

15. Mori R, Ochi M, Sakai Y, et al. Clinical significance of magnetic resonance imaging (MRI) for focal chondral lesions. *Magn Reson Imaging* 1999;17:1135–1140.

16. Potter HG, Linklater JM, Allen AA, et al. Magnetic resonance imaging of articular cartilage in the knee: an evaluation with use of fast-spin-echo imaging. *J Bone Joint Surg Am* 1998;80:1276–1284.

17. Recht MP, Piraino DW, Paletta GA, et al. Accuracy of fat-suppressed three-dimensional spoiled gradient echo FLASH MR imaging in the detection of patellofemoral articular cartilage abnormalities. *Radiology* 1996;198:209–212.

18. Sonin AH, Pensy RA, Mulligan ME, et al. Grading articular cartilage of the knee using fast spin-echo proton density-weighted MR imaging without fat suppression. *AJR Am J Roentgenol* 2002;179: 1159–1166.

19. Radin E, Pugh J, Rose R. Response of joints to impact loading. Relationship between trabecular microfractures and cartilage degenerations. *J Biomech* 1973;6:51–57.

20. Mankin HJ. The response of articular cartilage to mechanical injury. *J Bone Joint Surg Am* 1982;64:460–466.

21. Terzidis IP, Christodoulou AG, Ploumis AL, et al. The appearance of kissing contusion in the acutely injured knee in the athletes. *Br J Sports Med* 2004;38:592–596.

22. Alparslan L, Winalski CS, Boutin RD, et al. Postoperative magnetic resonance imaging of articular cartilage repair. *Semin Musculoskelet Radiol* 2001;5:345–363.

23. Brittberg M, Winalski CS. Evaluation of cartilage injuries and repair. *J Bone Joint Surg Am* 2003;85(Suppl 2):58–69.

24. Henderson IJ, Tuy B, Connell D, et al. Prospective clinical study of autologous chondrocyte implantation and correlation with MRI at three and 12 months. *J Bone Joint Surg Br* 2003;85:1060–1066.

25. Recht M, White LM, Winalski CS, et al. MR imaging of cartilage repair procedures. *Skeletal Radiol* 2003;32:185–200.

26. Sanders TG, Mentzer KD, Miller MD, et al. Autogenous osteochondral "plug" transfer for the treatment of focal chondral defects: postoperative MR appearance with clinical correlation. *Skeletal Radiol* 2001;30:570–578.

27. Tins BJ, McCall IW, Takahashi T, et al. Autologous chondrocyte implantation in knee joint: MR imaging and histologic features at 1-year follow-up. *Radiology* 2005;234:501–508.

28. Blevins FT, Steadman JR, Rodrigo JJ, et al. Treatment of articular cartilage defects in athletes: an analysis of functional outcome and lesion appearance. *Orthopedics* 1998;21:761–767.

29. Horas U, Pelinkovic D, Herr G, et al. Autologous chondrocyte implantation and osteochondral cylinder transplantation in cartilage repair of the knee joint: a prospective, comparative trial. *J Bone Joint Surg Am* 2006;85:185–192.

30. Knutsen G, Engebretsen L, Ludvigsen TC, et al. Autologous chondrocyte implantation compared with microfracture in the knee: a randomized trial. *J Bone Joint Surg Am* 2004;86:455–464.

31. Minas T. Autologous chondrocyte implantation in the arthritic knee. *Orthopedics.* 2003;26:945–947.

32. Peterson L, Minas T, Brittberg M, et al. Two- to 9-year outcome after autologous chondrocyte transplantation of the knee. *Clin Orthop* 2000;374:212–234.

33. Roberts S, McCall IW, Darby AJ, et al. Autologous chondrocyte implantation for cartilage repair: monitoring its success by magnetic resonance imaging and histology. *Arthritis Res Ther* 2003;5: R60–73.

34. Steadman JR, Briggs KK, Rodrigo JJ, et al. Outcomes of microfracture for traumatic chondral defects of the knee: average 11-year follow-up. *Arthroscopy* 2003;19:477–484.

35. Steadman JR, Rodkey WG, Rodrigo JJ. Microfracture: surgical technique and rehabilitation to treat chondral defects. *Clin Orthop* 2001;391:S362–369.

36. Hangody L, Kish G, Karpati Z, et al. Mosaicplasty for the treatment of articular cartilage defects: application in clinical practice. *Orthopedics* 1998;21:751–756.

37. Covey DC. Injuries of the posterolateral corner of the knee. *J Bone Joint Surg Am* 2001;83:106–118.

38. Munshi M, Pretterklieber ML, Kwak S, et al. MR imaging, MR arthrography, and specimen correlation of the posterolateral corner of the knee: an anatomic study. *AJR Am J Roentgenol* 2003;180:1095–1101.

39. Recondo JA, Salvador E, Villanua JA, et al. Lateral stabilizing structures of the knee: functional anatomy and injuries assessed with MR imaging. *Radiographics* 2000;20:91–102.

40. Sims WF, Jacobson KE. The posteromedial corner of the knee: medial-sided injury patterns revisited. *Am J Sports Med* 2004;32: 337–345.

41. Campos JC, Chung CB, Lektrakul N, et al. Pathogenesis of the Segond fracture: anatomic and MR imaging evidence of an iliotibial tract or anterior oblique band avulsion. *Radiology* 2001;219: 381–386.

42. Koulouris G, Connell D. Hamstring muscle complex: an imaging review. *Radiographics* 2005; 25:571–586.

43. Williams A. Understanding knee motion—the application of 'dynamic MRI.' *J Bone Joint Surg Br* 2004;86(Suppl IV):471.

44. Bashir A, Gray ML, Boutin RD, et al. Glycosaminoglycan in articular cartilage: in vivo assessment with delayed Gd(DPTA)^2-enhanced MR imaging. *Radiology* 1997;205:551–558.

45. Goodwin DW, Zhu H, Dunn JF. In vitro MR imaging of hyaline cartilage: Correlation with scanning electron microscopy. *AJR Am J Roentgenol* 2000;174:405–409.

46. Williams A, Gillis A, McKenzie C, et al. Glycosaminoglycan distribution in cartilage as determined by delayed gadolinium-enhanced MRI of cartilage (dGEMRIC): potential clinical applications. *AJR Am J Roentgenol* 2004;182:167–172.

Anterior Cruciate Ligament Reconstruction

8

J. Richard Steadman

■ INTRODUCTION 117

■ PATIENT SELECTION 117

■ SURGICAL TECHNIQUE 118
  Graft Choice 118
  The Two-Incision Technique 118
  Arthroscopic Evaluation and Notch Preparation 119
  Graft Harvest 119
  Graft Preparation 120
  Tibial Tunnel Placement 121
  Femoral Tunnel Placement 122
  Graft Passage 123
  Fixation 123
  Avoiding Anterior Knee Pain 124

■ POSTOPERATIVE MANAGEMENT 124
  Bracing 125

■ OUTCOMES 125

■ COMPLICATIONS 126

One of the most common knee injuries during sporting activities is a torn anterior cruciate ligament (ACL). Various treatments have been described in the literature through the years; however, the most common treatment has been the ACL reconstruction. Although several surgical techniques are currently in use, my personal choice is the two-incision bone-tendon-bone patellar tendon operation. More than 30 years of experience and 1,800 reconstructions have led to a repeatable technique with predictable outcomes. Several factors are required for success. These include patient selection, the timing of surgery, technical considerations, and postoperative rehabilitation.

The most common injury seen is the acute injury. If patients with these injuries are unwilling to modify their active lifestyle, then ACL surgery is recommended. In the chronic ACL-injured knee, an ACL is reconstructed if functional instability is interfering with sports or the patient's occupation. A reconstruction is also recommended for the patient who is experiencing giving way because this places the menisci and articular cartilage at risk of injury. Another option for treatment, the "healing response," is discussed in Chapter 10.

PATIENT SELECTION

There are many factors to consider in patient selection, one of which is age. In the skeletally immature patient, the possibility of epiphyseal injury must be considered. Although few cases of growth disturbances have been documented, a recent study that surveyed the ACL study group showed 15 disturbances.[1] *In my practice, the risk of even one growth disturbance limits the use of ACL reconstruction in the skeletally immature patient.*

ACL reconstruction in the older athlete has been controversial. In a review of a series of my patients, the increased age of a patient was not a factor if the patient met other patient selection criteria.[2] Older patients are given the choice of modifying their activity level. However, as "baby boomers" age, more and more people are staying active later in life. Also, if the patient has the appropriate injury pattern, the older patient is given the option of a less-invasive procedure, the healing response. This technique has also been used in treating the skeletally immature athlete.[3] Most patients whose exercise consists of cycling, swimming, and walking do not require a reconstruction. However, those patients participating in sports requiring more stability in the knee, such as skiing and change-of-direction sports, may need an ACL reconstruction.

The timing of surgery following injury has previously been debated.[4–9] In one study of my patients, we showed that there were no differences in the prevalence of arthrofibrosis between patients operated within 3 weeks of injury compared with patients operated at more than 3 weeks, if they met defined preoperative criteria.[10] The criteria for performing an ACL reconstruction on an acutely injured patient included (i) a minimum active range of motion of 0 to120 degrees, (ii) performing a straight-leg raise similar to the unaffected side with no loss of extension, and (iii) active quadriceps control demonstrated by quadriceps definition symmetric to the unaffected side, while performing quadriceps contraction. In recent years we have added a fourth criterion. *Only minimal temperature differential between the patient's knees is acceptable.* Increased temperature is an indication of inflammation and could predispose the knee to arthrofibrosis. The presence of a stable meniscal tear that is not locked is not a contraindication to aggressive range of motion. The physical environment around the knee is a more important factor to consider than the number of days since the injury.

Another important consideration in patient selection is the presence of injuries associated with the ACL injury. Some injuries may require changes in surgical technique or timing. If the patient has an unstable or locked meniscal tear, which is repairable, the repairs are done in two stages. The meniscus is repaired and rehabilitated prior to reconstruction. This is because of the required differences in rehabilitation. The meniscus repair is followed by 8 to 12 weeks of rehabilitation, which is followed by the ACL reconstruction.

Other injuries that may change patient selection include chondral injuries of the patellofemoral compartment, which may require that an allograft ACL reconstruction be done in order to place less pressure on the defect. If microfracture of the trochlea or patella is required, surgery may be done in two stages, with microfracture done first, and the reconstruction done after initial rehabilitation is completed. This takes approximately 3 months.

SURGICAL TECHNIQUE

The goal of ACL reconstruction is to re-create the constraints on motion supplied by the native ACL. To create success after ACL reconstruction, several conditions must be met.

1. The tunnels must be properly positioned to assure ideal graft length.
2. The graft must have adequate strength.
3. Impingement must be avoided for the reconstruction to be successful.
4. The fixation of the graft in the tunnels must allow for early range of motion.
5. The reconstruction must restore normal biomechanics of soft tissue.

The ACL can be reconstructed using a variety of techniques. My preference is the two-incision bone-tendon-bone patellar tendon.

Graft Choice

Patellar tendon bone-tendon-bone, semitendinosus or semitendinosus and gracilis, quadriceps tendon, and allograft can all replace the ACL.[11–13] My personal choice for graft is the patellar tendon bone-tendon-bone autograft or allograft with a two-incision technique. The patellar tendon provides adequate strength,[13] and allows for bone-to-bone fixation and healing,[14] and the tendon graft site regenerates. For any technique to be successful, it must be reproducible. The tunnel position must be correct 100% of the time. There must be no graft impingement, either medial to lateral or superior to inferior. The technique allows for reliable fixation. One must always have a backup plan if an unexpected complication occurs.

The use of allograft has increased because of improved graft testing for disease transmission and better preparation techniques, which have minimal effect on graft strength. This graft is used if there are patellofemoral problems in revisions, and if the patient has a preference after hearing the preoperative explanation. A recent study of our patients has shown that results from allograft reconstructions are similar to autograft results.

The Two-Incision Technique

The technical advantages of the two-incision technique include the reproducibility, the ability to check the posterior position and adjust the graft's position on the femur, and the flexibility of the anterior position. The fixation is predictable, and if complications occur a backup plan can be implemented. The two-incision technique also decreases the risk of potential pitfalls that exist with the single-incision technique.[15,16] The outside-in drilling on the femoral side allows the femoral position to be near the most posterior attachment of the native ACL.

TIP: If problems are encountered during a single-incision technique, this technique is an ideal option allowing for excellent fixation and anatomic placement.

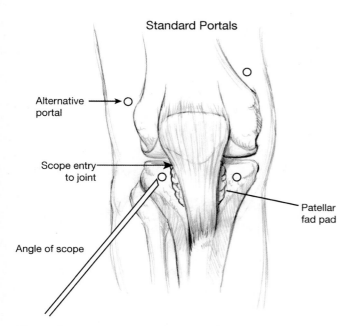

Figure 8.1   Three arthroscopic portals made in the superomedial, inferomedial, and high inferolateral positions.

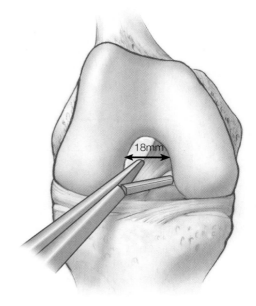

Figure 8.2   Pituitary rongeurs are used to measure the width of the anterior notch. The desired width is 18 mm, which is the width of most pituitary rongeurs when fully opened.

Arthroscopic Evaluation and Notch Preparation

Three arthroscopy portals are made in the superomedial, inferomedial, and high inferolateral positions. The high inferolateral portal (Fig. 8.1) is based lateral to the lateral patella, 0.5 cm proximal to the distal pole of the patella in a "soft spot." The 11-blade knife is angled 20 to 30 degrees cephalad. Care is taken to go through the capsule only, in order to avoid lacerating the articular cartilage of the patella or lateral condyle. The inflow cannula is placed through the superomedial portal, the camera is placed through the inferolateral portal, and the working instruments are shuttled in and out of the inferomedial portal. A diagnostic arthroscopy of the knee is performed. All compartments of the knee are examined to determine if any other injuries exist, which could be a contraindication to ACL reconstruction. The ACL rupture is examined arthroscopically.

An anterior notch width of at least 18 mm is desirable to help avoid lateral wall impingement (Fig. 8.2). Most arthroscopic pituitary rongeurs are 18 mm in width when fully opened, and can be used as a guide for notch size. A stenotic notch is widened using a curved osteotome and/or a motorized burr on the lateral wall. The posterior notch is also important. Using a 70-degree scope, the lateral wall is contoured to form an oval surface, avoiding impingement in this important area.

Graft Harvest

Along the central patellar tendon a longitudinal skin incision is made between a point 1 cm proximal to the inferior

pole of the patella and the tibial tubercle, with the knee passively flexed (Fig. 8.3). The subcutaneous tissue is dissected down to the level of the peritenon. The peritenon is incised and elevated as a distinct layer to allow closure after harvesting of the tendon is completed (Fig. 8.4). The peritenon is kept intact throughout its entirety. Dissection under the peritenon is performed until the medial and

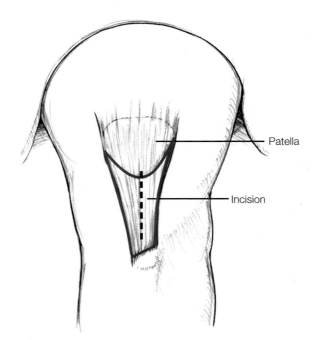

Figure 8.3   The skin incision for the harvest of the patellar tendon autograft. The incision is 1 cm proximal to the inferior pole of the patella and the tibial tubercle.

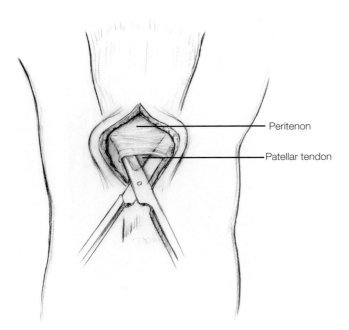

Figure 8.4 The elevated peritenon is excised as a distinct layer to allow for closure after harvesting is complete.

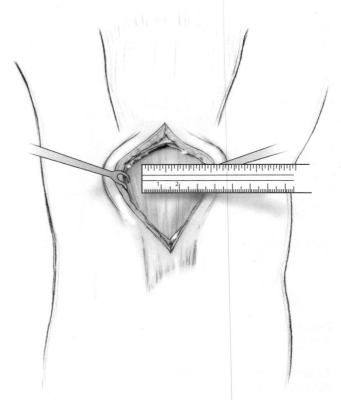

Figure 8.5 A ruler is used to measure the width of the tendon.

lateral borders of the tendon are defined. The width of the tendon is measured (Fig. 8.5). One third of the tendon is harvested, with a 10-mm graft usually chosen. If the width is less than 27 mm, a 9-mm graft is used. The tendon is divided in line with its fibers from the patella and down to the tubercle.

A 2-mm drill bit is used to weaken the distal attachments of the tibial bone block (Fig. 8.6), which is 30 to 40 mm in length. (If an oscillating saw is used at the corners, it could go past the point and leave a stress riser, making the area more susceptible to fracture.) Cuts perpendicular to the tibia are then made on the medial and lateral sides of the graft. A curved gouge connects the drill holes and the saw cuts. Two drill holes are placed through the bone plug and a number 5 FiberWire (Arthrex, Naples, FL) suture is placed through the holes. The tendon is freed from the underlying fat pad.

Next, a knife is used to outline a 25 × 10 mm area on the distal patella. On the patellar side, a 2-mm drill is used again to define the corners of the bone blocks and across the proximal edge of the patellar graft. The patellar block is about 25 × 10 mm. Lateral saw cuts are made at a 10-degree angle to make a more trapezoidal graft. A curved gouge is used to remove the bone piece (Fig. 8.7). A pick is used to make holes in the patella just posterior to the tendon, weakening the patella at the inferior pole so that the patellar bone block does not break into the joint on harvest.

Graft Preparation

Bone plugs are trimmed with scissor and bone rongeurs until they can be passed through a 9-mm graft sizer (Fig.

8.8). All bone that is removed is saved to fill the patellar and tibial defects on closure. *Maximizing the size of the bone plugs within the respective tunnels is important to obtain rigid fixation of the graft.* Two number 5 FiberWire sutures are placed in each bone block. The tibial block is generally

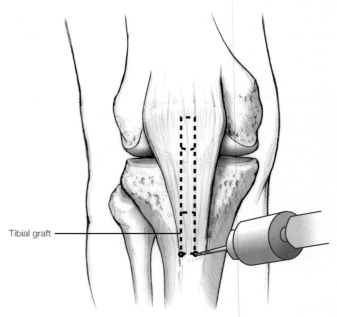

Figure 8.6 The distal attachments of the tibial bone block are weakened with drill holes. The tibial bone blocks are 30 to 40 mm in length.

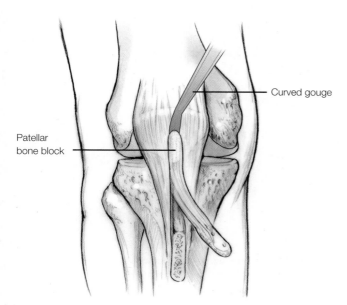

Figure 8.7 A curved gouge is used to remove the bone piece to make it easier to pass in the femoral tunnel.

35 mm in length × 10 mm, and the patellar block is usually 25 × 9 mm. If 25 mm represents more than one third of the length of the patella, a shorter graft is generally harvested instead. In this case, the minimum patella graft length is 20 mm.

Tibial Tunnel Placement

Correct tunnel position is important to allow for appropriate graft tension through full range of motion. The anterior aspect of the native ACL accommodates the anterior aspect of the intercondylar roof to avoid ligamentous impingement.[17] *Placing the tibial tunnel too far anteriorly increases graft tension in flexion and results in impingement of the graft on the intercondylar roof as the knee moves into extension.* Proper tunnel position avoids impingement, which weakens the graft. The position of the guide pin on the tibia is 6 mm lateral to the medial wall

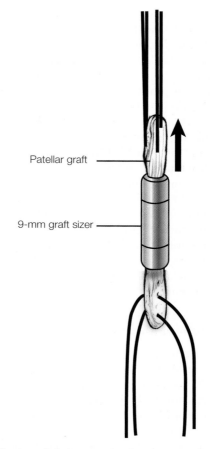

Figure 8.8 A graft being prepared to be passed thru a 9-mm graft sizer.

and 7 to 9 mm anterior to the posterior cruciate ligament (Fig. 8.9). The posterior tibial wall should not be lowered. Such placement minimizes the risk of impingement on the intercondylar roof and the lateral wall. The guide pin should enter the joint on a line drawn parallel to the anterior edge of the femoral condyles. *Because individual anatomy may vary, this secondary guide confirms correct placement of the guide pin.* A tibial tunnel guide with a variable

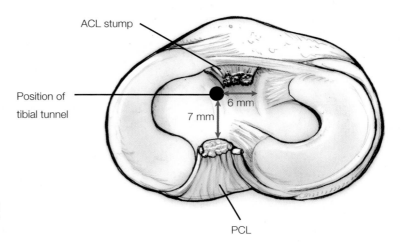

Figure 8.9 The position of tibial tunnel is 6 mm lateral to the medial wall and 7 to 9 mm anterior to the posterior cruciate ligament (PCL). ACL, anterior cruciate ligament.

arm is used with an angle of 45 degrees. A point is chosen for the entrance to the tibial tunnel at a position at least 1 cm medial to the medial edge of tibial tubercle. The tunnel must not be too far lateral in the notch in order to avoid impingement.

After the guide pin is passed, placement is confirmed by lifting the heel to passively extend the knee, while arthroscopically observing for pin impingement on the intercondylar roof. Once the pin is placed, it is overdrilled with a 10-mm drill. This type of drill allows bone fragments to exit at the distal tunnel and these fragments can be used to pack the defect in the tibia and femur after graft harvest. A chamfer is used to bevel the posterior edge of the tibia, if necessary, and a shaver is used to debride the soft tissue from the tibial tunnel site if needed. The chamfer can be used to make minor corrections to avoid impingement, taking care not to create a lateral position, which could impinge on the lateral wall. *If the tibial tunnel is too far medial or anterior, chamfer.*

Femoral Tunnel Placement

The femoral tunnel is established from the outside using the two-incision technique. The incision is begun at a level two fingerbreadths proximal to the superior pole of the patella and extended proximally for a distance of 3 to 4 cm (Fig. 8.10). The iliotibial band is split longitudinally about 5 mm from its anterior edge, exposing the vastus lateralis muscle. The vastus lateralis is dissected off of the intermuscular septum and retracted anteriorly to expose the lateral aspect of the distal femoral metaphysis (Fig. 8.11). Hemostasis is obtained at this point. The intermuscular septum is carefully divided from the over-the-top position to a point 3 cm proximal.

> **TIP: Curved Mayo scissors are used to divide the intermuscular septum. Care is taken not to go more than 2 mi deep into the septum to avoid vascular structures.**

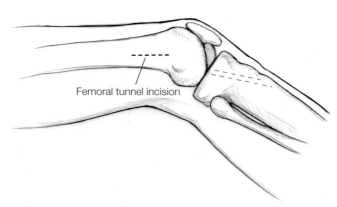

Figure 8.10 The lateral femoral tunnel incision is superior to the pole of the patella and extends proximal for a distance of 3 to 4 cm.

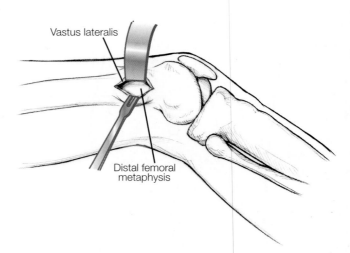

Figure 8.11 Retraction of the vastus lateralis muscle to expose the lateral aspect of the distal femoral metaphysis.

After the femur has been exposed, a 70-degree arthroscope is inserted through the anterior inferior lateral portal. The torn ACL remnant is debrided, exposing the lateral wall of the intercondylar notch. The posterior notch is examined, and an oval posterior wall is created using a burr.

> **TIP: An oval surface is created on the posterolateral wall to avoid impingement.**

A long, curved vascular clamp is inserted through the inferomedial portal. It is passed around the posterior aspect of the lateral femoral tunnel, through the over-the-top position. The clamp is used to perforate a hole in the posterior capsule to allow passage of the rear-entry femoral guide. As long as the clamp is passed laterally, adhering closely to the posterior aspect of the femur, no damage to the neurovascular tissues has been encountered. Once the septum has been perforated by the clamp, a curved hook passer is inserted through the inferomedial portal, along the over-the-top position and through the opened intermuscular septum into the lateral operative field. At this point, the rear-entry guide is hooked onto the eyelet at the distal tip of the curved passer. The passer is then withdrawn, pulling the rear-entry guide into the joint without danger to the neurovascular structures.

The femoral tunnel can then be established. The tip of the rear-entry drill guide is positioned at the back wall of the notch, 2 mm anterior to the back wall. The two-incision technique permits maximal posterior placement of the femoral tunnel because there is no concern over blowout of the posterior wall. The lateral incision site is planned so that it is 2 cm proximal to the patella and 5 mm below the iliotibial band. This allows the guide pin to enter at a 45- to 60-degree angle to the femur; a near anatomic angle. The 10:30 position or 1:30 position on the notch is chosen.[18] A guide pin is drilled from the lateral aspect of the femur into the tip of the drill guide in the joint, using an angle of approximately 45 to 60 degrees to the femur. The hole should enter anterior and distal to the tibial flair to allow for proper placement of the interference screw. A 1-cm bridge between the guide pin and the lateral flair of the condyle is needed to allow for placement of the screw. A 10-mm cannulated drill is used to create the femoral tunnel from the outside.

A suture is passed from the outside of the femoral tunnel, through the joint and through the tibial tunnel, and the knee is put through a range of motion from 0 to 90 degrees. The suture length change should be less than 2 mm in this range.

Graft Passage

Graft passage is accomplished using a "graft passer" (Depuy, Tracy, CA). A Hewson suture passer (Smith & Nephew, Andover, MA) is inserted through the femoral tunnel into the knee joint, and an arthroscopic grasper is used to retrieve the suture through the tibial tunnel. The plastic graft passer is tied to the suture and pulled through the tunnels from distal to proximal. The graft is then placed inside the plastic sleeve and pulled through the tunnels, and the plastic is removed. The graft can be pulled either proximally or distally to maximize graft-tunnel contact. In this way, the possibility of any graft-tunnel mismatch is eliminated. Do not twist the graft before fixation.

> **TIP: If the passer is difficult to remove as the graft is passed, pull the proximal block proximally, and manually pull the passer distally. This may be repeated several times. Care must be taken to avoid tearing the passer as it is pulled distally.**

Fixation

Correct fixation is important because early rehabilitation can affect the graft length if the fixation points do not solidly fix the graft. My preference is 9-mm interference, using interference screws placed along guide wires inserted parallel and posterior to the bone blocks. Guide wires decrease the possibility of screw divergence, which has been shown to weaken the initial fixation strength of ACL grafts. These guide wires should be removed when the screw is engaged in the femur, but before the final tightening. The femoral screw is generally placed first, leaving the proximal head of the screw at the level of the lateral femoral cortex (Fig. 8.12).

After femoral screw placement is performed, the knee is cycled 25 times with tension applied to the graft. If there is no retraction into the tibia of the distal bone block in

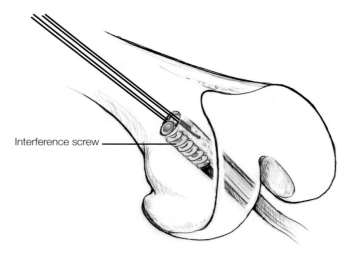

Figure 8.12 Illustration showing the placement of the femoral screw with the proximal head of the screw left at the level of the lateral femoral cortex.

extension, and with a posterior drawer applied to the tibia, the tibial interference screw is then placed with the knee in 30 degrees of flexion. *If the graft retracts with hyperextension, then the graft is fixed in extension.* The sutures used to pass the graft are left prominent after screw fixation to allow the screws to be located in the event of a revision reconstruction, even if there is bony overgrowth (Fig. 8.13). A proximal drain is applied.

> **TIP: Prior to passing the graft, 25 pick holes are made in the soft tissue portion of the graft to allow marrow from the tunnels to enter the graft.**

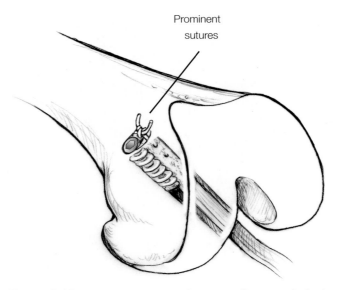

Figure 8.13 Prominent sutures after screw fixation, which allows for the screw to be located if a revision is necessary.

The anterior half of the patellar tendon is loosely closed with interrupted figure-of-eight no. 1 Vicryl sutures. The bone graft from the tunnel drilling is packed into the distal pole of the patella, as well as the proximal tibia. The peritenon is then closed with interrupted figure-of-eight no. 1 Vicryl sutures. The skin and portal sites are closed. A sterile cast padding, a Cryo-Cuff (Aircast, Vista, CA), a Sentry brace (Ossur, Aliso Viejo, CA), and TED hose (Kendall, Mansfield, MA) are placed on the lower leg.

Avoiding Anterior Knee Pain

The goal following harvest of the patellar tendon autograft is to avoid deficit in the donor site. When the patellar tendon is used for ACL reconstruction, weakness may be present early after the graft is taken. A brace with a flexion stop can avoid abrupt strain on the donor site. This abrupt strain may lead to graft rupture. *To avoid scarring after the graft is placed, the patient should avoid excessive strain early, up to 6 to 12 weeks.* To avoid scarring and joint stiffness, all patients undergo patellar mobilization exercises, in addition to early range of motion. Full extension and flexion is important. Strengthening exercises are avoided until range of motion and patellar mobility are achieved. Other solutions used to avoid anterior knee pain include bone grafting defects with bone from the tunnel drilling (Fig. 8.14), and loose partial-thickness closure of the patellar tendon (Fig. 8.15). Lateral retinacular decompression is also used. This consists of incising the lateral retinaculum from the lower

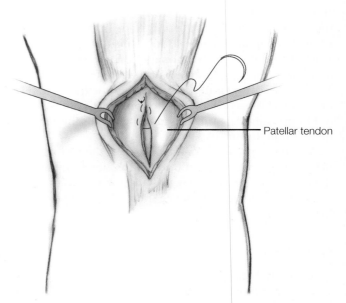

Figure 8.15 Loose partial-thickness closure of the patellar tendon.

patella to the superior patella. *Using this postoperative regimen, we have had graft-site morbidity of less than 3%.*

POSTOPERATIVE MANAGEMENT

Postoperative pain management begins with a femoral nerve block in most cases. If the block is successful, oral pain medications are usually enough to control postoperative pain. If the block is unsuccessful, intravenous analgesia can be used. Cold therapy is also helpful for pain and swelling.

As with most other arthroscopic knee surgeries, postoperative management and correct rehabilitation is crucial to success. Early rehabilitation is progressive in nature, with an emphasis on mobilization. Continuous passive motion in a 30- to 70-degree range is used for 1 to 7 days. *It is critical to maintain patellar mobility in all phases.* The therapist and patient work on medial-to-lateral and superior-to-inferior patellar motion, and range of motion (particularly extension) is also emphasized in early rehabilitation. If the patient has no patellar pain, active motion should be achieved using the stationary bike with little-to-no resistance. The stationary bike is used from postoperative day 4 to 7 to week 2 if an autograft was used, and at 4 weeks if an allograft was employed. Deep water rehabilitation programs are also added at 4 to 12 weeks if the patient has access to a pool.

Once again, it is important to achieve mobility in early rehabilitation. If good mobility and motion is obtained at 6 weeks, strengthening programs can begin. If a patient experiences stiffness and decreased range of motion at 6 weeks, additional surgery with scar release may

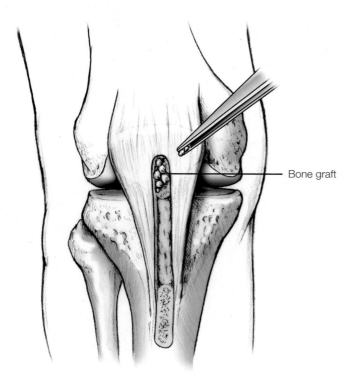

Figure 8.14 Bone grafting the site of the patellar tendon graft harvest site with bone from the tibial tunnel.

very likely be required later (at about 6 months). In the next stage of rehabilitation, the exercise intensity is increased. This phase includes the stationary bike with resistance and weightbearing exercises, starting with the elevated treadmill and progressing to the elliptical, and finally, to running. Agility exercise is emphasized at 4 to 6 months postoperatively. The final stage of rehabilitation is meant to simulate the patient's sport and improve agility. *Rehabilitation is not advanced unless motion, strength, and mobility are attained.* Return to sport varies, but is usually accomplished at 6 to 8 months. This time frame can be affected by the size of the patient and the intensity of the sport.

Bracing

We use bracing for the first 3 months. The first 6 weeks, a long leg brace is used with a range of 0 to 90 degrees. At 6 weeks a functional brace is applied with an extension stop at 10 degrees. Studies have questioned brace use, but it is my opinion that graft site protection is achieved with bracing. In addition, studies have shown that if looseness is present, a brace can prevent injury. With this in mind, I have recommended bracing with a functional brace postoperatively for up to one year. If the brace does not interfere with performance, bracing continues permanently.

OUTCOMES

A satisfied patient is one of the most important outcomes following any surgery. We studied factors that determine patient satisfaction following ACL reconstruction.[19] We looked at surgical variables, objective variables at the time of follow-up, as well as symptoms and function. We used the Lysholm knee score and the International Knee Documentation Committee scores. Patients were asked "How satisfied are you with the outcome of your surgery?" There were no associations between patient satisfaction that pertained to age, gender, chronicity, surgeon, or side of involvement. Patients were less satisfied with outcome if they lacked extension or flexion, had a pivot-shift, effusion, or tenderness at the medial joint line or patella. Independent determinants of patient satisfaction with outcome included Lysholm score, subjective knee function, range of motion, patellar tenderness, knee giving way, flexion contracture, and swelling.

The study concluded that specific surgical and objective variables were associated with patient satisfaction with the outcome after reconstruction of the ACL; however, the most robust associations were with subjective variables of symptoms and function. Clinically relevant groupings of variables affecting satisfaction included issues of stiffness, giving way, swelling, and patellofemoral symptoms. The study emphasized the importance of patient-dependent subjective assessment of symptoms and function.

ACL injuries in the elite athlete can result from various mechanisms of injury. In a review of Olympic-level skiers who were treated at our clinic, we found 41 individuals with ACL tears. These athletes had been on the United States Ski Team for an average of 6.4 years. Following ACL reconstruction, the skiers returned to skiing at an average of 6 months and returned to racing at 10 months. However, it did take 16 months for them to return to their preinjury level. At follow-up, all skiers reported normal to nearly normal activity and function according to the International Knee Documentation Committee score. All skiers had normal range of motion. Eight racers had reinjuries, other than ACL injuries, at an average of 40 months following ACL reconstruction.

In professional football players from the National Football League, 20 out of 21 players returned to the season following ACL reconstruction. Of the 20 who returned, 8 players required subsequent surgeries, 7 for scar removal and 1 for a new injury to the posterior cruciate ligament in the opposite knee. Patient satisfaction was high, and the average Lysholm score at follow-up was 94. In these elite-level athletes, the two-incision ACL reconstruction with patellar tendon autograft proved to be a reliable and effective construct for returning the high-demand athlete to play.

In the mature athlete, returning individuals to an active lifestyle is just as important. We looked at 72 of my patients who had an ACL reconstruction with patellar tendon graft.[2] The average age was 45 years, with the oldest patient being 60 years of age and the youngest being 40 years of age. Most patients were injured while participating in sports. At an average of 4.5 years following reconstruction, patients had significant improvement in their symptoms and function. No patient reported patellofemoral symptoms. Patients returned to bicycling at 4 months, jogging at 9 months, skiing at 10 months, and tennis at 12 months. All patients were satisfied with the results. Fourteen of the 72 patients needed an additional surgery. Most of these surgeries were for painful scar tissue, lack of mobility, and hardware issues. Of course, hardware technology has advanced since these surgeries were done (prior to 1993). We have also changed our rehabilitation protocol based on these results.

For patients who have patellofemoral degenerative changes, patellar tendon pathology, or revision ACL reconstruction, the bone-tendon-bone allograft is my primary alternative graft choice. Other cases in which allograft tissue is considered are multiple-ligament injuries or patients with narrow patellar tendons. We analyzed the outcome in a group of 42 patients who underwent ACL reconstruction using a bone-tendon-bone allograft. The average age of this group was 41 years, with a range of 18 to 67 years, and follow-up was collected at an average of 46 months. Patients were highly satisfied at follow-up with a satisfaction score of 9.1 (1 = not satisfied, 10 = very satisfied). The preoperative Lysholm mean was 45 and the postoperative Lysholm was 88. The postoperative Tegner score was 5.5. There was one failure in the allograft group. This study, in a difficult patient group, has made it possible to offer allografts (bone-tendon-bone) to all patients, emphasizing that the allograft results are almost equal to the autograft results.

COMPLICATIONS

Infections, contracture, anterior knee pain, and phlebitis have all been reported as possible complications following ACL reconstruction.[20-23] Anterior knee pain is a well-documented complication after arthroscopic ACL reconstruction, and has been reported as the most common complaint after ACL surgery.[20-27] Although the initial studies reported anterior knee pain after patellar tendon autograft reconstruction, recent work confirms a real incidence of anterior knee pain even after hamstring or allograft ACL reconstruction.[25] Consequently, the etiology of this anterior knee pain remains elusive and controversial.[28-30] In my referral practice, I have a large population of patients with recalcitrant anterior knee pain after ACL reconstruction (done elsewhere) who have failed conservative treatment and have alterations in patellar mobility with or without full range of flexion and extension. Chapter 12 provides a detailed description of our technique for anterior interval release. We also report on the clinical results of this arthroscopic release of pathologic adhesions in the pretibial recess (anterior interval release) to treat anterior knee pain.

REFERENCES

1. Kocher MS, Saxon HS, Hovis WD, et al. Management and complications of anterior cruciate ligament injuries in skeletally immature patients: survey of the Herodicus Society and The ACL Study Group. *J Pediatr Orthop* 2002;22:452–457.
2. Plancher KD, Steadman JR, Briggs KK, et al. Reconstruction of the anterior cruciate ligament in patients who are at least forty years old. A long-term follow-up and outcome study. *J Bone Joint Surg Am* 1998;80:184–197.
3. Steadman JR, Cameron-Donaldson ML, Briggs KK, et al. A minimally invasive technique ("healing response") to treat proximal ACL injuries in skeletally immature athletes. *J Knee Surg* 2006;19:8–13.
4. Fisher SE, Shelbourne KD. Arthroscopic treatment of symptomatic extension block complicating anterior cruciate ligament reconstruction. *Am J Sports Med* 1993;21:558–564.
5. Harner CD, Irrgang JJ, Paul J, et al. Loss of motion after anterior cruciate ligament reconstruction. *Am J Sports Med* 1992;20:499–506.
6. Nogalski MP, Bach BR Jr. A review of early anterior cruciate ligament surgical repair or reconstruction. Results and caveats. *Orthop Rev* 1993;22:1213–1223.
7. Shelboume KD, Johnson GE. Outpatient surgical management of arthrofibrosis after anterior cruciate ligament surgery. *Am J Sports Med* 1994;22:192–197.
8. Strum GM, Friedman MJ, Fox JM, et al. Acute anterior cruciate ligament reconstruction. Analysis of complications. *Clin Orthop* 1990;253:1184–1189.
9. Wasilewski SA, Covall DJ, Cohen S. Effect of surgical timing on recovery and associated injuries after anterior cruciate ligament reconstruction. *Am J Sports Med* 1993;21:338–342.
10. Sterett WI, Hutton KS, Briggs KK, et al. Decreased range of motion following acute versus chronic anterior cruciate ligament reconstruction. *Orthopedics* 2003;26:151–154.
11. Hamner DL, Brown CH Jr, Steiner ME, et al. Hamstring tendon grafts for reconstruction of the anterior cruciate ligament: biomechanical evaluation of the use of multiple strands and tensioning techniques. *J Bone Joint Surg Am* 1999;81:549–557.
12. Miller SL, Gladstone JN. Graft selection in anterior cruciate ligament reconstruction. *Orthop Clin North Am* 2002;33:675–683.
13. Noyes FR, Butler DL, Grood ES, et al. Biomechanical analysis of human ligament grafts used in knee-ligament repairs and reconstructions. *J Bone Joint Surg Am* 1984;66:344–352.
14. Rodeo SA, Arnoczky SP, Torzilli PA, et al. Tendon-healing in a bone tunnel. A biomechanical and histological study in the dog. *J Bone Joint Surg Am* 1993;75:1795–1803.
15. Lemos MJ, Albert J, Simon T, et al. Radiographic analysis of femoral interference screw placement during ACL reconstruction: endoscopic versus open technique. *Arthroscopy* 1993;9:154–158.
16. Sgaglione NA, Schwartz RE. Arthroscopically assisted reconstruction of the anterior cruciate ligament: initial clinical experience and minimal 2-year follow-up comparing endoscopic transtibial and two-incision techniques. *Arthroscopy* 1997;13:156–165.
17. Lintner DM, Dewitt SE, Moseley JB. Radiographic evaluation of native anterior cruciate ligament attachments and graft placement for reconstruction. A cadaveric study. *Am J Sports Med* 1996;24:72–78.
18. Loh JC, Fukuda Y, Tsuda E, et al. Knee stability and graft function following anterior cruciate ligament reconstruction: comparison between 11 o'clock and 10 o'clock femoral tunnel placement. 2002 Richard O'Connor Award paper. *Arthroscopy* 2003;19:297–304.
19. Kocher MS, Steadman JR, Briggs K, et al. Determinants of patient satisfaction with outcome after anterior cruciate ligament reconstruction. *J Bone Joint Surg Am* 2002;84:1560–1572.
20. Graf B, Uhr F. Complications of intra-articular anterior cruciate reconstruction. *Clin Sports Med* 1988;7:835–848.
21. Harner CD, Irrgang JJ, Paul J, et al. Loss of motion after anterior cruciate ligament reconstruction. *Am J Sports Med* 1992;20:499–506.
22. Phelan DT, Cohen AB, Fithian DC. Complications of anterior cruciate ligament reconstruction. *Instr Course Lect* 2006;55:465–474.
23. Strum GM, Friedman MJ, Fox JM, et al. Acute anterior cruciate ligament reconstruction. Analysis of complications. *Clin Orthop* 1990;253:184–189.
24. Aglietti P, Buzzi R, D'Andria S, et al. Patellofemoral problems after intraarticular anterior cruciate ligament reconstruction. *Clin Orthop* 1993;288:195–204.
25. Beynnon BD, Johnson RJ, Fleming BC, et al. Anterior cruciate ligament replacement: comparison of bone-patellar tendon-bone grafts with two-strand hamstring grafts. A prospective, randomized study. *J Bone Joint Surg Am* 2002;84:1503–1513.
26. Jackson DW, Schaefer RK. Cyclops syndrome: loss of extension following intra-articular anterior cruciate ligament reconstruction. *Arthroscopy* 1990;6:171–178.
27. Johnson RJ, Eriksson E, Haggmark T, et al. Five- to ten-year follow-up evaluation after reconstruction of the anterior cruciate ligament. *Clin Orthop* 1984;183:122–140.
28. Paulos LE, Wnorowski DC, Greenwald AE. Infrapatellar contracture syndrome. Diagnosis, treatment, and long-term followup. *Am J Sports Med* 1994;22:440–449.
29. Sachs RA, Daniel DM, Stone ML, et al. Patellofemoral problems after anterior cruciate ligament reconstruction. *Am J Sports Med* 1989;17:760–765.
30. Shelbourne KD, Trumper RV. Preventing anterior knee pain after anterior cruciate ligament reconstruction. *Am J Sports Med* 1997;25:41–47.

ACL Bone-Tendon-Bone Graft

Name: _____

Dr. _____ Date: _____

Howard Head
Sports Medicine Centers
A service of Vail Valley Medical Center

● = Do exercise for that week

Initial Exercises	WEEK	1	2	3	4	5	6	7	8	9	10	13	17	21	25
Extension/Flexion–wall slides		●	●	●	●	●	●	●	●	●	●				
Extension/Flexion–sitting		●	●	●	●	●	●	●	●	●	●				
Quad sets with straight leg raises		●	●	●	●	●	●								
Patellar mobilizations/quad-patellar tendon		●	●	●	●	●	●	●	●	●	●				
Hamstring sets		●	●	●	●	●	●								
Ankle pumps		●	●	●											
Sit and reach for hamstrings (towel)		●	●	●	●	●	●	●	●	●	●	●	●	●	●
Runners stretch for calf and achilles				●	●	●	●	●	●	●	●	●	●	●	●
Stork stand/quad stretching							●	●	●	●	●	●	●	●	●
Toe and heel raises			●	●	●	●	●								
1/3 knee bends				●	●	●	●								
Cardiovascular Exercises		1	2	3	4	5	6	7	8	9	10	13	17	21	25
Bike with single leg/single leg rowing		●	●	●	●	●	●								
Bike with both legs			●	●	●	●	●	●	●	●	●	●	●	●	●
Aquajogging				●	●	●	●	●	●	●	●	●	●	●	●
Treadmill–incline 7-12%								●	●	●	●	●	●	●	●
Swimming with fins								●	●	●	●	●	●	●	●
Elliptical trainer											●	●	●	●	●
Rowing											●	●	●	●	●
Stair stepper												●	●	●	●
Resisted Exercises		1	2	3	4	5	6	7	8	9	10	13	17	21	25
Double knee bends								●	●	●	●				
Carpet drags								●	●	●	●				
Gas pedal								●	●	●	●				
Leg press–double leg											●	●	●	●	●
Single knee bends											●	●	●	●	●
Balance squats											●	●	●	●	●
Forward/backward jogging												●	●	●	●
Side to side lateral agility												●	●	●	●
Agility Exercises		1	2	3	4	5	6	7	8	9	10	13	17	21	25
Running progression													●	●	●
Initial													●	●	●
Advanced														●	●
Functional Sports Test														●	●
High Level Activities		1	2	3	4	5	6	7	8	9	10	13	17	21	25
(After Cleared by Physician)															
Golf														●	●
Running														●	●
Skiing, basketball, tennis, football, soccer															●

ROM RESTRICTIONS
(full prom)
_____
_____
_____
_____

BRACE SETTINGS

0-90 x 6 weeks

WEIGHT BEARING STATUS

Partial 30% WB

X 1-2 weeks

TIME LINES
Week 1 (1-7POD)
Week 2 (8-14POD)
Week 3 (15-21POD)
Week 4 (22-28POD)

181 West Meadow Drive
Vail, Colorado 81657
970-476-1225
Fax 970-479-7193

7128

Therapist Name

Microfracture

J. Richard Steadman

9

■ INTRODUCTION 129

■ BASIC SCIENCE OF ARTICULAR CARTILAGE
INJURY 129
Biological and Physiological Backgrounds 130
Basic Science of Microfracture 132

■ THE ACUTE CHONDRAL INJURY 134
Indications and Contraindications 134
Preoperative Planning 135
Imaging 135
Surgical Technique 137

■ THE CHRONIC LESION 140
Nonoperative Treatment 140
Contraindications for Microfracture 141
Microfracture Procedure if Patient
Has No Contraindications 141
Postoperative Management 143

■ REHABILITATION 144
Rehabilitation Protocol for Patients with Lesions
on the Femoral Condyle or Tibial Plateau 144
Rehabilitation Protocol for Patients with
Patellofemoral Lesions 145

■ POTENTIAL COMPLICATIONS FROM
MICROFRACTURE 145

■ PATIENT OUTCOMES 145
Outcome Measures 146
Lysholm Score 146
Tegner Activity Scale 146
*Western Ontario and McMaster University Osteoarthritis
Index 146*
Patient Satisfaction 146

■ RESULTS OF MICROFRACTURE 147

Trauma to the articular cartilage of the knee is a common result of recreational and elite sport injuries. The poor capacity of articular cartilage to heal itself makes the treatment of these lesions challenging.[1] The microfracture technique (Fig. 9.1) has been shown to be an effective arthroscopic treatment for full-thickness chondral lesions of the knee.[2,3] This technique is cost-effective, not technically complicated, has an extremely low rate of associated patient morbidity, and does not present any hindrances to further treatment. Microfracture does not replace tissue; rather, it should be considered tissue repair. This technique relies on a "marrow-based" strategy to foster tissue repair. In order for tissue to regenerate, cells must be present. The creation of controlled "microfractures" through the subchondral bone promotes the release of marrow-based mesenchymal stem cells and growth factors (Fig. 9.2). A marrow clot is formed at the base of a prepared chondral lesion (Fig. 9.3). These cells proliferate and differentiate into cells with morphologic features of chondrocytes, and produce a cartilaginous repair tissue that fills the chondral defect.

BASIC SCIENCE OF ARTICULAR CARTILAGE INJURY

In a single event, the shearing forces of the femur on the tibia may result in trauma to the articular cartilage, causing the cartilage to fracture, lacerate, and separate from the underlying subchondral bone, or separate along with a piece of the subchondral bone (Fig. 9.4).[1,4,5] The articular surface may also fatigue and fail as a result of chronic repetitive loading beyond the tolerance of normal physiological levels. Younger patients usually experience a single event that leads to acute cartilage lesions (Fig. 9.5), whereas chronic degenerative lesions (Fig. 9.6) are seen in middle-aged and older members of the population.[1,4-6] Repetitive impacts can cause cartilage swelling, an increase in collagen

129

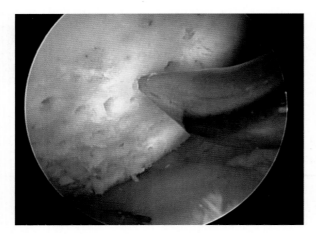

Figure 9.1 A microfracture awl creating microfractures in a full-thickness chondral defect of the femoral condyle of the knee.

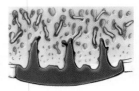

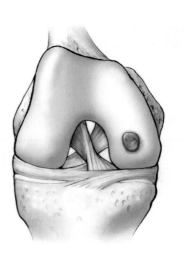

Figure 9.3 A marrow clot, or "super clot" as we refer to it, is formed at the base of the lesion following microfracture.

fiber diameter, and an alteration in the relationship between collagen and proteoglycans.[1,5] Thus, acute events may not result in full-thickness cartilage loss, but rather start a degenerative cascade that can lead to chronic full-thickness loss (Fig. 9.7A–D). The degenerative cascade typically includes early softening and fibrillation (grade I); fissures and cracks in the surface of the cartilage (grade II); severe fissures and cracks with a "crab meat" appearance (grade III); and, finally, exposure of the subchondral bone (grade IV).[1,4–6]

Biological and Physiological Backgrounds

Articular cartilage is maintained by the balanced coupling of the anabolic and catabolic processes of chondrocytes.

Much research has focused on defining the mechanism that regulates the anabolic/catabolic homeostasis seen in normal cartilage. In a degenerative process, matrix resorption is accelerated, causing degradation that outpaces the anabolic attempt of the chondrocyte to produce new matrix. Correcting this imbalance in cartilage metabolism or promoting the healing of damaged cartilage is necessary to stop the cascade of the degenerative lesion.

Various polypeptide mediators, such as transforming growth factor-β, insulinlike growth factor-1 (IGF-1), and basic fibroblast growth factor regulate the metabolic balance between anabolism and catabolism of articular cartilage.[7] Transforming growth factor-β has been shown to

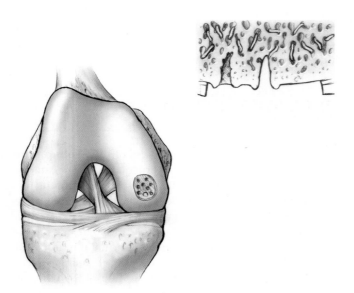

Figure 9.2 Marrow elements, which may contain stem cells and growth factors, are released from the marrow cavities formed by the microfractures.

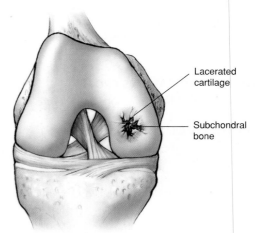

Lacerated cartilage

Subchondral bone

Figure 9.4 Illustration demonstrating fracture, laceration, and separation of articular cartilage following trauma.

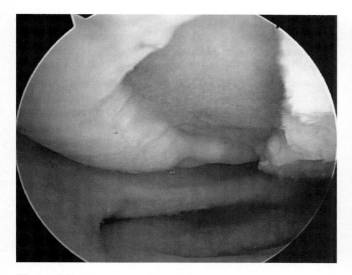

Figure 9.5 An acute cartilage lesion.

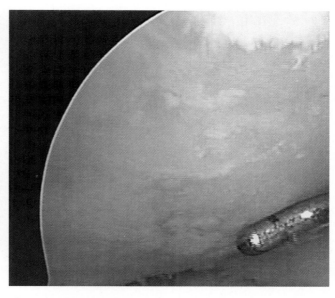

Figure 9.6 A degenerative cartilage lesion.

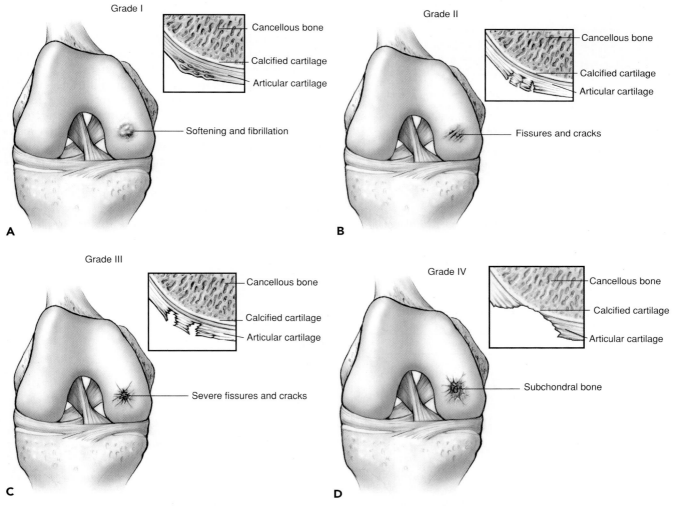

Figure 9.7 Illustration of degenerative cascade of acute cartilage loss to full-thickness loss. **A:** A grade I chondral lesion. **B:** A grade II chondral lesion. **C:** A grade III chondral lesion. **D:** A grade IV chondral lesion.

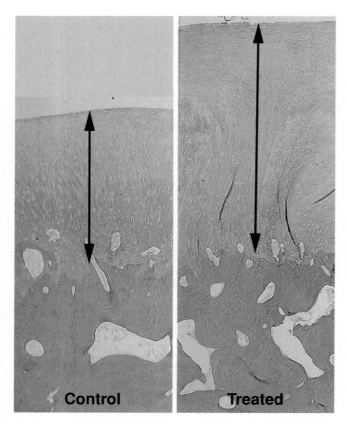

Figure 9.8 Computer image (×10; 5-mcm osteochondral section stained with hematoxylin and eosin). Repair tissue (between arrows) in a control and treated femorotibial joint defect. (Reprinted with permission from Frisbie DD, Trotter GW, Powers BE, et al. Arthroscopic subchondral bone plate microfracture technique augments healing of large osteochondral defects in the radial carpal bone and medial femoral condyle of horses. *J Vet Surg* 1999;28:242–255, Fig. 4.)

proliferation and the synthesis of aggrecan and hyaluronic acid.[10–12] IGF-1 can also decrease cartilage degradation by antagonizing interleukin-1 action.[13] Basic fibroblast growth factor is a potent mitogenic agent for chondrocytes and can stimulate chondrocytes to synthesize a cartilaginous matrix.[14] These results indicate a potential therapeutic application of exogenetic growth factors to enhance the healing of damaged cartilage.[15]

Chondrocytes may also respond to physical stimulation. Studies have shown that mechanical force can regulate the metabolic response of articular cartilage.[16–19] Immobilization or reduced loading of the joint was shown to result in a decrease in proteoglycan synthesis, whereas moderate exercise led to an increase in proteoglycan synthesis[16] and thickening of the cartilage matrix.[17] Severe mechanical loading resulted in a thinning of cartilage matrix and led to degenerative changes.[19] Dynamic loading has also been shown to affect glycosaminoglycan and DNA synthesis.[18]

Basic Science of Microfracture

Several animal studies have been done to assess the microfracture technique. In our experience, the equine model is the best model to use for cartilage research. The horse-human relationship research is described in Chapter 16.

Equine articular cartilage is similar in thickness to that of humans. In the horse, procedures (including relooks) can be done arthroscopically. The horse joint undergoes realistic biomechanical forces during gait, and its rehabilitation can also be controlled. Swimming allows horses to avoid full weightbearing exercise, and the treadmill can be used to control the intensity and duration of activity. The fact that horses must be immediately weightbearing following surgery is a disadvantage. Although partial weightbearing is impossible for the horse, this limitation provides an even more challenging environment in which to test cartilage repair. After surgery, the

stimulate the synthesis rate of matrix macromolecules, especially small glycosaminoglycans, and promote the repair of damaged cartilage.[8,9] IGF-1 can stimulate chondrocyte

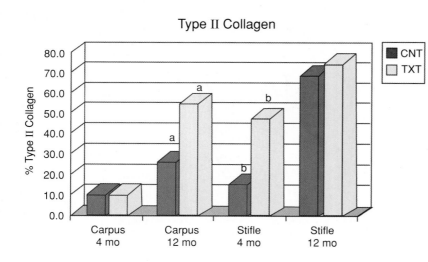

Figure 9.9 Type II collagen (%) by treatment group, joint, and time period. Like letters represent statistical difference ($p < 0.05$) between the comparison. CNT, control group; TXT, treatment group. (Reprinted with permission from Frisbie DD, Trotter GW, Powers BE, et al. Arthroscopic subchondral bone plate microfracture technique augments healing of large osteochondral defects in the radial carpal bone and medial femoral condyle of horses. *J Vet Surg* 1999;28:242–255, Fig. 9.)

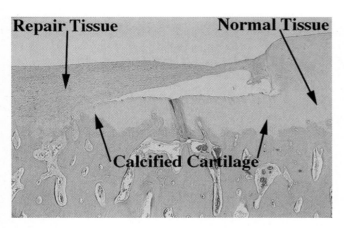

Figure 9.10 Computer image (×10; 5-mcm osteochondral section stained with hematoxylin and eosin). Good attachment of repair tissue to the subchondral bone in an area devoid of calcified cartilage and poor attachment in an area containing subchondral bone. (Reprinted with permission from Frisbie DD, Trotter GW, Powers BE, et al. Arthroscopic subchondral bone plate microfracture technique augments healing of large osteochondral defects in the radial carpal bone and medial femoral condyle of horses. *J Vet Surg* 1999;28:242–255, Fig. 6.)

antalgic quadruped gait provides some protection for the area of microfracture.

The first study on microfracture in the horse was to determine if microfracture produced more repair tissue than an untreated lesion.[20] Large chondral defects were created in the radial carpal bones and in both medial femoral condyles of the horses. One carpal bone and one femoral condyle of each horse were treated with microfracture and the others were left untreated. In five horses at 4 months, and five horses at 12 months, gross, histologic, and histomorphometric examinations of defect sites and repair tissues were performed. The repair tissues were also evaluated for collagen typing. The results showed a significant amount of repair tissue in the defects that were treated with microfracture (Fig. 9.8). An increase in Type II collagen (Fig. 9.9) and earlier bone remodeling, as documented by changes in porosity, was also seen in the defects treated with microfracture.

On histologic evaluation of these samples, it was noted that the presence of calcified cartilage impeded the growth of repair tissue (Fig. 9.10). This finding led to further analysis of defects treated by removing calcified cartilage and those with calcified cartilage intact. In this study, defects were made in mature horses on the axial weight-bearing portion of both medial femoral condyles.[21] The calcified cartilage layer was removed from one defect in each horse. At 4 months and 12 months, removal of calcified cartilage resulted in improved grade of overall repair tissue and increased histological filling of the defect. The study concluded that removal of calcified cartilage layers provided optimal amount and attachment of repair tissue. The results of this study led to changes in the technique. Removal of the calcified cartilage was determined to be an important step in the microfracture procedure (Fig. 9.11).

Another study in the horse was performed to assess key matrix component expression in early cartilage healing

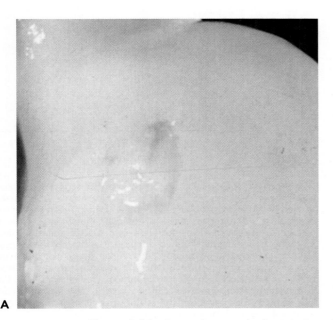
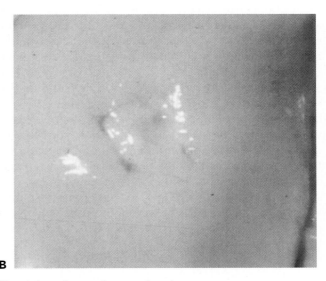

Figure 9.11 Gross photograph of repair tissue filling defects 1 year after creation. **A** represents removal of the calcified cartilage and **B** shows calcified cartilage remaining. (Reprinted with permission from Frisbie DD, Morisset S, Ho CP, et al. Effects of calcified cartilage on healing of chondral defects treated with microfracture in horses. *Am J Sports Med* 2006;34:1824–1831, Fig. 4.)

with microfracture.[22] Microfracture and control samples were collected at 2, 4, 6, and 8 weeks. Analyses included determining qualitative impression of cellular and molecular changes. Comparisons of histomorphometric data and molecular and protein expression of critical cartilage components were performed at 8 weeks. The results demonstrated a gradual and significant increase in mRNA content for both Type II collagen and aggrecan over the 8-week period (Fig. 9.12). The Type II collagen expression was enhanced with microfracture. This enhancement of Type II collagen protein after microfracture was supported by the previous long-term study.[20] In this study, aggrecan expression did not appear to be influenced by microfracture treatment, whereas another critical matrix component was enhanced (Type II collagen).

The study by Frisbie et al.[22] confirmed that microfracture significantly increases Type II collagen expression as early as 8 weeks after treatment (Fig. 9.13). However, microfracture did not alter other key components of the matrix (aggrecan and Type I collagen). The quest for additional improvement in repair tissue character after the use of this technique continues.

THE ACUTE CHONDRAL INJURY

Indications and Contraindications

General indications for microfracture include full-thickness defect, unstable cartilage that overlies the subchondral bone, and a partial-thickness lesion in which cartilage simply scrapes off the bone when probed. Other considerations for use of the microfracture procedure include the patient's age, acceptable biomechanical alignment of the knee, activity level, his or her willingness to accept rehabilitation protocol, and the individual's expectations (Fig. 9.14).[3,23–25] If all of these criteria are met, microfracture should be considered as a treatment option.

Patient age is not a specific contraindication. Our studies have shown that patients younger than 35 years of age with acute lesions have greater improvement, while older patients show some improvement. The size of the lesion is also not a contraindication for microfracture.[2,3] In previous studies, we have shown that large acute lesions respond well to microfracture; however, lesions less than 400 mm[2] (Fig. 9.15) tend to respond better to microfracture than those lesions greater than 400 mm[2], but we have not observed this difference to be statistically significant.[2,3]

Specific contraindications for microfracture include axial malalignment (Fig. 9.16; as described in Chapter 13), patients unwilling or unable to follow the required strict and rigorous rehabilitation protocol, partial-thickness

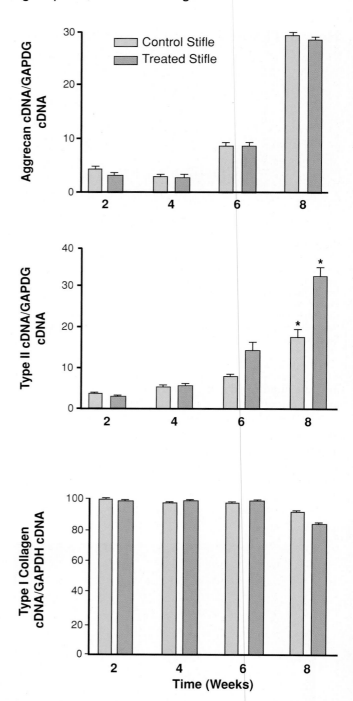

Figure 9.12 The results of the reverse transcription coupled polymerase chain reaction of repair tissue are shown. An increase is seen in the expression level of Type II and aggrecan with time, whereas the expression levels of Type I collagen and Type III collagen (not shown) remained relatively constant related to glyceraldehyde 3-phosphate dehydrogenase (GAPDH). An enhancement in Type II collagen expression in repair tissue was observed as early as 6 weeks after treatment with microfracture. An asterisk indicates statistically significant difference in values ($p < 0.05$) between treatment groups. (Reprinted with permission from Frisbie DD, Oxford JT, Southwood L, et al. Early events in cartilage repair after subchondral bone microfracture. *Clin Orthop* 2003;407: 215–227, Fig. 3.)

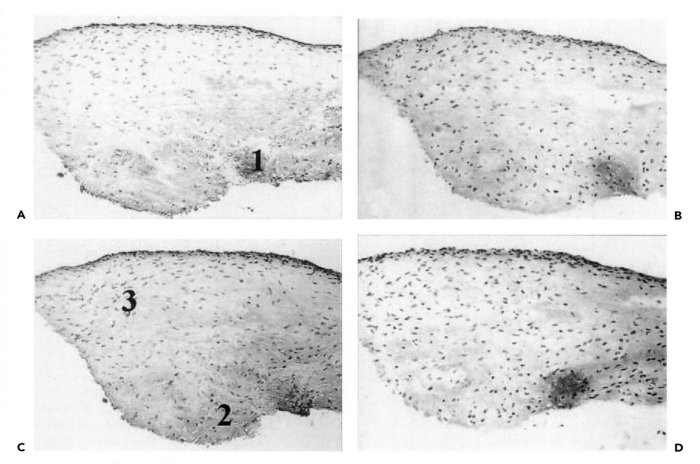

Figure 9.13 The distribution of Type II collagen and aggrecan peptides in 8-week repair tissue are shown. **A:** Immunohistochemistry was used to detect Type II collagen antibody. **B:** Antibody preabsorbed with antigen and aggrecan also was detected by immunohistochemistry. **C:** Aggrecan antibody peptides are shown as detected by immunohistochemistry. **D:** Also shown are antibodies reabsorbed with antigen peptides. (1) Calcified tissue, (2) fibrocartilage, and (3) fibrouslike tissue also were detected. The original magnification is ×4. (Reprinted with permission from Frisbie DD, Oxford JT, Southwood L, et al. Early events in cartilage repair after subchondral bone microfracture. *Clin Orthop* 2003;407:215–227, Fig. 6A–D.)

defects, and inability to use the opposite leg for weight-bearing during the minimal or nonweightbearing period.[2,26]

Preoperative Planning

Initial evaluations of patients who present with knee joint pain include a thorough physical and orthopaedic examination, as well as an evaluation of their symptoms. These symptoms may include pain, swelling, stiffness, and mechanical symptoms. It is important on the initial evaluation to determine the patient's activity level and expectations. Identification of point tenderness over a femoral condyle or tibial plateau is a useful finding, but in itself is not diagnostic. If compression of the patella (Fig. 9.17)

elicits pain, this finding may be indicative of a patellar or trochlear lesion. At times, physical diagnosis can be difficult and elusive, especially if only an isolated chondral defect is present.

Imaging

We use long standing radiographs to determine angular deformity and joint-space narrowing, which is often indicative of articular cartilage loss (Fig. 9.18). We also obtain standard anteroposterior and lateral radiographs of both knees, as well as weightbearing views with the knees flexed to 30 or 45 degrees (Fig. 9.19). Patellar views are also useful to evaluate the patellofemoral joint. Magnetic resonance imaging, which employs newer diagnostic

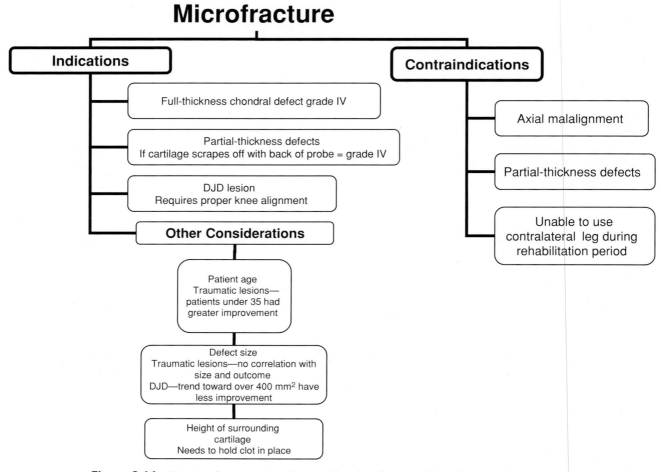

Figure 9.14 Diagram demonstrating the considerations for use of the microfracture procedure. DJD, degenerative joint disease.

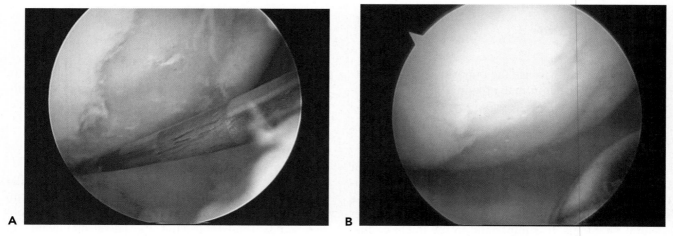

Figure 9.15 **A:** A large chondral lesion prepared for microfracture. **B:** The same large lesion 6 months following microfracture.

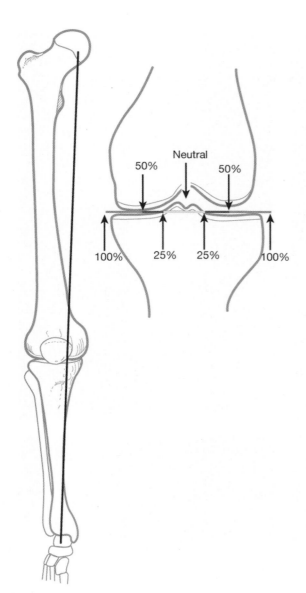

Figure 9.16 With a line from the center of the hip to the center of the ankle, the weightbearing-line across the tibial plateau determines patient alignment.

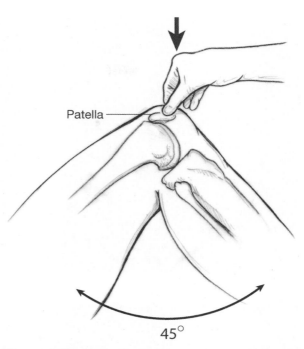

Figure 9.17 Illustration of compression of the patella during physical examination. Arrow indicates direction of pressure applied.

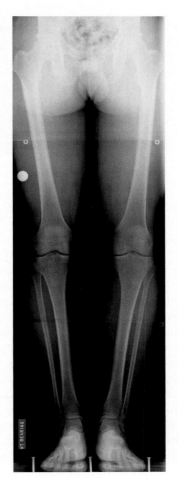

Figure 9.18 Long standing radiographs.

sequences specific for articular cartilage, has become a mainstay of our diagnostic workup of patients with suspected chondral lesions (Fig. 9.20). Imaging is described in detail in Chapter 7.

Surgical Technique

A thorough diagnostic arthroscopic examination of the knee is performed through three portals (inflow cannula, arthroscope, and working instruments) (Fig. 9.21). We typically do not use a tourniquet during the microfracture procedure; rather, we vary the arthroscopic fluid

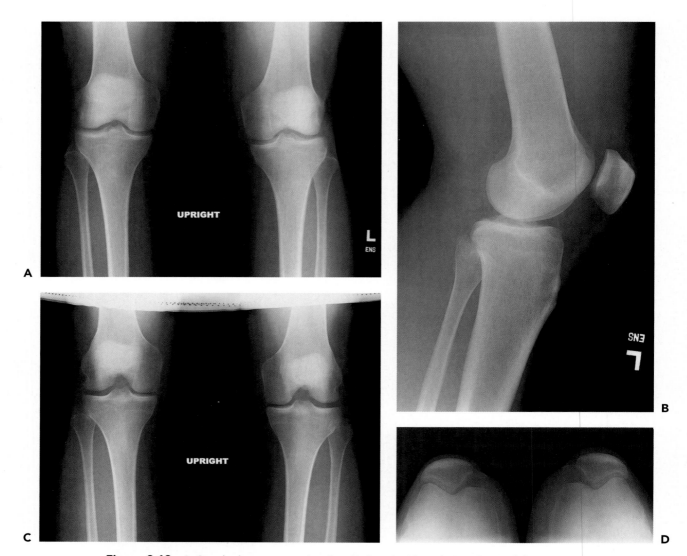

Figure 9.19 A: Standard anteroposterior view. **B:** Standard lateral view. **C:** Weightbearing view with knee flexed. **D:** Patellar view.

pump pressure to control bleeding. All geographic areas of the knee are inspected. This includes the suprapatellar pouch, the medial and lateral gutters, the patellofemoral joint, the intercondylar notch and its contents, and the medial and lateral compartments, including the posterior horns of both menisci. Particular attention is paid to plicae (Fig. 9.22) and the lateral retinaculum, which have the potential to increase compression between cartilage surfaces.[2,23,25–28] Microfracture is the final intra-articular procedure performed. This is to help prevent loss of marrow elements when blood and fat droplets enter the knee joint, and to avoid dislodging the marrow clot.

After identification of the full-thickness articular cartilage lesion, all remaining unstable cartilage is removed. A hand-held curved curette and a full radius resector can be used to remove the loose or marginally attached cartilage back to a stable rim of cartilage (Fig. 9.23). The calcified cartilage layer that remains as a cap to many lesions must be removed, usually with a curette (Fig. 9.24). Thorough and complete removal of the calcified cartilage layer is extremely important based on animal studies we have completed.[20–22] The integrity of the subchondral plate should be maintained (Fig. 9.25). It is important that the defect, if debrided, be deep enough to remove the calcified cartilage layer but not so deep as to damage the subchondral plate. This prepared lesion, with a stable perpendicular edge of healthy, well-attached, viable cartilage surrounding the defect, provides a pool that helps contain the marrow clot, ("super clot," as we call it), as it forms.

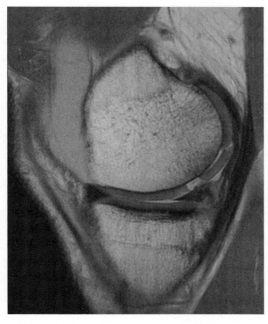

Figure 9.20 Magnetic resonance image of a suspected chondral lesion. (From Chapter 7, Courtesy Dr. Charles Ho.)

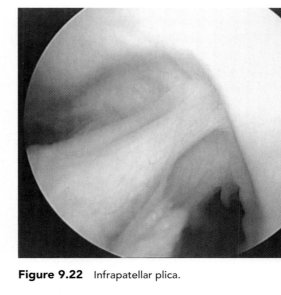

Figure 9.22 Infrapatellar plica.

After preparation of the lesion, arthroscopic awls are used to make multiple holes, or "microfractures" (Fig. 9.26). An angled awl, typically 30 or 45 degrees, permits the tip to be perpendicular to the bone as it is advanced. A 90-degree awl is used for the patella if an angle cannot be created to accommodate the 45-degree awl. If the 90-degree pick is used, the subchondral plate must be prepared with a shaver or abrader to permit manual use of the 90-degree instrument. It is important that it only be advanced manually, with no use of a mallet. Starting at the periphery, microfracture holes are made, with holes toward the center of the defect made last (Fig. 9.27). The holes are made (Fig. 9.28) close to each other, but not so close that one breaks into another, damaging the

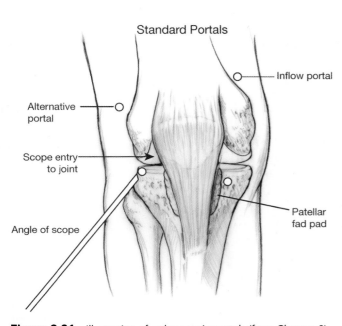

Figure 9.21 Illustration of arthroscopic portals (from Chapter 8).

Standard Portals

Inflow portal

Alternative portal

Scope entry to joint

Angle of scope

Patellar fad pad

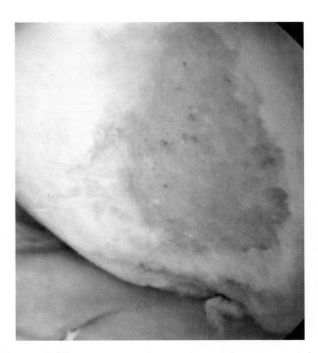

Figure 9.23 Stable rim of a cartilage defect prepared for microfracture.

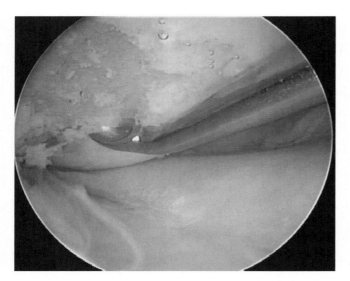

Figure 9.24 Curette removing the calcified cartilage layer of a defect.

subchondral plate between them. When the appropriate depth (approximately 2 to 4 mm) has been reached, fat droplets can be seen coming from the marrow cavity (Fig. 9.29). After we have determined that an appropriate number of holes have been made, the irrigation fluid pump pressure is reduced so the release of marrow fat droplets and blood from the microfracture holes into the subchondral bone can be seen (Fig. 9.30). We then remove all instruments from the knee and evacuate the fluid from the joint. Intra-articular drains should not be used because the goal is for the surgically induced marrow clot, which is rich in marrow elements, to form and stabilize while covering the lesion.[20,22] *The key to the microfracture procedure is to establish the marrow clot effectively (Fig. 9.31).* This provides the optimal environment for the body's mesenchymal stem cells or progenitor cells to differentiate into stable tissue within the lesion.[20,22]

Microfracture creates a rough surface on the subchondral bone. This surface allows for the marrow clot to adhere more easily, while the integrity of the subchondral plate is maintained for joint surface shape (Fig. 9.32). We believe that the success of the entire procedure depends on the effective establishment of the marrow clot. No shaving is done after the microstructure is completed.

THE CHRONIC LESION

Nonoperative Treatment

Degenerative joint disease in a knee that has correct axial alignment is another common indication for microfracture. Performing an adequate microfracture is more difficult in the chronic degenerative chondral lesions because of the eburnated bone and bony sclerosis with thickening of the subchondral plate (Fig. 9.33).[3,6] Patients with chronic or degenerative chondral lesions are often treated nonoperatively (conservatively) for at least 12 weeks after the initial diagnosis. This treatment regimen includes activity modification, physical therapy, nonsteroidal anti-inflammatory

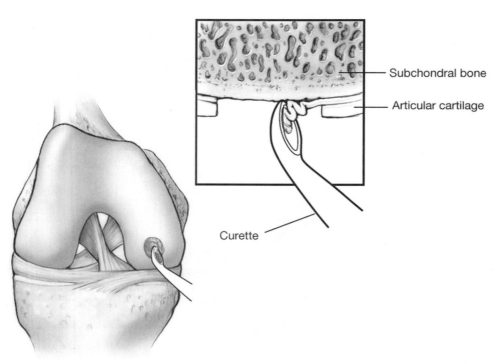

Subchondral bone

Articular cartilage

Curette

Figure 9.25 Illustration showing the subchondral plate maintained beneath the calcified cartilage layer.

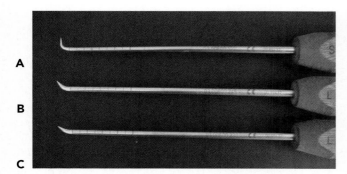

Figure 9.26   The three microfracture awls used: 30 degree (**A**), 45 degree (**B**), and 90 degree (**C**).

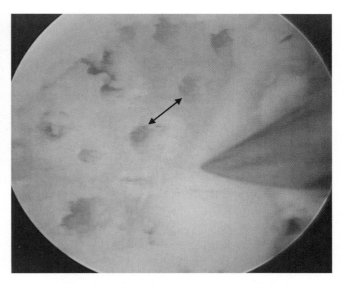

Figure 9.28   Double-headed arrow shows distance between microfracture holes in the lesion.

drugs, joint injections, and perhaps dietary supplements that may have cartilage-stimulating properties. If nonoperative treatment is not successful, then a surgical approach is considered.[2,23,25–30]

Contraindications for Microfracture

In the treatment of chronic degenerative lesions with microfracture, correct axial alignment is essential. In addition to the contraindications mentioned in the acute section, other specific contraindications include any systemic immune-mediated disease, disease-induced arthritis, or cartilage disease. A relative contraindication exists for patients older than 65 years because the author has observed that it is difficult for some patients older than 65 years to use crutches and properly perform the required rigorous rehabilitation.[24,26] Other contraindications to microfracture include global degenerative osteoarthrosis or cartilage surrounding the lesion that is too thin to establish a perpendicular rim to hold the marrow clot (Fig. 9.34).[3,24,26]

Microfracture Procedure if Patient Has No Contraindications

If the patient meets the criteria, the lesion is debrided of all remaining unstable cartilage with a shaver and curette in order to create a circumferentially stable shoulder to the defect (Fig. 9.35). A few microfracture holes are made to

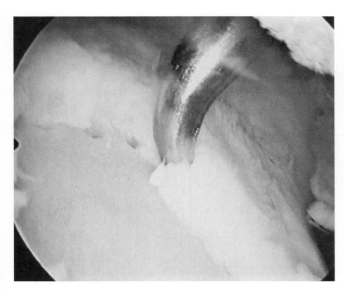

Figure 9.27   Microfracture holes being performed at the edge of the lesion.

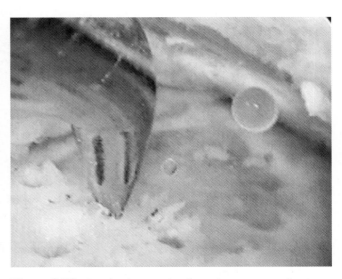

Figure 9.29   Fat droplets coming from the marrow cavity.

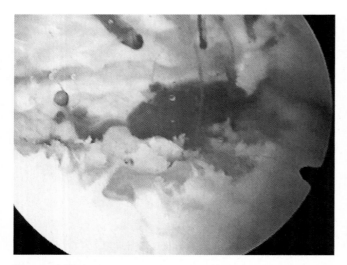

Figure 9.30 Fat droplets and blood coming from the microfracture holes when the irrigation fluid pump pressure is reduced.

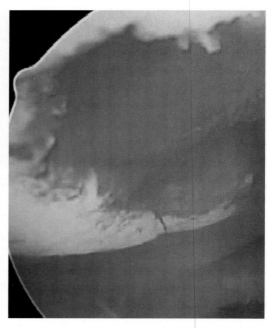

Figure 9.31 A marrow clot established in a defect caused by microfracture.

assess the thickness of the subchondral plate. A motorized burr can be used to remove the sclerotic bone until punctate bleeding is seen (Fig. 9.36). After the bleeding appears uniformly over the surface of the lesion, a microfracture procedure can be performed as previously described (Fig. 9.37).[3,24] Cartilage surrounding the defect must be thick enough to contain the marrow clot (Fig. 9.38). Patients having thin cartilage, such as in advanced degenerative lesions, are less appropriate candidates for microfracture.[3,24] It should be noted that patients who have degenerative joint disease rarely have a calcified cartilage layer sufficient

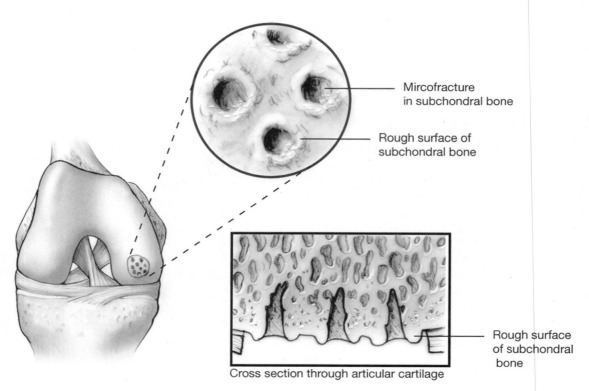

Mircofracture in subchondral bone

Rough surface of subchondral bone

Rough surface of subchondral bone

Cross section through articular cartilage

Figure 9.32 Illustration of the rough surface and the subchondral plate in relation to the joint surface shape.

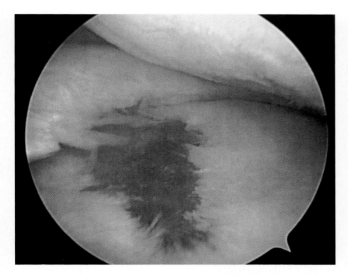

Figure 9.33 A degenerative chondral defect with sclerotic bone.

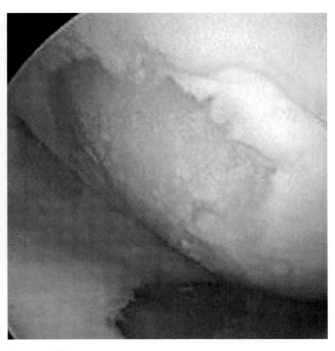

Figure 9.35 A stable shoulder on a degenerative lesion.

for microfracture. Preparation involves a process that Johnson[6] described in abrasion arthroplasty. Arthroscopic treatment as described in Chapter 12 is added to improve the joint environment.

Postoperative Management

The postoperative program is designed to promote the ideal physical environment in which the newly recruited mesenchymal stem cells from the marrow can differentiate into the appropriate articular cartilage-like cell lines.[2,23,24, 26,31] These differentiation and maturation processes must occur slowly but consistently.[31,32] Our animal studies have confirmed that both cellular and molecular changes are an essential part of the development of durable repair tissue.[20,22]

Patients are carefully counseled so they understand that they may not experience improvement in their knees for at least 6 months after microfracture. It has been our experience, supported by our clinical research data, that improvement can be expected to occur slowly and steadily for at least 2 years.[2,23,29,30] During this protracted period, the repair tissue matures, pain and swelling resolve, and patients

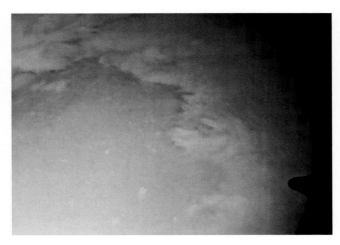

Figure 9.34 A cartilage defect with a rim too thin to maintain a marrow clot.

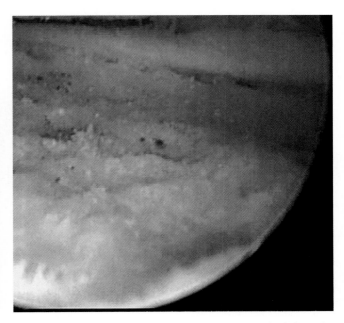

Figure 9.36 Punctate bleeding following removal of the sclerotic bone with a motorized burr.

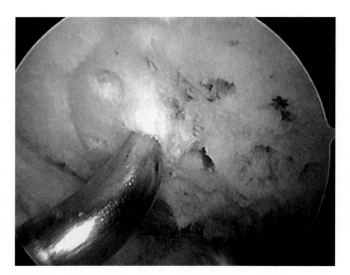

Figure 9.37 Microfracture of a degenerative lesion following adequate preparation.

regain confidence and comfort in their knees during increased levels of activity.[2]

REHABILITATION

To optimize the results of microfracture, the rehabilitation program should be followed closely. The rehabilitation protocol promotes the optimal physical environment for the mesenchymal stem cells to differentiate and produce new extracellular matrix, which eventually matures into durable repair tissue. The surgically induced marrow clot provides the basis for the most ideal chemical environment

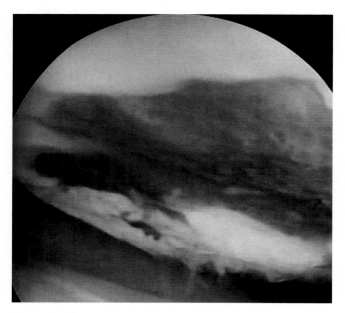

Figure 9.38 Marrow clot held in place in a degenerative lesion by the surrounding cartilage.

to complement the physical environment.[20,22] This newly proliferated repair cartilage then fills the original defect.

The postoperative rehabilitation program after microfracture requires special consideration.[24,26,31] The specific protocol recommended depends on both anatomic location and the size of the defect. These two factors are critical to the design of the ideal postoperative plan. For example, if other intra-articular procedures are done concurrently with microfracture, such as anterior cruciate ligament reconstruction, we do not hesitate to alter the rehabilitation program as necessary. All of the possible variations of the rehabilitation program are not within the scope of this chapter, but in the following paragraphs we describe two different protocols.

Rehabilitation Protocol for Patients with Lesions on the Femoral Condyle or Tibial Plateau

After microfracture of lesions on the weightbearing surfaces of the femoral condyles or tibial plateaus, we commence immediately with a continuous passive motion (CPM) machine in the recovery room. Typically, the initial range of motion (ROM) is 30 to 70 degrees, and can be increased as tolerated by the patient. The rate of the machine is usually one cycle per minute, but the rate can be varied based on patient preference and comfort. Many patients tolerate use of the CPM machine at night. For those who do not, we have observed that intermittent use during the day is probably as beneficial. Regardless of when the CPM machine is used, the goal is to have the patient in the CPM machine for 6 to 8 hours every 24 hours. If the patient is unable to use the CPM machine, then instructions are given for passive flexion and extension of the knee with 500 repetitions three times per day. We encourage patients to gain full passive ROM of the injured knee as soon as possible after surgery.

We also prescribe cold therapy for all patients postoperatively. Our experience and observations indicate that cold helps control pain and inflammation, and most patients state that the cold provides overall postoperative pain relief. Cold therapy generally is used for 1 to 7 days postoperatively, but can be used throughout the treatment period.[33]

We prescribe crutch-assisted touch-down weightbearing ambulation for 6 to 8 weeks, depending on the size of the lesion. For most patients, 6 to 8 weeks seems to be an adequate time to limit weightbearing; however, for patients with small lesions (less than 1 cm diameter), weightbearing may begin a few weeks earlier. Patients with lesions on the femoral condyle or tibial plateau rarely use a brace during the initial postoperative period; however, we now prescribe an unloading type of brace when the patient becomes more active and the postoperative swelling has resolved.

As mentioned mobilization begins immediately after surgery, with an emphasis on ROM of the knee, patella, and patellar tendon motion. Patients are touch-down weight-bearing, placing 10% of their body weight on the injured leg during weightbearing. One to 2 weeks after microfracture, patients begin stationary biking without resistance and a deep-water exercise program. The deep-water exercises include use of a flotation vest for deep-water running. *It is critical and imperative that the foot of the injured leg not touch the bottom of the pool during this exercise.* Patients progress to full weightbearing after about 8 weeks and begin more vigorous biking with increasing resistance. Biking is the key exercise between 8 and 16 weeks. Patients also begin knee flexion exercises at approximately the same time. An elastic resistance cord is added to the exercise regimen at about 12 weeks. A detailed description of use of the cord and the exercises has been published.[31]

According to our observations, the ability to achieve predetermined maximum levels for sets and repetitions of elastic resistance cord exercises is an excellent indicator for beginning weight training. We permit free or machine weights when the patient has achieved the early goals of the rehabilitation program, but not before 16 weeks after microfracture. We strongly emphasize the importance of proper technique when beginning a weight program. The decision to return to sport is based on several factors: clinical examination, the size of the patient, the sport, and the size of the lesion. We usually recommend that patients do not return to sports that involve pivoting, cutting, or jumping until at least 6 to 9 months after microfracture.

Rehabilitation Protocol for Patients with Patellofemoral Lesions

All patients treated by microfracture for patellofemoral lesions must use a brace set at 0 to 20 degrees for at least 8 weeks. This brace limits compression of the regenerating surfaces of the trochlea or patella, or both. We allow passive motion with the brace removed, but otherwise the brace must be worn at all times. Patients with patellofemoral lesions are placed into a CPM machine immediately postoperatively. (The brace is removed for CPM treatment and replaced following CPM.) The CPM is set for a range of zero to fifty degrees. We also use cold therapy as previously described. With this regimen, patients typically obtain a pain-free, full passive ROM soon after surgery.

For patients with patellofemoral joint lesions, we carefully observe joint angles at the time of arthroscopy to determine where the defect comes into contact with the patellar facet or the trochlear groove. We make certain we avoid these areas during strength training for approximately 4 months. This avoidance allows for immediate training in the 0 to 20 degree range postoperatively because there is minimal compression of these chondral surfaces with such limited motion.

Patients with lesions of the patellofemoral joint treated by microfracture are allowed weightbearing as tolerated in their brace 2 weeks after surgery. *It is essential for patients to use a brace that prevents placing excessive shear force on the maturing marrow clot in the early postoperative period.* We routinely lock the brace between 0 and 20 degrees ROM to prevent flexion past the point where the median ridge of the patella engages the trochlear groove. After 8 weeks, we gradually open the knee brace before its use is discontinued. When the brace is discontinued, patients are allowed to advance their training progressively. Stationary biking is allowed 2 to 6 weeks postoperatively, with increased resistance added at 8 weeks after microfracture. At 12 weeks after microfracture, the exercise program is the same one used for femorotibial lesions.

POTENTIAL COMPLICATIONS FROM MICROFRACTURE

Complications are rare following the microfracture technique. Some patients present with mild, transient pain, most frequently following microfracture in the patellofemoral joint. Small changes in the articular surface of the patellofemoral joint may be characterized as a grating or "gritty" sensation in the joint, especially when a patient discontinues use of the knee brace and begins normal weightbearing through full ROM. Patients rarely complain of pain at this time, and this grating sensation usually resolves spontaneously in a few days or weeks. Patients may also notice "catching" or "locking" as the apex of the patella rides over the patellofemoral lesion during joint motion, if a steep perpendicular rim was made in the trochlear groove. These symptoms may be reported when the patients uses the CPM machine. In our experience, these symptoms usually dissipate within 3 months. If this perceived locking is painful, the patient is advised to limit weightbearing and avoid the symptomatic joint angle for an additional period.[24,26]

Swelling and joint effusion typically resolve within 8 weeks after microfracture.[2] Occasionally, a recurrent effusion develops between 6 and 8 weeks after microfracture, usually when a patient begins to bear weight on the injured leg after microfracture for a defect on the femoral condyle. Although this effusion may mimic the preoperative or immediate postoperative effusion, usually it is painless. We treat this type of painless effusion conservatively. It usually resolves within several weeks after onset. Rarely has a second arthroscopy been required for recurring effusions.

PATIENT OUTCOMES

The Steadman ♦ Hawkins Research Foundation Clinical Research Database currently has data on more than 15,000 arthroscopic knee procedures. Of these surgical procedures, 2,804 knees underwent microfracture (Table 9.1). This database includes preoperative physician and patient subjective assessments, findings at arthroscopy and treatments, and postoperative physician and patient subjective

TABLE 9.1

DISTRIBUTION OF LOCATIONS OF GRADE IV CHONDRAL LESIONS TREATED WITH MICROFRACTURE IN STEADMAN♦HAWKINS CLINICAL RESEARCH DATABASE (N = 2,804)

Area	% of Patients
MFC	19
LFC	10
MTP	4
LTP	5
TG	13
PAT	4
MFC and MTP	17
LFC and LTP	10
TG and PAT	2
Other	16

MFC, medial femoral condyle; LFC, lateral femoral condyle; MTP, medial tibial plateau; LTP, lateral tibial plateau; TG, trochlear groove; PAT, patella.

assessments. At the time of first examination, the patients are asked to complete a self-administered questionnaire. Patients are then sent the questionnaire yearly for evaluation of symptoms, function, return to sports, activities of daily living, and satisfaction. All patient information is stored anonymously in a database. Database files are linked and queried to obtain desired data. Data analysis is performed using an SPSS (SPSS Inc., Chicago, IL) software package. All statistics are reviewed by an independent statistician.

Outcome Measures

Lysholm Score

We use the Lysholm knee score to measure knee function. The scale of Lysholm and Gillquist[34]consists of eight domains related to function of the knee: walking with a limp, support, locking, instability, pain, swelling, stair-climbing, and squatting. Pain and instability receive the highest point allocation, followed by locking, swelling, and stair climbing. A total score of 95 to 100 points is associated with normal function; 84 to 94 points indicates symptoms related to vigorous activity, and less than 84 points suggests symptoms related to activities of daily living.

Kocher et al.[35] determined the reliability, validity, and responsiveness of the Lysholm score for the treatment of chondral defects. These psychometric properties were analyzed in a group of 1,657 patients with chondral disorders of the knee. Reliability of the score was determined by test-retest, which entailed the same patient completing the questionnaire twice within 4 weeks to determine the reproducibility of the score between patients. Validity of the score, which included content validity, criterion validity,

and construct validity, was also measured. To determine if the score can assess change, the responsiveness was determined. There was acceptable test-retest reliability for the overall Lysholm scale and six of the eight domains. Internal consistency was acceptable. There were acceptable floor (0%) and ceiling (0.7%) effects for the overall Lysholm scale. High floor effects for the domain of squatting and high ceiling effects for the domains of limp, instability, support, and locking were evident. There was acceptable criterion validity with significant ($p < 0.05$) correlations between the overall Lysholm scale and the physical functioning domain of the Short Form (SF)-12 scale; the pain, stiffness, and function domains of the Western Ontario and McMaster University Osteoarthritis Index (WOMAC) scale; and the Tegner activity scale. Construct validity and responsiveness to change for the overall Lysholm scale (effect size = 1.16; standardized response mean = 1.10) were acceptable. This study showed that the overall Lysholm score performed acceptably for the assessment of outcome following treatment of chondral disorders. Some individual domains of the score, however, did not perform as well.[35]

Tegner Activity Scale

In our database, we recorded the measured activity by using the Tegner activity scale.[36] With the Tegner scale, a numerical value, 0 to 10, is assigned to specific activities. An activity level of 10 represents competitive sports, including soccer, football, and rugby at the elite level; an activity level of 6 represents recreational sports; and a level of zero represents a person on sick leave or disability pension because of knee problems. Activity levels of 5 to 10 can be achieved only if the patient participates in recreational or competitive sports. The Tegner activity scale is easy to use; however, not all sports are represented in the categories.[36]

Western Ontario and McMaster University Osteoarthritis Index

In studies documenting the outcomes of patients with osteoarthritis of the knee, we use the WOMAC score in addition to the Lysholm and Tegner scores. The WOMAC[37] is a general musculoskeletal instrument for patients who have osteoarthritis of the hip or knee. It has been validated in randomized clinical trials and has been shown to be a responsive tool in measuring outcomes following treatments for osteoarthritis of the knee. The WOMAC has three domains: pain (5 items), stiffness (2 items), and physical functioning (17 items). The questions are ranked on a five-point Likert scale (0 = none, 1 = slight, 2 = moderate, 3 = severe, 4 = extreme). The score is reported as the sum of the scores for each domain.

Patient Satisfaction

As health care becomes more patient-driven, assessing patient satisfaction is a major objective of our data collection. Our goals are to evaluate patient satisfaction with treatment outcome and to identify parameters that are related to that satisfaction. With determinants of patient satisfaction from these studies, we can identify the elements that are most important to the patients following surgery. We measure satisfaction with outcome of treatment using a scale of 1 to 10, with 10 being very satisfied and 1 being dissatisfied.

RESULTS OF MICROFRACTURE

In 2003, the first long-term outcomes article was published on the microfracture technique.[2] This study followed 72 patients an average of 11 years following microfracture, with the longest follow-up being 17 years. This study included only knees with no joint-space narrowing, no degenerative arthritis, and no ligament or meniscus pathology that required treatment. All patients were younger than 45 years of age. The microfracture technique used on these patients did not include recent improvements in the technique as described in the Acute Chondral Injury—Surgical Technique section of this chapter. With a 95% follow-up rate, the results showed a decrease in symptoms and improved function. Patients reported decreased pain and swelling at postoperative year 1, which continued to decrease at year 2, and the clinical improvements were maintained over the study period (Fig. 9.39). The majority of patients indicated good-to-excellent results on the SF-36 and

WOMAC scoring systems at final follow-up. The study identified age as the only independent predictor of Lysholm improvement. Patients more than 35 years of age improved less than patients younger than 35 ($p = 0.048$); nonetheless both groups showed improvement.[2]

In summary, we found that arthroscopically performed microfracture for isolated full-thickness chondral defects in patients younger than 45 years of age led to significant improvement as measured by the Lysholm scoring system. Given pain relief ($p < 0.001$), improvement in function ($p < 0.01$), and no perioperative complications, we recommend that the arthroscopically performed microfracture procedure be the initial treatment for traumatic, full-thickness chondral defects of the knee.

Recently, a study compared the outcomes of autologous chondrocyte implantation with microfracture treatment in a randomized trial.[38] Forty patients were treated in each group. At 2 years, both groups showed significant improvement on Lysholm scale and, in particular, pain, with no difference between the groups. However, the microfracture group had more improvement in the SF-36 physical component score. A high physical functioning score corresponds to a person who performs all types of physical activities, including the most vigorous, without limitations related to health. The authors theorized that this difference may be because microfracture is one arthroscopic procedure, compared with autologous chondrocyte implantation, which

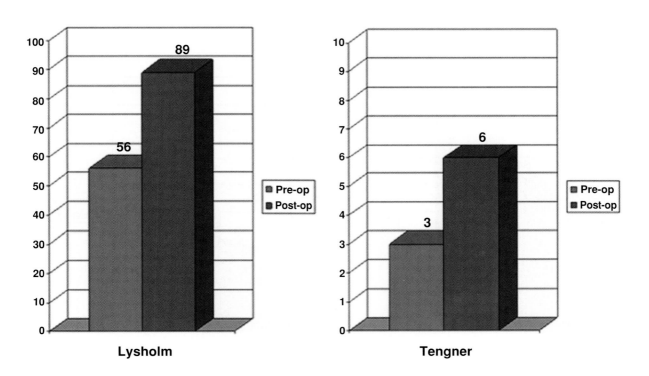

Average follow-up 11 years (range, 7 to 17 years)

Figure 9.39 Graph showing patient outcome 11 years following microfracture. Pre-op, preoperative; post-op, postoperative.

TABLE 9.2
AVERAGE FUNCTIONAL SCORES OF ALL PATIENTS

Lesions Studied (Ref.)	Patient Age Range (years)	Lysholm	Tegner
Traumatic lesions[2] (Arthroscopy, 2003)	13–45	89	6
Traumatic lesions[38] (J Bone Joint Surg, 2004)	18–45	76	4
NFL players[28] (J Knee Surg, 2003)	22–36	90	9
Degenerative knees[3] (J Knee Surg, 2003)	40–70	83	4.5
HTO and microfracture* (Am J Sports Med, 2004)	34–79	78	5

NFL, National Football League; HTO, high tibial osteotomy.
*Sterett WI, Steadman JR. Am J Spots Med 204;32:1243–1249.

requires two procedures, one arthroscopic and one open procedure.

This study also found age to be a predictor of improvement with microfracture. Activity level and lesion size were also identified as predictors of clinical results. Histologic evaluations showed no differences between the groups. Based on these results and other studies (Table 9.2) that indicate that microfracture outcomes are similar to autologous chondrocyte implantation, we believe that microfracture should be the recommended initial treatment for isolated chondral defects.

Cartilage injuries are common in high-impact sports. We documented the outcome of microfracture in patients who played professional football in the United States.[28] Twenty-five active National Football League players were treated with microfracture between 1986 and 1997. The study found that 76% of players returned to play the next football season. Following return to play, those same players played an average of 4.6 additional seasons. All players showed decreased symptoms and improvement in function. Of those players who did not return to play, most had pre-existing degenerative changes of the knee.[28]

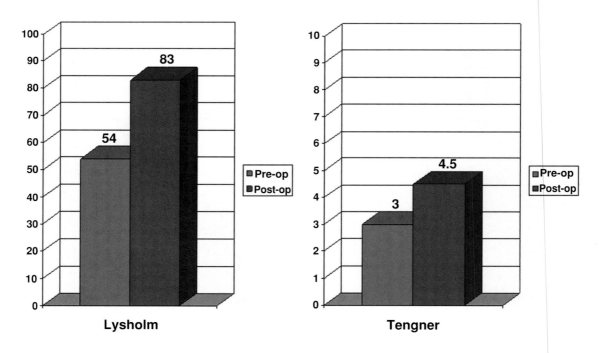

Average follow-up 2.5 years (range, 2 to 6 years)

Figure 9.40 Graph showing outcome following microfracture for degenerative chondral defects. Pre-op, preoperative; post-op, postoperative.

Outcomes following microfracture in the degenerative knee have been reported in a recent study.[3] We documented the outcome at 2 years in patients with degenerative chondral lesions treated with microfracture. Patients showed improvement in their function and had decreased symptoms. Proper surgical technique, including removal of the sclerotic bone, as well as patient compliance with a well-defined rehabilitation program were critical in this population. Lysholm score improved from 54 to 83 and mean Tegner Activity Scale at follow-up was 4.5 (Fig. 9.40). Factors that were associated with less Lysholm improvement included bipolar lesions, lesions more than 400 mm^2, and knees with absent menisci. Repeat arthroscopy was reported in 15.5% of these patients. Failures, as defined by revision microfracture or total knee replacement, were documented in 6% of the patients. These results confirm excellent short-term outcomes. We will continue to follow these patients to determine how long the results last.

REFERENCES

1. Mankin HJ. The response of articular cartilage to mechanical injury. *J Bone Joint Surg Am* 1982;64:460–465.
2. Steadman JR, Briggs KK, Rodrigo JJ, et al. Outcomes of microfracture for traumatic chondral defects of the knee: average 11-year follow-up. *Arthroscopy* 2003;19:477–484.
3. Miller BS, Steadman JR, Briggs KK, et al. Patient satisfaction and outcome after microfracture of the degenerative knee. *J Knee Surg* 2004;17:13–17.
4. Buckwalter JA. Articular cartilage: injuries and potential for healing. *J Orthop Sports Phys Ther* 1998;28:192–202.
5. Mankin HJ. Reaction of articular cartilage to injury and osteoarthritis. *N Engl J Med* 1974;291:1335–1340.
6. Johnson LL. The sclerotic lesion: pathology and the clinical response to arthroscopic abrasion arthroplasty. In: Ewing JW, ed. *Articular Cartilage and Knee Joint Function: Basic Science and Arthroscopy*. New York: Raven Press; 1990:319–333.
7. Morales TI, Hascall VC. Factors involved in the regulation of proteoglycan metabolism in articular cartilage. *Arthritis Rheum* 1989;32:1197–1201
8. Morales TI, Roberts AB. Correlated metabolism of proteoglycans and hyaluronic acid in bovine cartilage organ cultures. *J Biol Chem* 1988;263:12828–12831.
9. Joyce ME, Roberts AB, Sporn MB, Bolander ME. Transforming growth factor-β and the initiation of chondrogenesis and ostogenesis in the rat femur. *J Cell Biol* 1990;110:2195–2207.
10. Guenther Hl, Guenther HE, Froesch ER, Fleisch H. Effect of insulin-like growth factor-1 on collagen and glycosaminoglycan synthesis by rabbit articular chondrocytes in culture. *Experientia* 1982;38:979–980.
11. McQuillan DJ, Handley CJ, Campbell MA, et al. Stimulation of proteoglycan biosynthesis by serum and insulin-like growth factor-1 in cultured bovine articular cartilage. *Biochem J* 1986;240: 423–430.
12. Schalkwijk J, Joosten LAB, van den Berg WB, van de Putter LBA. Insulin-like growth factor stimulation of chondrocyte proteoglycan synthesis by human synovial fluid. *Arthritis Rheum* 1989;32: 66–67.
13. Tyler JA. Insulin-like growth factor-1 can decrease degradation and promote synthesis of proteoglycan in cartilage exposed to cytokines. *Biochem J* 1986;260:543–548.
14. Kato Y, Gospodarowicz D. Sulfated proteoglycan synthesis by confluent cultures of rabbit costal chondrocytes grown in the presence of fibroblast growth factor. *J Cell Biol* 1985:100;477–485.
15. van den Berg WB, van der Kraan P, Scharstuhl A, van Beuningen HM. Growth factors and cartilage repair. *Clin Orthop* 2001;391: S244–S250.
16. Caterson B, Lowther DA. Changes in metabolism of the proteoglycans from sheep articular cartilage in response to mechanical stress. *Biochim Biophys Acta* 1978;540:412–422.
17. Helminen HJ, Kiviranta I, Saamanen AM, et al. Effect of motion and load on articular cartilage in animal models. In: Kuettner K, ed. *Articular Cartilage and Osteoarthritis*. New York: Raven Press, 1992;503–510.
18. Li, KW, Williamson AK, Wang AS, Sah RL. Growth responses of cartilage to static and dynamic compression. *Orthopedics* 2001; 391:S34–S48.
19. Radin EL, Martin RB, Burr DB, et al. Effects of mechanical loading on the tissues of the rabbit knee. *J Orthop Res* 1984;2:221–234.
20. Frisbie DD, Trotter GW, Powers BE, et al. Arthroscopic subchondral bone plate microfracture technique augments healing of large osteochondral defects in the radial carpal bone and medial femoral condyle of horses. *J Vet Surg* 1999;28:242–255.
21. Frisbie DD, Morisset S, Ho CP, et al. Effects of calcified cartilage on healing of chondral defects treated with microfracture in horses. *Am J Sports Med* 2006;34:1824–1831
22. Frisbie DD, Oxford JT, Southwood L, et al. Early events in cartilage repair after subchondral bone microfracture. *Clin Orthop* 2003; 407:215–227.
23. Steadman JR, Rodkey WG, Rodrigo JJ. "Microfracture": surgical technique and rehabilitation to treat chondral defects. *Clin Orthop* 2001;391S:S362–S369.
24. Steadman JR, Rodkey WG, Briggs KK. Microfracture chondroplasty: indications, techniques, and outcomes. *Sports Med Arthrosc Rev* 2003;11:236–244.
25. Steadman JR, Rodkey WG, Singleton SB, et al. Microfracture procedure for treatment of full-thickness chondral defects: technique, clinical results and current basic science status. In: Harner CD, Vince KG, Fu FH, eds. *Techniques in Knee Surgery*. Media, PA: Williams & Wilkins; 1999;23–31.
26. Steadman JR, Rodkey WG, Briggs KK. Microfracture to treat full-thickness chondral defects. *J Knee Surg* 2002;15:170–176.
27. Steadman JR, Rodkey WG. Microfracture in the pediatric and adolescent knee. In: Micheli LJ, Kocher M, eds. *The Pediatric & Adolescent Knee*. Philadelphia: WB Saunders; 2005:308–311
28. Steadman JR, Karas SG, Miller BS, et al. The microfracture technique in the treatment of full-thickness chondral lesions of the knee in National Football League players. *J Knee Surg* 2003;16:83–86.
29. Blevins FT, Steadman JR, Rodrigo JJ, et al. Treatment of articular cartilage defects in athletes: an analysis of functional outcome and lesion appearance. *Orthopedics* 1998;21:761–768.
30. Rodrigo JJ, Steadman JR, Silliman JF, et al. Improvement of full-thickness chondral defect healing in the human knee after debridement and microfracture using continuous passive motion. *Am J Knee Surg* 1994;7:109–116.
31. Hagerman GR, Atkins JA, Dillman C. Rehabilitation of chondral injuries and chronic degenerative arthritis of the knee in the athlete. *Oper Tech Sports Med* 1995;3:127–135.
32. Irrgang JJ, Pezzullo D. Rehabilitation following surgical procedures to address articular cartilage lesions of the knee. *J Orthop Sports Phys Ther* 1998;28:232–240.
33. Ohkoshi Y, Ohkoshi M, Nagasaki S, et al. The effect of cryotherapy on intraarticular temperature and postoperative care after anterior cruciate ligament reconstruction. *Am J Sports Med* 1999;27: 357–362.
34. Lysholm J, Gillquist J. Evaluation of knee ligament surgery with special emphasis on use of a scoring scale. *Am J Sports Med* 1982;10:150–154.
35. Kocher MS, Steadman JR, Briggs KK, et al. Reliability, validity, and responsiveness of the Lysholm knee scale for various chondral disorders of the knee. *J Bone Joint Surg Am* 2004;86:1139–1145.
36. Tegner Y, Lysholm J. Rating systems in the evaluation of knee ligament injuries. *Clin Orthop* 1985;198:43–49.
37. Bellamy N, Buchanan WW, Goldsmith CH, et al. Validation study of WOMAC: a Health Status Instrument for measuring clinically important patient relevant outcomes to antirheumatic drug therapy in patients with osteoarthritis of the hip or knee. *Rheumatology* 1988;15:1833–1840.
38. Knutsen G, Engebretsen L, Ludvigsen TC, et al. Autologous chondrocyte implantation compared with microfracture in the knee. *J Bone Joint Surg Am* 2004;86:455–464.

Microfracture / Trochlear Groove

Howard Head Sports Medicine Centers
A service of Vail Valley Medical Center

Name: _____

Dr. _____ Date: _____

● = Do exercise for that week

ROM RESTRICTIONS

_____
_____
_____
_____

BRACE SETTINGS

0-20 x 6-8 weeks

WEIGHT BEARING STATUS

Partial 30% WB
x 2 weeks

TIME LINES

Week 1 (1-7POD)
Week 2 (8-14POD)
Week 3 (15-21POD)
Week 4 (22-28POD)

Initial Exercises — WEEK	1	2	3	4	5	6	7	8	9	10	13	17	21	25
Extension/Flexion–wall slides	●	●	●	●	●	●	●	●	●	●				
Extension/Flexion–sitting	●	●	●	●	●	●	●	●	●	●				
Quad sets with straight leg raises	●	●	●	●	●	●	●	●	●	●				
Patellar mobilizations/quad-patellar tendon	●	●	●	●	●	●	●	●	●	●				
Hamstring sets	●	●	●	●	●	●	●	●	●	●				
Ankle pumps	●	●	●	●										
Sit and reach for hamstrings (towel)	●	●	●	●	●	●	●	●	●	●	●	●	●	●
Runners stretch for calf and achilles		●	●	●	●	●	●	●	●	●	●	●	●	●
Stork stand/quad stretching									●	●	●	●	●	●
Toe and heel raises			●	●	●	●	●	●	●	●				
1/3 knee bends									●	●				

Cardiovascular Exercises	1	2	3	4	5	6	7	8	9	10	13	17	21	25
Bike with single leg/single leg rowing	●	●	●	●	●	●								
Bike with both legs			●	●	●	●	●	●	●	●	●	●	●	●
Aquajogging									●	●	●	●	●	●
Treadmill–incline 7-12%										●	●	●	●	●
Swimming with fins											●	●	●	●
Elliptical trainer											●	●	●	●
Rowing											●	●	●	●
Stair stepper												●	●	●

Resisted Exercises	1	2	3	4	5	6	7	8	9	10	13	17	21	25
Double knee bends											●	●		
Carpet drags									●	●	●			
Gas pedal									●	●	●			
Leg press–double leg											●	●	●	●
Single knee bends											●	●	●	●
Balance squats											●	●	●	●
Forward/backward jogging												●	●	●
Side to side lateral agility												●	●	●

Agility Exercises	1	2	3	4	5	6	7	8	9	10	13	17	21	25
Running progression													●	●
Initial													●	●
Advanced														●
Functional Sports Test														●

High Level Activities	1	2	3	4	5	6	7	8	9	10	13	17	21	25
(After Cleared by Physician)														
Golf												●	●	●
Running														●
Skiing, basketball, tennis, football, soccer														●

181 West Meadow Drive
Vail, Colorado 81657
970-476-1225
Fax 970-479-7193

* 7 1 1 9 *

Therapist Name

Microfracture: Femoral Condyle / Tib Plateau

Name: _____

Dr. _____ Date: _____

Howard Head
Sports Medicine Centers
A service of Vail Valley Medical Center

● = Do exercise for that week

ROM RESTRICTIONS
(full prom)

_____

_____

_____

_____

BRACE SETTINGS

(no brace)

WEIGHT BEARING STATUS

Touch Down WB
x 6-8 weeks

TIME LINES
Week 1 (1-7POD)
Week 2 (8-14POD)
Week 3 (15-21POD)
Week 4 (22-28POD)

Initial Exercises WEEK	1	2	3	4	5	6	7	8	9	10	13	17	21	25
Extension/Flexion–wall slides	●	●	●	●	●	●	●	●	●	●				
Extension/Flexion–sitting	●	●	●	●	●	●	●	●	●	●				
Quad sets with straight leg raises	●	●	●	●	●	●	●	●						
Patellar mobilizations/quad-patellar tendon	●	●	●	●	●	●	●	●	●	●				
Hamstring sets	●	●	●	●	●	●	●	●						
Ankle pumps	●	●	●	●										
Sit and reach for hamstrings (towel)	●	●	●	●	●	●	●	●	●	●	●	●	●	●
Runners stretch for calf and achilles									●	●	●	●	●	●
Stork stand/quad stretching									●	●	●	●	●	●
Toe and heel raises									●	●				
1/3 knee bends									●	●	●			
Cardiovascular Exercises	1	2	3	4	5	6	7	8	9	10	13	17	21	25
Bike with single leg/single leg rowing	●	●	●	●	●	●								
Bike with both legs			●	●	●	●	●	●	●	●	●	●	●	●
Aquajogging			●	●	●	●	●	●	●	●	●	●	●	●
Treadmill–incline 7-12%									●	●	●	●	●	●
Swimming with fins									●	●	●	●	●	●
Elliptical trainer											●	●	●	●
Rowing											●	●	●	●
Stair stepper												●	●	●
Resisted Exercises	1	2	3	4	5	6	7	8	9	10	13	17	21	25
Double knee bends											●	●		
Carpet drags									●	●	●			
Gas pedal									●	●	●			
Leg press–double leg											●	●	●	●
Single knee bends											●	●	●	●
Balance squats											●	●	●	●
Forward/backward jogging												●	●	●
Side to side lateral agility												●	●	●
Agility Exercises	1	2	3	4	5	6	7	8	9	10	13	17	21	25
Running progression												●	●	●
Initial												●	●	●
Advanced													●	●
Functional Sports Test													●	●
High Level Activities	1	2	3	4	5	6	7	8	9	10	13	17	21	25
(After Cleared by Physician)														
Golf												●	●	●
Running														●
Skiing, basketball, tennis, football, soccer														●

Copyright ©2006 Rehabilitation and Performance Center at Vail

181 West Meadow Drive
Vail, Colorado 81657
970-476-1225
Fax 970-479-7193

* 7 1 1 8 *

Therapist Name

10

The Healing Response Technique: A Minimally Invasive Procedure to Stimulate Healing of Anterior Cruciate Ligament Injuries Using the Microfracture Technique

J. Richard Steadman   *William G. Rodkey*

■ **INTRODUCTION 153**

■ **BASIC SCIENCE STUDIES 154**
   Gross Observations 155
   Histologic Findings 156
   Biochemical Changes 156

■ **CLINICAL USE AND OUTCOME STUDIES 157**
   Preoperative Considerations 157
   Operative Technique 157
   Postoperative Rehabilitation 157
   Outcome Studies 159

■ **SUMMARY 160**

Defects in the anterior cruciate ligament (ACL) rarely heal spontaneously. The torn ACL sometimes scars to the poste-

rior cruciate ligament (PCL), but this aberrant healing probably does not result in any significant biomechanical function. ACL injuries continue to present a difficult problem for orthopaedic surgeons because it is difficult to predict whether such injuries will cause severe disability or only minimal impairment.

Primary repair of cruciate ligament injuries has often produced less than rewarding results.[1–4] Both clinical and experimental studies have demonstrated poor healing of these intra-articular ligaments.[1–11] This failure to heal completely is thought to be because of the inhibitory effects of the intra-articular environment (poor hematoma formation and a lack of cytokine stimulation) and the inherent inability of the cruciate ligament cells themselves to mount a significant reparative response.[1,7,12,13] Several studies have shown that cruciate ligament cells are less responsive to cytokine stimulation (chemotaxis, mitogenesis, and metabolic activity) than cells from extra-articular ligaments (i.e., medial collateral ligament).[1,5,12,14] Furthermore, the lack of an additional source of reparative cells in the intra-articular environment may further limit the healing response of these intra-articular ligaments.

A similar problem exists in articular cartilage injuries. The inability of chondrocytes to mount a reparative response and the lack of adjacent reparative cells naturally migrating into the wound make the treatment of these lesions very challenging. However, clinical and experimental studies have shown that accessing mesenchymal cells, as well as an array of cytokines, through surgically created connections to the underlying bone marrow ("microfracture" technique), stimulates a "healing response" sufficient enough to repair the defect.[15-23] The efficacy of the microfracture technique to treat articular cartilage defects has been demonstrated both experimentally and clinically.[16-18,20,22] Theoretically, using this same technique to access bone marrow elements might be useful to stimulate intra-articular ligament healing. Hence, a direct extension of the microfracture procedure involves the use of a surgical awl to produce between three and ten microfracture holes in the cortical bone at the femoral footprint of the origin of the injured ACL, or other ligaments intra-articularly, as well as making numerous perforations in the injured ligament itself. In this way, a marrow clot is surgically induced. The clot, which forms after the bone perforations are made, captures the ends of the damaged ligament and provides a rich environment for tissue repair. Previous reports describe the use of microfracture to treat chondral lesions,[16-18,20,22] but until recently there have been no reports on use of the microfracture technique to treat intra-articular ligament injuries.[24,25]

The *healing response*, the term given by the senior author (JRS) who developed this procedure to treat intra-articular ligament injuries, is partly a response to findings by Daniel and coworkers,[26,27] who reported the increased risk of degenerative arthritis following ACL reconstruction. They concluded that a large group of patients with ACL disruption would not benefit from intra-articular reconstruction of the ligament. In fact, such procedures may be detrimental in certain patients. Laboratory studies in primates by McCarthy et al.[28] supported the clinical observations by Daniel and associates.[26,27] Although historically, it has been stated that intra-articularly injured ligaments are not expected to heal,[1,2,4,7-10] use of the microfracture procedure to stimulate healing may be an alternative to intra-articular ligament reconstruction.

This healing response procedure was originally conceived especially for proximal-third ACL injuries, the type frequently seen in skiers. Nonetheless, it has proven its utility in many types of ACL injuries regardless of the injury mechanism. We believe that the healing response procedure has significant advantages that outweigh the potential disadvantages. It is a technically easy procedure for the surgeon to perform, with minimal downside risk. We recently completed a canine study to investigate the morphologic,

cellular, and molecular events that occur within the surgically induced clot and ligament during the healing process.[24] With this new understanding of the basic science of the healing response technique, we were able to assess and better understand our observations in clinical patients.[25]

BASIC SCIENCE STUDIES

These studies were carried out in adult laboratory dogs. After medial parapatellar arthrotomies, we exposed the femoral attachment of the PCL, and a partial-thickness lesion (75% of the PCL width) was made through the PCL adjacent to its bony attachment (Fig. 10.1). We used the PCL in this study because of its ease of access and because the dog is less dependent on this ligament for joint stability.[6] Thus, should a complete rupture have occurred, it would have been less likely to debilitate the animal to the extent that would occur with rupture of the ACL.[6] In one limb of each dog the lacerated PCL was treated with the healing response technique by making six microfracture holes (approximately 2 to 3 mm diameter and 3 to 4 mm deep) in the cortical bone at the femoral origin of the injured ligament with a surgical awl (Fig. 10.2). Bleeding from these holes was observed immediately when the awl penetrated into the marrow space, and a clot formed *in situ* within a few minutes. This surgically induced marrow clot was composed of blood and marrow components as evidenced by the presence of small droplets of fat in the blood. The clot filled the space between the detached ligament and its bony insertion.

As a part of this procedure, the portion of the ligament distal to the lesion was also perforated with the awl

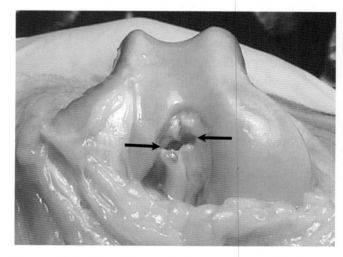

Figure 10.1 Gross photograph of a canine knee (stifle) illustrating the lesion produced in the posterior cruciate ligament (PCL) (delineated by *arrows*). Approximately 75% of the width of the PCL was sharply transected.

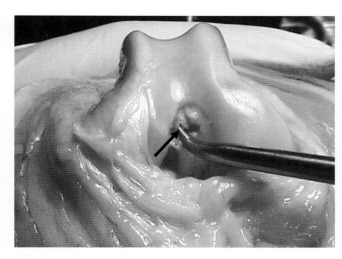

Figure 10.2 Gross photograph illustrating microfracture holes being made into the marrow cavity at the femoral attachment of the posterior cruciate ligament with a surgical awl *(arrow)*.

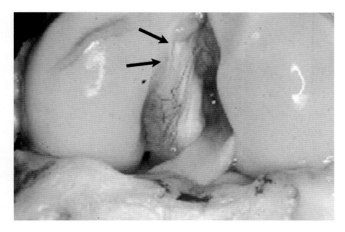

Figure 10.3 Gross photograph of a marrow-stimulated posterior cruciate ligament lesion at 12 weeks. Note the glistening, white repair tissue *(arrows)* that has completely spanned and filled the lesion.

multiple times over its entire length to aid marrow clot invasion. Care was taken to assure that the lacerated end of the ligament was in the correct anatomic location prior to wound closure. No further manipulation or fixation of the ligament or the marrow clot was done. The lacerated PCL in the contralateral limb was not treated with the healing response or any other intervention, and served as a control. Closure of the arthrotomies was done in a routine manner. Joints were not immobilized, and animals were allowed unrestricted activity in individual indoor runs and were observed daily for lameness or other gait abnormalities.[24]

Animals were euthanized after 12 weeks, and healing in both treated and untreated control ligament lesions was evaluated grossly. The character of the repair tissue was also examined using descriptive histology. After formalin fixation of the knee, the PCL with a block of bone incorporating the femoral origin of the ligament, was harvested. The ligament-bone sections were prepared for histologic evaluation. Following staining with hematoxylin and eosin, the sections were examined under light and polarized light. The repair tissue, if present, was characterized in terms of cellularity and extracellular matrix organization.[24]

Gross Observations

The animals had no apparent untoward effects from the surgical procedures and were actively weightbearing immediately postoperatively. No lameness or clinical evidence of joint instability was noted in any of the animals throughout the 12-week period. At harvest, the healing response-treated ligaments showed 81% to 100% healing in five of ten animals, 61% to 80% healing in three of ten animals, and 0% to 20% healing in two of ten animals. Conversely, the nonstimulated control group showed 81% to 100% healing in no animals, 61% to 80% healing in two

of ten animals, 41% to 60% healing in two of ten animals, and 0% to 20% healing in six of ten animals. In the treated ligaments the repair tissue appeared homogeneous, white, and glistening (Fig. 10.3), and it appeared smooth and was contiguous with the substance of the ligament and its femoral attachment. On palpation it felt like normal ligament tissue, and it appeared to tighten and relax like a native PCL when the joint was taken through a range of motion. In the majority of control animals, the portion of the transected PCL distal to the lesion site appeared contracted and rounded off (Fig. 10.4). Although new tissue was present in some of these animals, the PCL attachment to the femur was not completely re-established in any animal. The tissue did not have the same functional appearance as the tissue from the treated knees. Based on these observations, healing response resulted in a statistically significant

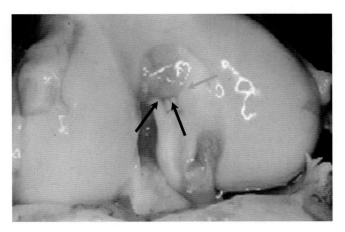

Figure 10.4 Gross photograph of a control posterior cruciate ligament (PCL) lesion at 12 weeks. Although some new tissue is present *(green arrow)*, the majority of the transected PCL has retracted and appears rounded off ends in a ball of scar *(black arrows)*.

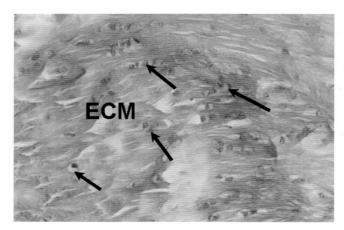

Figure 10.5 The repair tissue in the healing response group demonstrates an abundance of cells *(arrows)* surrounded by a dense extracellular matrix (ECM).

(p <0.05) improvement in ligament healing in this study.[24]

Histologic Findings

The repair tissue in the healing response group always demonstrated an abundance of cells surrounded by a dense extracellular matrix (Fig. 10.5). This dense, regularly oriented connective tissue was mainly composed of fibroblasts and collagen bundles, which always appeared to originate from the marrow access holes and blend into the collagen bundles of the ligament (Fig. 10.6). We also observed excellent integration of the repair tissue into both the treated ligament and its bony insertion.

Conversely, in the untreated controls, the repair tissue (when present) was always characterized as loosely woven connective tissue with limited cellularity and an absence of

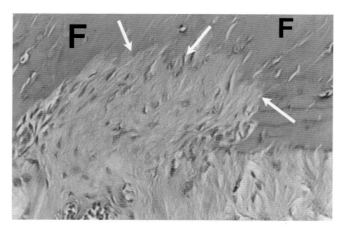

Figure 10.6 Photomicrograph of a longitudinal section of the femoral (F) insertion of the posterior cruciate ligament in a marrow-stimulated specimen. Dense, regularly oriented repair tissue can be seen originating from one of the surgical awl holes *(white arrows)*. (Hematoxylin-eosin stain, original magnification ×200.)

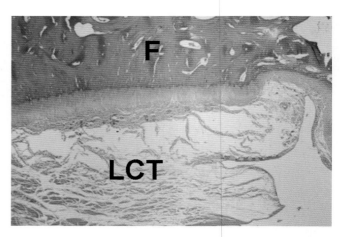

Figure 10.7 Photomicrograph of a longitudinal section of the femoral (F) insertion of the posterior cruciate ligament (PCL) in a control specimen. Disorganized loose connective tissue (LCT) with limited cellularity and poor collagen content can be seen overlying the femoral origin of the PCL. (Hematoxylin-eosin stain, original magnification ×100.)

dense collagen bundles (Fig. 10.7). There was no apparent organization to this repair tissue, and it did not appear contiguous with either the substance of the ligament or its bony insertion.[24]

Biochemical Changes

In another study (as yet unpublished) changes in the tissue concentrations of two growth factors, transforming growth factor-β1 (TGF-β1) and insulinlike growth factor-1 (IGF-1), in the surgically induced marrow clot correlated with gross and histologic changes observed in the forming tissue using the same animal model. These two growth factors were chosen for study because they are abundant in bone and marrow tissue[29–33] and are thought to play key roles in many wound repair settings,[34–36] including ligament healing.[32,37] The joints were harvested at 1, 4, or 7 days so that half the specimens were analyzed grossly and histologically and the remaining half were analyzed biochemically for the two growth factors. The concentration of TGF-β1 in the surgically induced marrow clots was 36.0 ng on day 1 and decreased significantly to 24.0 ng on day 4 and 12.7 ng on day 7 (p <0.05). A different pattern of change was observed in IGF-1 concentrations. The concentration of IGF-1 in the surgically induced marrow clots was 38.2 ng on day 1 and increased significantly to 70.0 ng on day 4 and 78.0 ng on day 7 (p <0.05).

These findings confirm that TGF-β1 and IGF-1 were present in the initial clot, but the respective temporal changes in concentration that they undergo suggest that they play very different roles in the development of new tissue during ligament healing in this model. TGF-β1 likely plays a role in the initial recruitment of macrophages and fibroblasts to the clot, similar to its function in dermal wound healing.[35] The increase with time in the levels of IGF-1 in the clot suggests that this growth factor plays a prominent role in the later stages of the healing process. For example, neovascularization of the surgically induced clots is a delayed event that may be related to increased IGF-1 levels. Regardless of their specific roles, both TGF-β1 and IGF-1 are anabolic and would be expected to play a pivotal role in the recruitment and enlargement of the cell population and in the stimulation of matrix formation by cells during ligament healing.[12,32]

CLINICAL USE AND OUTCOME STUDIES

Preoperative Considerations

The healing response technique was originally conceived as a minimally invasive treatment for proximal-third ACL injuries; however, the indications have broadened with use and long-term experience. The technique is now frequently used in partial tears of the ACL as well as in more severe multiligamentous injuries in which a major reconstruction might be contraindicated early when other stabilization procedures are first undertaken. Even if the healing response is unsuccessful in such a situation, it does not "burn bridges," and a formal reconstruction can be performed under more elective circumstances.

Knees are examined in the clinic, and objective data, including Lachman and pivot shift measurements, are recorded according to the International Knee Documentation Committee score format (Med Metric Corp, San Deigo, CA). A KT1000 measurement is performed preoperatively in those patients in whom the diagnosis of ACL injury is uncertain based on physical examination alone. Standard radiographs are taken in all patients. In young patients, special attention is directed to the status of the physes. All patients also undergo magnetic resonance imaging examination to determine associated injuries, status of the menisci, and tear location of the ACL (Fig. 10.8).

Operative Technique

The healing response is an all-arthroscopic technique.[24,25] The procedure consists of using an arthroscopic microfracture awl with an angle that allows the tip of the awl to be perpendicular to the femoral attachment site of the ACL (Fig. 10.9). With the awl, six to ten holes (approximately 2 to 3 mm diameter and 3 to 4 mm deep) are made into the cortical bone at the origin of the disrupted ligament (Fig. 10.10). The distal stump of the ligament is also perforated with the awl multiple times over its entire length to aid blood clot invasion (Fig. 10.11). Care is taken to assure that the disrupted end of the ligament is

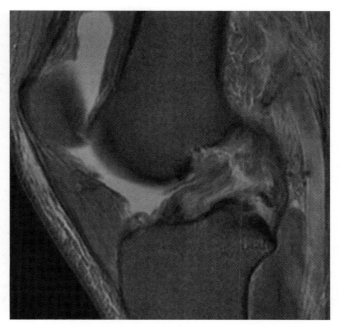

Figure 10.8 Magnetic resonance image of a proximal tear of the anterior cruciate ligament.

manipulated into the correct anatomic location with a probe prior to wound closure. No further manipulation of the ligament or the marrow clot is done, and no fixation is used.

The marrow clot surrounds the end of the ligament and holds it in place[24] (Fig. 10.12). *Extreme caution should be exercised to assure that an open growth plate is not penetrated with the microfracture awl.* Furthermore, if the physis is open, the awl is advanced through the cortex only to avoid impaction injury to the growth plate (Fig. 10.13).

Postoperative Rehabilitation

All patients are placed in a postoperative brace immediately upon completion of the surgical procedure.[25] The brace is locked in full extension to help stabilize the ligament end in the marrow clot. Patients continue to wear the postoperative brace for at least 6 weeks, and thereafter they may be transitioned into a functional ACL brace. Crutch-assisted walking with gradually increasing weightbearing is continued for 2 to 6 weeks. Physical therapy begins within 24 hours postoperatively. Passive range of motion (ROM) exercises are carried out three to four times daily with the brace removed. For days 1 through 3, passive ROM is limited to 0 to 30 degrees only. For days 4 through 7, the passive ROM is 0 to 60 degrees, and it is increased to 0 to 90 degrees for days 8 through 14. From day 15 onward, active full ROM is permitted as tolerated by the patient.

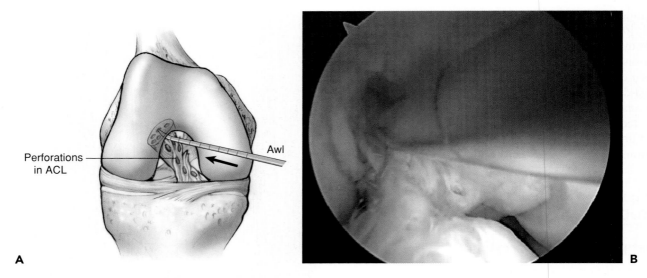

A

B

Figure 10.9 **A:** Illustration demonstrating an arthroscopic microfracture awl with an angle. The tip of the awl is perpendicular to the femoral attachment site of the anterior cruciate ligament. **B:** Arthroscopic view of awl.

For other physical therapy, week 1 is focused on quadriceps control, gait training, and swelling control. During weeks 2 through 6, patients begin isometrics and low-resistance closed kinetic chain activities. Crutches may be discontinued after 2 to 6 weeks. Weeks 6 through 12 involve progressive strengthening, eccentric loading, and initiation of open chain range of motion exercises, with special focus on avoiding patellofemoral pain. Stationary bicycling also may begin at 6 weeks. Weeks 12 through 24 emphasize strengthening, sport-specific conditioning, agility, and proprioceptive training.

Patients are allowed to return to full activity as tolerated after 24 weeks. Ongoing use of the functional ACL brace during athletic activities is recommended postoperatively through at least the first year to further protect the maturing healing site.

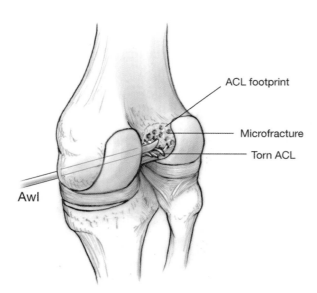

Figure 10.10 Illustration of six to ten holes into the cortical bone at the origin of the disrupted ligament. ACL, anterior cruciate ligament.

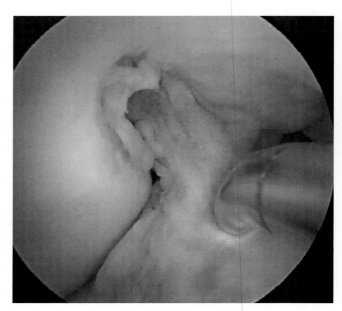

Figure 10.11 The awl is used to perforate the distal stump of the ligament multiple times over its entire length to aid blood clot invasion.

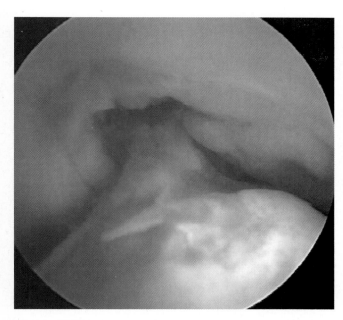

Figure 10.12 A completed healing response with blood at the femoral attachment and in the holes in the ligament.

Outcomes Studies

Between 1992 and 1998, 24 skeletally immature athletes presented with an ACL tear. Of these 24 patients, 13 met the criteria for this study. The inclusion criteria included skeletally immature as defined by open physes on radiographs, a disruption of the ACL in the proximal-third area, and patients who underwent a healing response procedure. Exclusion criteria were patients with previous ACL surgery, other concurrent ligament pathology, and/or complete midsubstance ACL tears. Average preoperative KT1000 manual maximum difference for all patients was 5 mm (range, 3 to 10 mm). Preoperatively, all patients had a

1+ or 2+ pivot shift, and all patients reported knee function as abnormal or severely abnormal. Patients were followed prospectively with clinical examinations, KT1000 testing, and subjective questionnaires.[25]

Three of 13 patients (23%) had fully recovered, but each reinjured her ACL and underwent an ACL reconstruction at 30 months, 40 months, or 55 months status after healing response, respectively. One patient was hurt by contact injuries while playing competitive soccer, one while skiing at a national level, and one patient was injured while performing ballet at the international level. They had continued athletically and epiphyseal closure was complete, allowing standard ACL reconstruction to be performed. Subjective follow-up on the remaining ten patients at an average of 69 months (range, 26 to 113 months) postoperatively confirmed that no patients experienced pain or giving way, and all considered their knee function normal. Average Lysholm score was 96, Tegner score was 8.5 (range, 7 to 10), and patient satisfaction at follow-up was 9.9 (1 = very dissatisfied and 10 = very satisfied).

Clinical examination at least 1 year postoperatively was performed on seven of ten patients at 35 months (range, 12 to 63 months). Five patients had a negative pivot shift and two had a 1+ pivot shift. KT1000 measurements improved to 2 mm (range, 0 to 3 mm). Survivorship analysis showed 92% survivorship at 2 or more years and 70% survivorship at 5 or more years. The end point for survivorship analysis was defined as ACL reconstruction following the healing response procedure. *No patient in this series experienced any growth disturbance after undergoing the healing response procedure.*

Based on these results, we conclude that in athletically active, skeletally immature patients, the healing response procedure can restore stability and knee function. In this study group, patients were very satisfied with the procedure and returned to a high level of sports and other activities.[25]

In another study (unpublished data) of patients more than 40 years of age, the healing response procedure was performed acutely on 198 patients with an average age of 50 years (range, 40 to 74 years). The average time from injury to surgery was 13 days (range, 1 to 42 days). The healing response was performed only on complete proximal-third ACL tears in patients included in the present study. Complete midsubstance ACL tears were excluded. The surgical procedure and rehabilitation were as previously described.

Five patients (2.5%) reinjured their involved ACL and underwent full ACL reconstruction. Two patients died of unrelated causes. Of the remaining 191 patients, 169 (88%) had a minimum 2-year subjective follow-up. Average subjective follow-up was 41 months (range, 24 to 116 months). At the most recent follow-up, 155 patients (92%) experienced no or minimal pain, 165 (98%) had no or minimal swelling, and 161 (95%) had no giving way. Average Lysholm scores improved from 63 to 94.

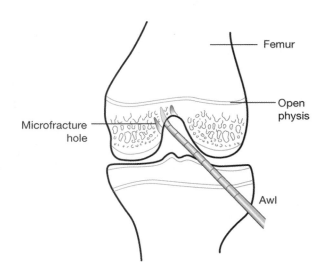

Figure 10.13 Illustration of the open physis and the location of the awl during the healing response.

Activities of daily living scores improved from 4.6 to 8.7 (10 = normal function). One hundred fifty-nine patients (94%) considered their knee function to be normal or nearly normal. Average patient satisfaction at the latest follow-up was 9.1 (on a 1 to 10 scale). Clinical examinations were performed at 2 or more years after healing response on 122 of 191 patients (64%). Average clinical follow-up was done at 45 months (range, 24 to 116 months). The clinical examinations revealed that 85 patients (70%) had a negative pivot shift, 30 (25%) had a 1+ and 7 (5%) had a 2+. The KT1000 manual maximum difference testing improved from an average of 5.0 mm preoperatively to 1.9 mm postoperatively, a mean difference of 3.1 mm ($p < 0.05$).

These data confirm that the healing response technique restored ligament stability and knee function in patients more than 40 years of age with torn ACLs in the proximal-third of the ligament. The healing response technique is an effective alternative to restore structural integrity to the proximally torn ACL.

SUMMARY

The healing response procedure, an all-arthroscopic, minimally invasive method to treat the torn ACL, is a direct extension of the microfracture technique to treat chondral lesions. It was originally conceived especially for proximal-third ACL injuries, the type frequently seen in skiers. Nonetheless, it has proven its utility in many types of ACL injuries regardless of the injury mechanism. The healing response procedure has been proven to have significant advantages that outweigh the potential disadvantages. It is a technically easy procedure for the surgeon to perform with minimal downside risk. The findings reported here, both basic science and clinical data, support the hypothesis that the surgically induced marrow clot that results from the healing response procedure supports progressive development of functionally competent healing tissue at the site of the ligament injury. The marrow clot appears to provide an enriched milieu conducive to ligament healing.

REFERENCES

1. Amiel D, Kuiper S, Akeson WH. Cruciate ligaments. Response to injury. In: Daniel DM, Akeson WH, O'Connor JJ, eds. *Knee Ligaments. Structure, Function, Injury, and Repair.* New York: Raven Press; 1990:365–377.
2. Andersson C, Odensten M, Gillquist J. Knee function after surgical or nonsurgical treatment of acute rupture of the anterior cruciate ligament: a randomized study with a long-term follow-up period. *Clin Orthop* 1991;164:255–263.
3. Feagin JA, Curl WW. Isolated tears of the anterior cruciate ligament: five year followup study. *Am J Sports Med* 1976;4:95–100.
4. Steadman JR, Rodkey WG. Role of primary anterior cruciate ligament repair with or without augmentation. *Clin Sports Med* 1993;12:685–695.
5. Arnoczky SP. Physiologic principles of ligament injuries and healing. In: Scott WN, ed. *Ligament and Extensor Mechanism Injuries of the Knee: Diagnosis and Treatment.* St. Louis, MO: CV Mosby; 1991:67–81.
6. Arnoczky SP, Marshall JL. The cruciate ligaments of the canine stifle: an anatomical and functional evaluation. *Am J Vet Res* 1977;38:1807–1814.
7. Arnoczky SP, Rubin RM, Marshall JL. Microvasculature of the cruciate ligaments and its response to injury. An experimental study in dogs. *J Bone Joint Surg Am* 1979;61:1221–1229.
8. Bonamo JJ, Fay C, Firestone T. The conservative treatment of the anterior cruciate ligament deficient knee. *Am J Sports Med* 1990;18:618–623.
9. Buss DD, Min R, Skyhar M, et al. Nonoperative treatment of acute anterior cruciate ligament injuries in a selected group of patients. *Am J Sports Med* 1995;23:160–165.
10. Hawkins RJ, Misamore GW, Merritt TR. Followup of the acute nonoperated isolated anterior cruciate ligament tear. *Am J Sports Med* 1986;14:205–210.
11. O'Donoghue DH, Rockwood CA Jr, Frank GR, Jack SC, Kenyon R. Repair of the anterior cruciate ligament in dogs. *J Bone Joint Surg Am* 1966;48:503–519.
12. Amiel D, Nagineni CN, Choi SH, Lee J. Intrinsic properties of ACL and MCL cells and their responses to growth factors. *Med Sci Sports Exerc* 1995;27:844–851.
13. Murray MM, Martin SD, Martin TL, Spector M. Histological changes in the human anterior cruciate ligament after rupture. *J Bone Joint Surg Am* 2000;82:1387–1397.
14. Andriacchi TP, Sabiston P, DeHaven KE, et al. Ligament: Injury and repair. In: Woo S L-Y, Buckwalter JA, eds. *Injury and Repair of the Musculoskeletal Soft Tissues.* Park Ridge, IL: American Academy of Orthopaedic Surgeons; 1988:103–128.
15. Frisbie DD, Oxford JT, Southwood L, et al. Early events in cartilage repair after subchondral bone microfracture. *Clin Orthop* 2003;407:215–227.
16. Frisbie DD, Trotter GW, Powers BE, et al. Arthroscopic subchondral bone plate microfracture technique augments healing of large osteochondral defects in the radial carpal bone and medial femoral condyle of horses. *J Vet Surg* 1999;28:242–255.
17. Rodrigo JJ, Steadman JR, Silliman JF, Fulstone HA. Improvement of full-thickness chondral defect healing in the human knee after debridement and microfracture using continuous passive motion. *Am J Knee Surg* 1994;7:109–116.
18. Steadman JR, Briggs KK, Rodrigo JJ, et al. Outcomes of patients treated arthroscopically by microfracture for traumatic chondral defects of the knee: average 11-year follow-up. *Arthroscopy* 2003;19:477–484.
19. Steadman JR, Rodkey WG, Briggs KK. Microfracture to treat full thickness chondral defects. Surgical technique, rehabilitation and outcomes. *J Knee Surg* 2002;15:1–7.
20. Steadman JR, Rodkey WG, Briggs KK. Microfracture chondroplasty: Indications, techniques, and outcomes. *Sports Med Arthrosc* 2003;11:236–244.
21. Steadman JR, Rodkey WG, Rodrigo JJ. Microfracture: Surgical technique and rehabilitation to treat chondral defects. *Clin Orthop* 2001;391S:S362–S369.
22. Steadman JR, Rodrigo JJ, Briggs KK, et al. Debridement and microfracture ("Pick Technique") for full-thickness articular cartilage defects. In: Insall JN, Scott WN, eds. *Surgery of the Knee.* 3rd ed. New York: Churchill Livingstone; 2001:361–373.
23. Steadman JR, Rodkey WG, Singleton SB, et al. Microfracture procedure for treatment of full-thickness chondral defects: Technique, clinical results and current basic science status. In: Harner CD, Vince KG, Fu FH, eds. *Techniques in Knee Surgery.* Media, PA: Williams & Wilkins; 1999:23–31.
24. Rodkey WG, Arnoczky SP, Steadman JR. Healing of a surgically created partial detachment of the posterior cruciate ligament using marrow stimulation: an experimental study in dogs. *J Knee Surg* 2006;19:14–18.
25. Steadman JR, Cameron-Donaldson ML, Briggs KK, Rodkey WG. A minimally invasive technique ("healing response") to treat proximal ACL injuries in skeletally immature athletes. *J Knee Surg* 2006;19:8–13.

26. Daniel DM, Stone ML, Dobson, et al. Fate of the ACL-injured patient. A prospective outcome study. *Am J Sports Med* 1994;22: 632–644.

27. Daniel DM. Selecting patients for ACL surgery. In: Jackson DW, Arnoczky SP, Frank CB, et al., eds. *The Anterior Cruciate Ligament: Current and Future Concepts.* New York, Raven Press; 1993: 31–55.

28. McCarthy JA, Howe Z, Lippiello L, et al. The effect of ACL deficiency and reconstruction on knee articular cartilage. *Trans Orthop Res Soc* 1993;18:355.

29. Linkhart TA, Keffer MJ. Differential regulation of insulin-like growth factor-1 (IGF-1) and IGF-II release from cultured neonatal mouse calvaria by parathyroid hormone, transforming growth factor-β, and 1,25-dihydroxyvitamin D3. *Endocrinology* 1991;128: 1511–1518.

30. Linkhart TA, Mohan S, Baylink DJ. Growth factors for bone growth and repair: IGF, TGF beta and BMP. *Bone* 1996;19(1 Suppl): 1S–12S.

31. Schmid C. Insulin-like growth factors. *Cell Biol Int* 1995;19: 445–457.

32. Woo SL, Hildebrand K, Watanabe N, et al. Tissue engineering of ligament and tendon healing. *Clin Orthop* 1999;367(Suppl): S312–S323.

33. Zhang RW, Supowit SC, Xu X, et al. Expression of selected osteogenic markers in the fibroblast-like cells of rat marrow stroma. *Calcified Tissue Int* 1995;56:283–291.

34. Greenhalgh DG. The role of growth factors in wound healing. *J Trauma* 1996;41:159–167.

35. Wahl SM, Hunt DA, Wakefield LM, et al. Transforming growth factor beta induces monocyte chemotaxis and growth factor production. *Proc Natl Acad Sci U S A* 1987;84:5788–5792.

36. Wong MEK, Hollinger JO, Pinero GJ. Integrated processes responsible for soft tissue healing. *Oral Surg Oral Med Oral Pathol* 1996;82:475–492.

37. Liu SH, Yang R-S, Al-Shaikh R, et al. Collagen in tendon, ligament, and bone healing. *Clin Orthop Relat Res* 1995;318:265–278.

ACL Healing Response

Name: _____

Dr. _____ Date: _____

Howard Head
Sports Medicine Centers
A service of Vail Valley Medical Center

● = Do exercise for that week

ROM RESTRICTIONS

_____

_____

_____

_____

_____

BRACE SETTINGS

0-0 x 6 weeks

WEIGHT BEARING STATUS

Partial 30% WB
x 1-2 weeks

TIME LINES
Week 1 (1-7POD)
Week 2 (8-14POD)
Week 3 (15-21POD)
Week 4 (22-28POD)

Initial Exercises	WEEK	1	2	3	4	5	6	7	8	9	10	13	17	21	25
Extension/Flexion–wall slides		●	●	●	●	●	●	●	●	●	●				
Extension/Flexion–sitting		●	●	●	●	●	●	●	●	●	●				
Quad sets with straight leg raises		●	●	●	●	●	●								
Patellar mobilizations/quad-patellar tendon		●	●	●	●	●	●	●	●	●	●				
Hamstring sets		●	●	●	●	●	●								
Ankle pumps		●	●	●	●										
Sit and reach for hamstrings (towel)		●	●	●	●	●	●	●	●	●	●	●	●	●	●
Runners stretch for calf and achilles				●	●	●	●	●	●	●	●	●	●	●	●
Stork stand/quad stretching								●	●	●	●	●	●	●	●
Toe and heel raises			●	●	●	●	●								
1/3 knee bends								●	●	●					

Cardiovascular Exercises	1	2	3	4	5	6	7	8	9	10	13	17	21	25
Bike with single leg/single leg rowing	●	●	●	●	●	●								
Bike with both legs			●	●	●	●	●	●	●	●	●	●	●	●
Aquajogging							●	●	●	●	●	●	●	●
Treadmill–incline 7-12%							●	●	●	●	●	●	●	●
Swimming with fins							●	●	●	●	●	●	●	●
Elliptical trainer									●	●	●	●	●	●
Rowing									●	●	●	●	●	●
Stair stepper											●	●	●	●

Resisted Exercises	1	2	3	4	5	6	7	8	9	10	13	17	21	25
Double knee bends							●	●	●	●				
Carpet drags							●	●	●	●				
Gas pedal							●	●	●	●				
Leg press–double leg									●	●	●	●	●	●
Single knee bends										●	●	●	●	●
Balance squats										●	●	●	●	●
Forward/backward jogging											●	●	●	●
Side to side lateral agility											●	●	●	●

Agility Exercises	1	2	3	4	5	6	7	8	9	10	13	17	21	25
Running progression												●	●	●
Initial												●	●	●
Advanced													●	●
Functional Sports Test													●	●

High Level Activities	1	2	3	4	5	6	7	8	9	10	13	17	21	25
(After Cleared by Physician)														
Golf													●	●
Running													●	●
Skiing, basketball, tennis, football, soccer														●

181 West Meadow Drive
Vail, Colorado 81657
970-476-1225
Fax 970-479-7193

7132

Therapist Name

Arthrofibrosis of the Knee: Diagnosis and Management

11

Peter J. Millett

■ **INTRODUCTION 163**

■ **PATHOPHYSIOLOGY 163**
Contributing Factors 163
  Prior Surgery 164
  Anterior Cruciate Ligament Nodule 164
  Graft Malposition 164
  Prolonged Immobilization 166
  Infection 166
  Anterior Interval/Extensor Mechanism Scarring 166

■ **DIAGNOSIS 166**

■ **TREATMENT 167**
Nonoperative Treatment 167
Surgical Treatment 167
  Surgical Treatment When Infection Is Suspected 169
  Surgical Treatment When Infection Is Not Likely 169
Arthroscopic Treatment 169
  Capsular Distention 169
  Suprapatellar Pouch 170
  Medial and Lateral Gutters 170
  Anterior Interval/Pretibial Recess 171
Combined Arthroscopic and
  Open Surgical Treatment 171
Open Surgical Treatment 171
  Open Debridement and Releases 171
  Medial Release 172
  Extensor Mechanism Release and Patellar Eversion 172
  Ligament and Capsular Releases 173

■ **POSTOPERATIVE MANAGEMENT 173**

■ **OUTCOMES 174**

■ **CONCLUSION 174**

Arthrofibrosis of the knee is a difficult clinical problem that usually manifests as knee pain and loss of motion. There are a variety of definitions and causes of arthrofibrosis. In the majority of patients, early recognition and treatment can effectively restore motion and alleviate pain. Successful treatment also allows patients to restore function and to improve their activity level. In order to treat arthrofibrosis appropriately, the clinician must understand the pathoanatomic causes of motion loss so that treatment can be targeted appropriately. The purpose of this chapter is to review the diagnosis and management of arthrofibrosis of the knee.

PATHOPHYSIOLOGY

Contributing Factors

Arthrofibrosis in the knee is a complex, multifactorial process with a variety of causative factors. Simple mechanical blocks to extension or flexion cause the most obvious types of motion problems,[1] although more subtle types that involve the extensor mechanism may be more common but more difficult to diagnose. In order to develop effective preventive, diagnostic, and treatment strategies, it is important to understand the myriad causes of motion loss.

Arthrofibrosis is a process in which abnormal scar tissue forms in the knee in response to injury or surgery. The process usually manifests itself as joint stiffness or loss of motion. Sometimes the findings are more subtle and only present as pain. Because the causes for motion loss are broad, in our practice we find it useful to subdivide them into problems that cause loss of flexion and problems that cause loss of extension (Table 11.1). When an individual presents with a motion problem that involves both flexion and extension, it is important to identify the causes of the motion loss. The goals of treatment should be to attempt to re-establish full extension first and then to restore flexion, because the loss of flexion is usually better tolerated and is also easier to treat.[2,3] There are also types of arthrofibrosis that affect only the extensor mechanism and do not result in loss of motion. These are more subtle forms of the disease that will also be discussed in this chapter.

Prior Surgery

Prior surgery is a common cause of knee stiffness. Historically, arthrofibrosis and motion problems were relatively common after ligament surgery, particularly anterior cruciate ligament (ACL) surgery. Fortunately, the incidence of clinically relevant motion loss after ACL reconstruction has decreased with a better understanding of risk factors, with improvements in surgical technique, and with better rehabilitation programs.[4-11] In the literature, the incidence of motion problems after ligament injury or surgery has been variable.[3-5,8,9,12] Some of this variability may have been the result of inconsistencies across studies in how the injuries were defined, in how the injuries were treated both surgically and rehabilitatively, and in how the motion loss was

defined within each study. Shelbourne and Rask[13] defined motion loss very strictly and stressed the importance of using the contralateral knee as the norm for comparison. In their report, any deviation in motion from that of the normal, contralateral limb was considered abnormal or arthrofibrotic. Other authors have defined arthrofibrosis as a deviation of 5 degrees from full extension.[10]

In our practice, we consider loss of motion to be a deviation in flexion or extension from the contralateral side. Furthermore, we even recognize that there are more subtle forms of arthrofibrosis in which the flexion and extension arcs are symmetrical, but because of loss of mobility in the extensor mechanism (patella, patellar tendon, quadriceps tendon) or because of stiffness in the joint capsule, the patients are considered to have arthrofibrosis. Loss of mobility in the extensor mechanism, although less recognized, can have relevant clinical manifestations most commonly presenting as anterior knee pain. This type of arthrofibrosis can be particularly troubling for high-level athletes. In most instances, arthrofibrosis becomes more clinically relevant as the degree of motion loss increases, with significant disability occurring when the side-to-side difference in extension is greater than 10 degrees.

Anterior Cruciate Ligament Nodule

In cases of motion loss following ACL reconstruction, a fibroproliferative scar nodule (ACL nodule or cyclops lesion) can occur, which typically results in pain during knee extension. This localized form of arthrofibrosis usually begins to manifest itself clinically at about 2 to 3 months postoperatively. ACL nodules are most commonly located anterolateral to the tibial tunnel[3,14,15] and are typically attached to the ACL graft, as well as to the soft tissue overlying the tibia (Fig. 11.1). The nodules are composed of dense fibrous tissue with a central area of granulation tissue. As the knee moves into extension, impingement occurs between the ACL nodule and the intercondylar notch, blocking terminal extension. Hypertrophy of the graft or other soft tissue scarring in the notch can cause a similar block to extension.[16,17]

Graft Malposition

Technical factors such as graft malposition can also contribute to postoperative loss of motion.[3,18,19] Although technically not a form of arthrofibrosis, it is important to consider graft malpositioning in the differential diagnosis of patients who present with motion loss of the knee. Proper graft positioning is essential to prevent graft impingement (Fig. 11.2) and to allow normal knee kinematics. ACL grafts that are placed in the wrong position can obviously interfere with normal knee motion.[20,21] Graft position must be accurate in both the coronal and sagittal planes to ensure that the graft functions correctly and does not cause limited motion.

When the cruciate ligaments are reconstructed, the tibial and femoral attachment sites must be anatomically accurate

TABLE 11.1
CAUSES OF MOTION LOSS

Loss of Extension	Loss of Flexion
Malpositioned or nonisometric graft (anterior tibial tunnel, anterior femoral tunnel)	Suprapatellar adhesions
Notch impingement	Patellar entrapment
ACL nodule	Medial and lateral gutter adhesions or fibrosis
Infrapatellar contracture syndrome	Improper graft position
Captured joint capsule after meniscal repair	Infrapatellar contracture syndrome
Posterior capsular scarring	Reflex sympathetic dystrophy
Hamstring tightness	Soft tissue calcifications of capsule or MCL
MCL calcification	Postinfection
Postoperative infection	Quadriceps contracture or myositis
Reflex sympathetic dystrophy	

ACL, anterior cruciate ligament; MCL, medial collateral ligament.

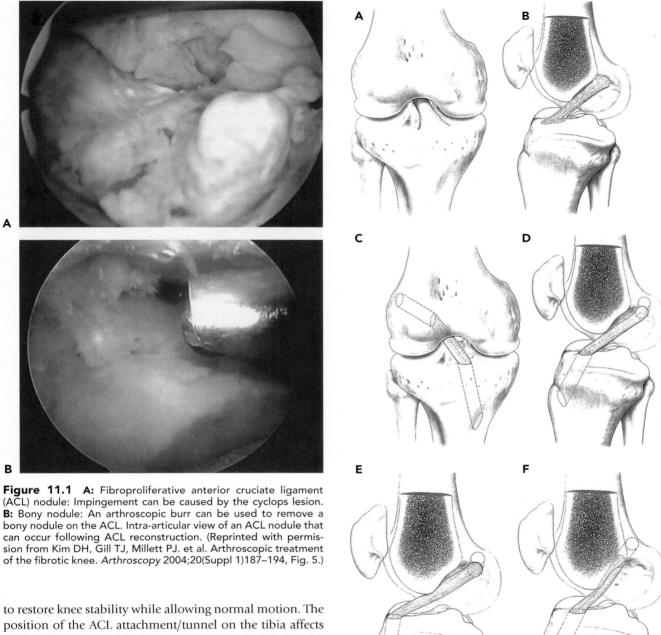

Figure 11.1 A: Fibroproliferative anterior cruciate ligament (ACL) nodule: Impingement can be caused by the cyclops lesion. **B:** Bony nodule: An arthroscopic burr can be used to remove a bony nodule on the ACL. Intra-articular view of an ACL nodule that can occur following ACL reconstruction. (Reprinted with permission from Kim DH, Gill TJ, Millett PJ. et al. Arthroscopic treatment of the fibrotic knee. *Arthroscopy* 2004;20(Suppl 1)187–194, Fig. 5.)

to restore knee stability while allowing normal motion. The position of the ACL attachment/tunnel on the tibia affects both range of motion and impingement in the intercondylar notch.[22] Malposition can cause excessive stress on the graft, development of an ACL nodule, or graft failure. In our experience, a tibial tunnel that is placed too far anterior results in limited flexion because of excessive graft tension and also limited extension from graft impingement (Fig. 11.2E). The graft must also be placed in the correct coronal plane position with enough obliquity across the joint to re-establish the normal rotational stability and to prevent persistent rotational instability.

Improper placement of the femoral tunnel can also be a cause for loss of motion. In the sagittal plane, the ideal femoral tunnel is placed in the posterior wall of the femoral notch, leaving 1 to 2 mm of posterior wall remaining.[20] An anterior femoral tunnel can lead to loss of

Figure 11.2 Proper tunnel placement is essential to prevent graft impingement and motion loss. **A, B:** Normal ACL anatomy; **C,D:** Proper anterior cruciate ligament graft position; **E:** The effects of anterior tibial tunnel placement. Notice the impingement of the graft in the intercondylar notch during terminal extension. **F:** The effects of anterior femoral tunnel placement. Notice the impingement of the graft in the intercondylar notch with extension. This results in loss of extension or graft failure. (Reprinted with permission from Millett PJ, Wickiewicz TL, Warren RF. Motion loss after ligament injuries to the knee. *Am J Sports Med* 2001;29:664–675, Fig. 1.)

motion, graft failure, or both (Fig. 11.2F). Coronal plane abnormalities of the femoral tunnel, most commonly an excessively vertical tunnel, are more commonly associated with persistent rotational instabilities. When using a transtibial drilling technique for ACL reconstruction it is important to recognize that the femoral tunnel position is influenced by the tibial tunnel position.

Overtensioning of the graft has been proposed as a potential cause of motion loss,[23] but we believe that excessive graft tension in a properly positioned graft will not, in and of itself, cause motion loss because of the viscoelastic properties of the ligament when the knee is moved through a full range of motion.

Prolonged Immobilization

Many studies have demonstrated the detrimental effects of prolonged immobilization on periarticular cartilage, bone, and soft tissues. Through the years, joint immobility has been one of the more common causes of arthrofibrosis and motion loss.[24–26] Fortunately, with modern rehabilitation programs that stress early motion and weightbearing, there are fewer reports of motion problems and better outcomes.[9,10,27–30] Our current rehabilitation programs after ACL reconstruction, meniscus repair, or cartilage restoration focus on early motion to prevent arthrofibrosis. A more recent addition to our program is patellar mobilization to prevent scarring around the patella and patellar tendon.

Infection

Infection should always be considered a cause or contributing factor to arthrofibrosis. Unrecognized or untreated infections will cause an inflammatory response that results in scarring and loss of tissue compliance. This results in pain and stiffness. Although fulminant infections with highly virulent organisms may be easily recognized, more subtle infections with organisms of low virulence may be completely missed. Infection must always be considered in the diagnosis of arthrofibrosis and must always be considered a potential cause of the disease until proven otherwise. The workup of suspected infection is discussed later in this chapter.

Anterior Interval/Extensor Mechanism Scarring

Paulos et al.[25] were among the first researchers to describe the infrapatellar contracture syndrome as a cause of posttraumatic knee stiffness with patellar entrapment and patella infera (baja). Patients who develop infrapatellar contracture syndrome have a combination of restricted knee extension and flexion associated with patellar entrapment. This is another localized form of arthrofibrosis that is caused by an exaggerated pathologic fibrous hyperplasia in the anterior fat pad.[25,32–36] Prolonged immobility and lack of extension, particularly after intra-articular ACL reconstruction, seem to be contributing factors. The fat pad becomes densely adherent to the underlying tibia, resulting in diminished excursion of the patella and loss of motion.

In more subtle cases of anterior interval scarring, flexion and extension arcs may be full, but the infrapatellar fat pad and patellar tendon adhere to the anterior tibial cortex below the inferior pole of the patella. The normal pretibial recess of the knee is obliterated, and the anterior interval adhesions prevent normal motion of the intermeniscal ligament over the tibial plateau during flexion and extension. Furthermore, the anterior horn of the medial meniscus fails to glide anteriorly and posteriorly with flexion and extension. These observations can be made at the time of arthroscopy.[32–36]

DIAGNOSIS

Usually, the correct diagnosis may be made from a careful history and physical examination. When patients are initially evaluated, a complete knee examination should be performed. If the chief complaint is stiffness, then goniometric measurements of knee flexion and extension angles should be performed. Patellar mobility in four directions, superior, inferior, medial, and lateral should also be assessed (Fig 11.3). The presence or absence of an effusion or a temperature differential between knees should also be noted. By monitoring active flexion and extension and palpating for crepitus or a "clunk," the clinician may be able to detect an ACL nodule.[34] The clinician should be alerted to the possibility of reflex sympathetic dystrophy when patients have pain out of proportion to examination, allodynia, and trophic or sudomotor changes.

A large, persistent hemarthrosis in the knee postoperatively causes a reflex inhibition of the quadriceps and can lead to motion problems. The effusion induces a quadriceps muscle avoidance gait pattern even in healthy persons.[35] Research from our laboratory has demonstrated the

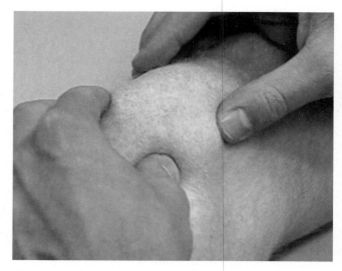

Figure 11.3 Assessment of patellar mobility.

negative effect that an effusion has on quadriceps activity.[35] Effusions not only cause the knee to be held in a flexed position (the greatest volume and least tension on the joint capsule) but can also cause an extension lag because of the quadriceps inhibition. Prevention of hemarthroses postoperatively is a key step that will allow for a more comfortable return of knee motion and will help prevent quadriceps muscle shutdown. When a large hemarthrosis occurs, it is sometimes prudent to evacuate it to prevent the adverse effects.

Radiographs may be useful to assess tunnel placement and patellofemoral alignment in the appropriate settings. Patella baja or graft malposition can be determined. When loss of patellar motion is noted on physical examination, we carefully assess patellar height, tilt, and subluxation on the radiographs. Previous hardware or old fractures can also be assessed by the radiographs when necessary. If we have questions or if the specific cause of the arthrofibrosis is unclear, we obtain a magnetic resonance image (MRI) to evaluate the soft tissues. An ACL nodule, fat pad scarring, anterior interval scarring, or graft malposition can be seen on the MRI (Fig. 11.4). Because excessive scarring can cause increased compression on articular cartilage,[36] in more severe cases, we also carefully evaluate the chondral surfaces with MRI.

Infection is among the most common causes of arthrofibrosis, so it is critical to be alert to any sign of infection. If there is any suspicion of infection, routine blood screening tests should be obtained. These typically include a complete blood count, an erythrocyte sedimentation rate, and a C-reactive peptide. Although these are nonspecific markers of inflammation, they are quite sensitive. If they are positive, we assume there is an occult infection that is contributing to the arthrofibrosis. In such instances, consultation with an infectious disease specialist is encouraged.

Further tests and evaluations, including an arthrocentesis, may be warranted. If the organism is not identified preoperatively and infection is suspected, the surgeon should withhold preoperative antibiotics so that intraoperative cultures can be obtained. Cultures from multiple samples will increase both the sensitivity and specificity in the event that it is a low virulent organism.

TREATMENT

The treatment of arthrofibrosis after soft tissue injury or surgery to the knee should be targeted to the specific cause. Preventive strategies include appropriate patient selection, technically correct surgery, and early rehabilitation that is focused on restoring and maintaining joint mobility. Prevention of motion loss is obviously the best strategy; however, when this fails and motion problems occur, early detection and treatment can help prevent severe sequelae. A careful and systematic approach should be used to establish the correct diagnosis, and once the cause of the motion loss is established, treatment can be targeted accordingly. We have developed a treatment algorithm for use in patients with loss of motion (Fig. 11.5).[31]

Nonoperative Treatment

Many patients in whom motion loss has developed can be treated nonoperatively. When concerns about motion loss or arthrofibrosis occur, our nonoperative protocol includes (a) early and appropriate rehabilitation with a skilled therapist; (b) anti-inflammatory medications; (c) rest, ice, compression, and elevation to alleviate swelling and decrease pain; and (d) aspiration of large joint effusions. The goal is to avoid creating more swelling or more inflammation. On occasion, patients are placed on crutches and therapy is stopped to allow the time for the joint to recover. This is particularly helpful in the early postoperative period when the joint is hot or warm or severely swollen. Ongoing stretching and rehabilitation in such settings is likely to create more injury. Other times when flexion or extension is lacking in the early postoperative period, dynamic bracing is used. This is most effective when there has been no progression with manual techniques and there are no signs of ongoing joint inflammation.

Surgical Treatment

Arthroscopic or open surgical treatments are indicated when nonoperative measures have failed or when there is a surgically correctable cause of motion loss. Operative intervention is not used alone; surgical treatment is always combined with specific rehabilitation and pain-management protocols. Our surgical treatment evaluates and treats all the anatomic areas that can be involved in the process of arthrofibrosis.[27]

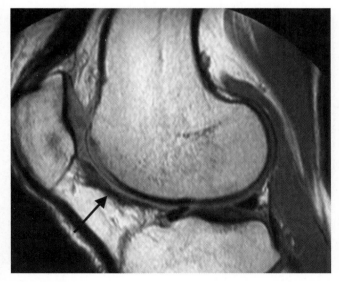

Figure 11.4 Magnetic resonance image demonstrating anterior interval scarring (*arrow*).

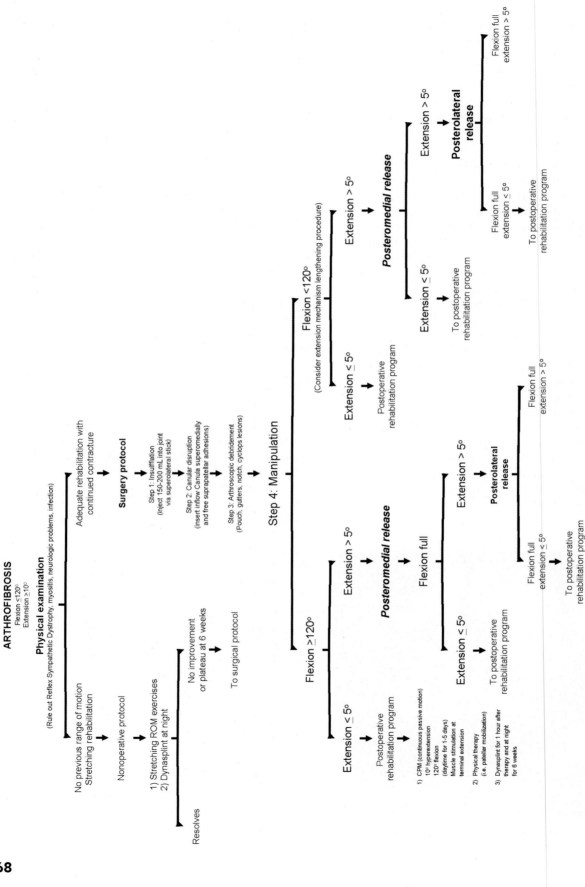

Figure 11.5 Treatment algorithm for patients with loss of motion.

ARTHROFIBROSIS
Flexion ≤120°
Extension ≥10°

Physical examination
(Rule out Reflex Sympathetic Dystrophy, myositis, neurologic problems, infection)

No previous range of motion
Stretching rehabilitation

Adequate rehabilitation with
continued contracture

Nonoperative protocol

Surgery protocol

1) Stretching ROM exercises
2) Dynasplint at night

Step 1: Insufflation
(inject 150-200 mL into joint
via superolateral stick)

Step 2: Canular disruption
(insert inflow Canula superomedially
and free suprapatellar adhesions)

No improvement
or plateau at 6 weeks

Step 3: Arthroscopic debridement
(Pouch, gutters, notch, cyclops lesions)

To surgical protocol

Step 4: Manipulation

Resolves

Flexion ≥120°

Flexion <120°
(Consider extension mechanism lengthening procedure)

Extension ≤ 5°

Extension > 5°

Extension ≤ 5°

Extension > 5°

Postoperative
rehabilitation program

Posteromedial release

Postoperative
rehabilitation program

Posteromedial release

1) CPM (continuous passive motion)
10° hyperextension
120° flexion
(daytime for 1-5 days)
Muscle stimulation at
terminal extension

Flexion full

Extension ≤ 5°

Extension > 5°

Flexion full
extension ≤ 5°

Extension > 5°

2) Physical therapy
(i.e. patellar mobilization)

3) Dynasplint for 1 hour after
therapy and at night
for 6 weeks

Extension ≤ 5°

Extension > 5°

To postoperative
rehabilitation program

**Posterolateral
release**

To postoperative
rehabilitation program

**Posterolateral
release**

Flexion full
extension ≤ 5°

Flexion full
extension > 5°

Flexion full
extension ≤ 5°

Flexion full
extension > 5°

To postoperative
rehabilitation program

To postoperative
rehabilitation program

Surgical Treatment When Infection Is Suspected

In cases in which there are signs of an infection as the cause of arthrofibrosis, urgent or emergent treatment is recommended. We recommend a preoperative evaluation that includes a complete history and physical examination with careful evaluation to exclude the possibility of a synchronous site of infection, the blood work previously mentioned, an MRI to exclude the possibility of an abscess or osteomyelitis, and a preoperative consultation with an infectious disease specialist. Arthrocentesis can be performed preoperatively in the office using sterile technique if there is an effusion. When surgery is needed, preoperative antibiotics should be withheld so that there will be a good chance of isolating the organism from operative culture specimens. Multiple samples should be obtained for culture to increase the chance of making an accurate diagnosis of the offending organism. In many instances of arthrofibrosis, the cause will be infection with organisms of low virulence. If multiple microbiology culture specimens become positive with the same organism, the likelihood is increased that that specific organism is actually the cause of the problem and is not simply a contaminant. Empiric antibiotics can be administered after the cultures are obtained and then postoperatively until the cultures come back to guide therapeutic antibiotics. In such cases, the first priority should be to eradicate the infection by surgical and medical treatment. Once the infection is cured, a second or third staged surgery may be needed to restore knee mobility.

Surgical Treatment When Infection Is Not likely

Anesthesia and Postoperative Analgesia

All patients generally receive regional epidural anesthesia or regional anesthesia with femoral nerve blocks. After surgery, catheters should be left in place for patient-controlled analgesia. We believe that this type of anesthesia provides better postoperative pain control and therefore allows more intensive physical therapy in the immediate postoperative period. The standard pain-control protocol involves fentanyl citrate and mepivacaine hydrochloride with a low-dose continuous infusion and a patient-controlled rescue dose, up to a maximum of four doses per hour.[27] Patients are routinely assessed by separate pain-management teams who titrate analgesics individually. When significant releases are performed, it is important that patients are monitored for excessive swelling to prevent missing a compartment syndrome by excessive analgesia.

Arthroscopic Treatment

Capsular Distention

We have found that capsular distention with saline at the time of arthroscopy is an important adjunct in the arthroscopic treatment of loss of motion of the knee.[31] The normal knee has a volume of approximately 180 mL, and we attempt to introduce that volume of saline into knees that are

being treated surgically for motion problems. Capsular distention re-establishes the effective joint space, which makes the insertion of arthroscopic instruments easier and safer. Furthermore, visualization is enhanced because scarred joint spaces have been separated and there is a relative tamponade of any vessels. Capsular distention also safely stretches the capsule in those regions, particularly the posterior capsule, that are not easily reached with standard arthroscopic portals. In our experience, this decreases the need for additional portals or incisions to release the posterior structures.[31]

With the patient under anesthesia, the patient's knee joint with loss of motion is palpated prior to arthroscopy. Severe scarring can make it difficult to identify the various surface landmarks. Under sterile conditions, normal saline is injected into the suprapatellar pouch from the lateral side. As the fluid is injected we carefully watch and feel the joint distention to ensure that the fluid is entering the true joint space. A 60-mL syringe and an 18-gauge needle are used.

In patients with significant adhesions or compartmentalization of the suprapatellar pouch, care must be taken to verify that the fluid is entering the true joint space, and not the quadriceps musculature. As the capsule is distended, care should be taken to avoid rupturing the joint capsule, allowing the capsule to stretch over time. Preservation of the true joint capsule prevents extravasation of the fluid during the arthroscopy and facilitates visualization. After the knee is maximally distended with saline, we insert the arthroscopic instruments. We prefer to make a high midlateral portal first as this allows one to see the anterior interval of the knee, a common location for scarring (Fig. 11.6). To date, we have had no complications from the adjunctive use of capsular distention. We routinely use this technique on arthrofibrotic knees.

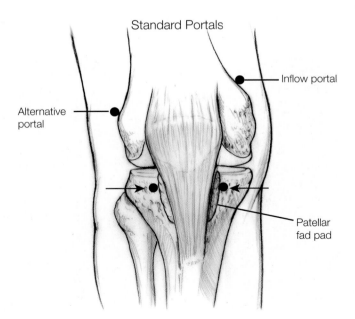

Figure 11.6 Location of a high midlateral portal, which allows for visualization of the anterior interval of the knee.

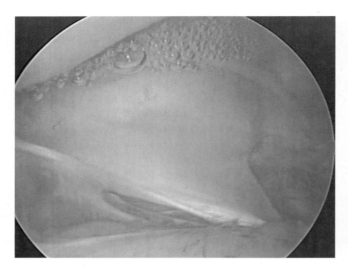

Figure 11.7 A scarred suprapatellar pouch.

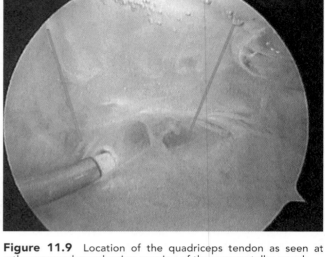

Figure 11.9 Location of the quadriceps tendon as seen at arthroscopy when releasing scarring of the suprapatellar pouch.

Suprapatellar Pouch

Although we normally prefer to perform a complete three-compartment diagnostic evaluation before we perform operative treatment, in arthrofibrotic knees it is often necessary to establish a working space so that visualization is achieved. In cases of arthrofibrosis, particularly severe cases, we prefer to re-establish the suprapatellar pouch first so we can obtain adequate visualization. The scar tissue is removed with radiofrequency ablation, a suction punch, and a shaver.

Adhesions in the suprapatellar pouch typically limit patellar mobility and can restrict knee flexion (Fig 11.7). The proximal extent of the pouch should be approximately 3.5 cm from the superior pole of the patella. A foreshortened pouch can lead to a further loss of knee flexion. In the suprapatellar pouch we use an electrocautery to lyse adhesions and release scarring to re-establish the pouch. It is

important to remember that the pouch is quite large and should extend 3 to 4 cm proximal to the patella and releases should continue until this is achieved (Fig. 11.8). Care should be taken to avoid injuring the quadriceps tendon (Fig. 11.9).

Medial and Lateral Gutters

The medial and lateral gutters are important locations for scar tissue. It is important to look for adhesions in this region. Often one can see adhesions that have formed between the capsule and the femoral condyles (Fig. 11.10). A suction punch or electrocautery can be used to remove adhesions from the lateral gutter. In severe cases, the retinacula are released to restore patellar mobility. Care should be taken when performing retinacular releases to avoid destabilizing the patella or incising the muscles of the quadriceps.

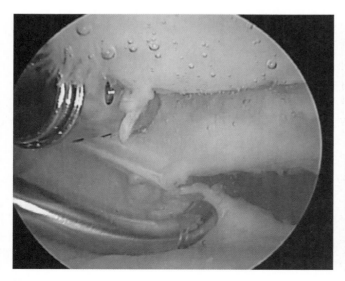

Figure 11.8 An electrocautery is used to lyse adhesions and release scarring to re-establish the suprapatellar pouch.

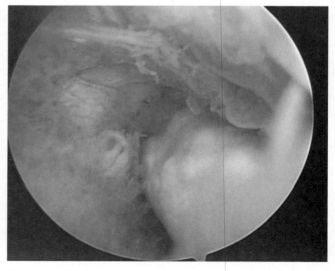

Figure 11.10 Adhesions located in the lateral gutter.

Anterior Interval/Pretibial Recess

The interval between the patellar fat pad and anterior tibia is released to re-establish the pretibial recess. For an anterior interval release, the arthroscope is placed in an inferolateral portal relative to the patella and the working instruments in an inferomedial portal. The inferolateral viewing portal should be placed at the level of the patella with the knee in full extension. This high portal was originally described by Patel.[37] It is approximately 1 cm proximal to the standard inferolateral arthroscopy portal and provides clear visualization of the anterior soft tissues in the retropatellar and pretibial regions.

An anterior interval release should be performed by releasing this scar tissue (Fig. 11.11) from medial to lateral, just anterior to the peripheral rim of the anterior horn of each meniscus. The release can be performed with either electrocautery or a thermal ablation device (Arthrocare; Arthrocare Corporation, Sunnyvale, CA). The release also should proceed from proximal (at the level of the meniscus) to approximately 1 cm distal along the anterior tibial cortex. Great care should be taken to avoid cauterizing or causing thermal necrosis to bone of the anterior tibia or the patellar tendon. Meticulous hemostasis should be obtained in the infrapatellar fat pad to prevent a postoperative effusion or recurrent scarring.

Combined Arthroscopic and Open Surgical Treatment

In certain refractory cases, a posteromedial or posterolateral release, or both, may be necessary. This can be performed in conjunction with an arthroscopic procedure.[31]

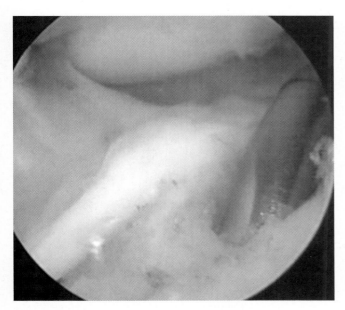

Figure 11.11 Scar tissue released at the anterior interval. Tissue is released medial to lateral just anterior to the peripheral rim of the anterior horn of each meniscus.

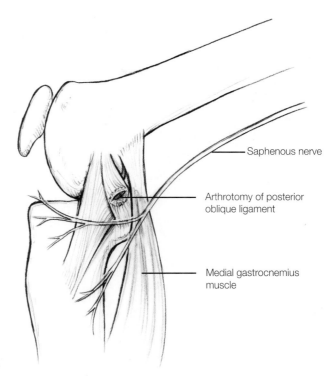

Saphenous nerve

Arthrotomy of posterior oblique ligament

Medial gastrocnemius muscle

Figure 11.12 A posteromedial limited arthrotomy is used to release the posterior oblique ligament. This arthrotomy can also be used to release the posterior capsule in severe cases.

Usually arthroscopic releases are performed first and then, if persistent stiffness that is attributable to a tight posterior capsule remains, a limited open procedure is added. A limited posteromedial arthrotomy can be performed, releasing the posterior oblique ligament (Fig. 11.12). Placing a hemostat into the joint allows the surgeon to identify the medial collateral ligament and to palpate the joint line and posterior oblique ligament so that the incision and release can be performed through a limited incision. In severe cases, a posterolateral arthrotomy can also be added to release to posterior capsule completely (Fig. 11.13). Care should be taken on the lateral side to avoid the popliteal nerve.

Open Surgical Treatment

Open Debridement and Releases

A small subset of patients will either fail nonoperative and arthroscopic techniques to restore motion or will have such severe scarring that arthroscopic surgery is technically impossible. In some patients, severe periarticular and intra-articular fibrosis can make arthroscopic techniques futile, while in others, obvious extra-articular contractures or graft malpositioning may destine arthroscopic techniques to failure. In such instances, an open procedure becomes the logical alternative to restore motion and normal kinematics to the knee. To restore flexion, releases may need to be performed for severe intra-articular fibrosis that, in some

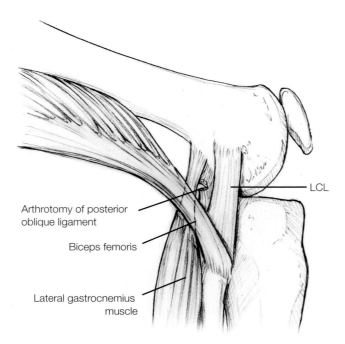

Figure 11.13 A posterolateral arthrotomy. LCL, lateral collateral ligament.

cases, can be several centimeters thick. To restore extension, anterior fibrosis, posterior capsular scarring, and graft-notch problems should be addressed.

Medial Release

The subcutaneous tissues should first be dissected in order to visualize the extensor mechanism. Undermining of soft tissue flaps is avoided. A medial parapatellar arthrotomy is performed through the medial aspect of the quadriceps tendon and the medial retinaculum, over the medial aspect of the patella, and down onto the anterior tibia (Fig. 11.14). A medial release should be performed by careful subperiosteal dissection of the soft tissues over the medial tibial cortex. The periosteum can be elevated to the level of the posterior tibial plateau, and the subperiosteal dissection can include the deep medial collateral ligament and the semimembranosus tendon (Fig. 11.15).[38] This release will help in mobilizing the tibia and regaining extension. Care should be taken to maintain a medial soft tissue sleeve and to preserve the superficial medial collateral ligament.

To re-establish the medial and lateral gutters, a combination of blunt and sharp dissection will be required to remove the dense adhesions and fibrosis. Using sharp dissection, the anterior joint capsule and intra-articular adhesions/fibrosis should be thoroughly debrided.

Extensor Mechanism Release and Patellar Eversion

Scar tissue is universally encountered in the infrapatellar fat pad and pretibial recess. This should be carefully removed, preserving the intermeniscal ligament. The patellar tendon should be mobilized from the anterosuperior border of the tibia. Particular care must be taken to preserve the insertion of the patellar tendon into the tibial tubercle, avoiding excessive tension on the patellar tendon. A release of the lateral retinaculum can be performed to assist in eversion of the patella and to gain additional exposure (Fig. 11.16). The release is typically performed using an inside-out technique. Care should be taken to identify and preserve the

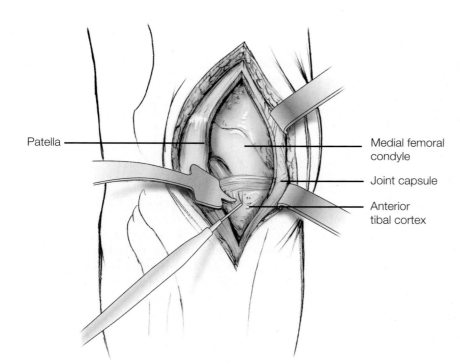

Figure 11.14 A medial parapatellar arthrotomy from the medial aspect of the quadriceps tendon and the medial retinaculum over the medial aspect of the patella, and down onto the anterior tibia.

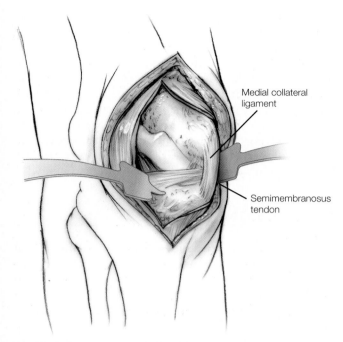

Figure 11.15 Dissection of the subperiosteal, including the deep medial collateral ligament and the semimembranosus tendon.

superior lateral geniculate vessels. When eversion of the patella is not possible, the arthrotomy should be extended proximally, and more extensor mechanism scar tissue must be removed until the patella can be everted. In particularly tight knees, moving the tibia anteriorly while rotating externally is a maneuver that can be helpful with exposure. To be able to mobilize the patients immediately after surgery and to avoid further disruption of the extensor mechanism,

quadriceps-plasties, such as rectus snips, V-Y plasties, and patellar turndowns, should be avoided.

The undersurface of the extensor mechanism and all peripatellar scar tissue are then excised until the patella is freely mobilized. Patellofemoral tracking can be assessed at intervals throughout each procedure.

Ligament and Capsular Releases

After mobilization of the extensor mechanism, release of the anterior structures, and excision of intra-articular adhesions, passive flexion and extension should be assessed. If the individual has had prior ligament surgery, the grafts can be assessed for malposition or impingement. If necessary, the ACL can be excised along with any associated fixation hardware. The tibia can now be subluxated anteriorly so that the posterior collateral ligament (PCL) and posterior aspect of the knee can be explored.

The knee should be passively extended to check for PCL or capsular impingement. The capsule is inspected first. If there is a posterior capsular contracture that is contributing to extension loss, a generous posterior capsular release can be performed. The "femoral peel," as advocated by Windsor and Insall,[38] will help restore extension in knees with severe flexion contractures. The femoral attachment of the posterior capsule can be safely "peeled" away from the posterior femur, effectively skeletonizing the femur and eliminating flexion contractures. The medial and lateral collateral ligaments should be protected. The posterior capsule can also be debrided of any thickened scar tissue. In the event that the PCL is malpositioned, impinges, or blocks motion, it may be excised. Instability postoperatively is not typically seen.[39]

If a flexion contracture persists after these releases, one may consider releasing the posterior from the proximal tibia using a periosteal elevator or a large curette, although one should be cautious of the neurovascular structures that may also be encased in the scar. This subperiosteal dissection can be carried distally until full extension is achieved or it is unsafe to proceed. Thus, in severe cases, both the posterior femur and tibia can be skeletonized in a single posterior layer.

POSTOPERATIVE MANAGEMENT

To take advantage of the analgesic properties provided by the indwelling epidural catheter or femoral nerve block, patients are typically hospitalized for 48 hours. Our rehabilitation is based on the specific procedure that was performed and a continuous re-evaluation of the patient.[40] In the immediate postoperative period, patients are placed in a continuous passive motion (CPM) machine for at least 8 to 10 hours a day to maintain the range of motion obtained in the operating room. CPM is less effective than manual mobilization for the terminal ranges of motion. Home CPM is continued for 2 to 3 weeks. Most patients remain

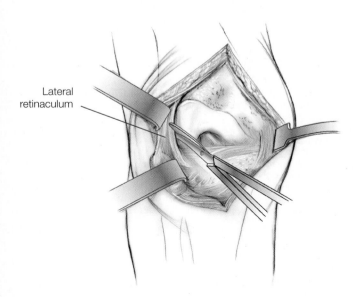

Figure 11.16 The release of the lateral retinaculum assists with the eversion of the patella and additional exposure.

on crutches with protected weightbearing for a few days; in more severe cases they may remain on crutches for 10 to 14 days until the swelling resolves.

Dynamic bracing can be used to help maintain full extension, although these devices are occasionally not well tolerated. Patellar mobility exercises, extensor mechanism exercises, and full passive and active-assisted range of motion exercises are all essential components of therapy, which begin on the first postoperative day. Daily outpatient physical therapy visits start when patients are discharged and should continue for 6 to 8 weeks. Stationary bicycling may begin immediately, whereas aquatherapy and resistance exercises are begun at 2 weeks, if range of motion is maintained and swelling is controlled.

OUTCOMES

There have been several reports on the outcomes of arthroscopic treatment of arthrofibrosis. Most reports have been on arthrofibrosis following ACL reconstruction.[1-3,6,10,16,41,42] The "cyclops" lesion after ACL reconstruction was first described by Jackson and Schaefer.[3] They reported on 13 patients who underwent arthroscopic debridement with knee manipulation. The patients' extension improved on average 12 degrees. Marzo et al.[41] reported on 21 patients who improved extension an average of 11 degrees after arthroscopic removal of fibrous nodules in the intercondylar notch. Other studies have also shown improvements in function and symptoms with arthroscopic debridement of anterior scar formation in combination with aggressive rehabilitation and serial extension casting.[16,42,43]

In our experience, most patients following arthroscopic treatment for loss of motion return to a high level of function and activity. In a group of patients with loss of motion who underwent arthroscopic treatment, we found 6% required a second arthroscopy at an average of 2.8 years (range, 0.5 to 7 years). Of the patients who did not require surgery, at an average follow-up of 4.2 years, patients had an average satisfaction of 8 (range, 2 to 10) (1 = very unsatisfied; 10 = very satisfied with outcome). The average Tegner activity level was 5 (range, 1 to 10). The average Lysholm score was 82 (range, 18 to 100).

Outcomes in patients following open knee debridement showed improvement in range of motion and function.[39] This study looked at a small group of patients with severely restricted motion. Following open debridement and soft tissue release, the patients gained more than 40 degrees of flexion and more than 17 degrees of extension. The Lysholm improved 35 points. However, at follow-up, patellofemoral arthrosis was commonly seen on radiographs. The patellar tendon was also shortened, which the authors stated was indicative of ongoing extensor mechanism problems.[39]

The most effective treatment for arthrofibrosis is prevention by delaying ACL reconstruction. In our practice, the criteria for performing an ACL reconstruction on either an acutely injured patient or a chronic ACL-deficient patient includes (a) a minimum active range of motion of 0 to 120 degrees, (b) ability to perform a straight-leg raise similar to the unaffected side with no loss of extension, and (c) active quadriceps control demonstrated by quadriceps definition symmetric to the unaffected side while performing quadriceps contraction. Based on these criteria, we have experienced a very low rate of arthrofibrosis and no increased incidence of decreased range of motion when an ACL reconstruction was performed within 3 weeks of injury.[44]

CONCLUSION

Loss of knee motion has a variety of causes and for optimal outcomes treatment should be targeted at the specific cause. Our arthroscopic approach allows the surgeon to systematically address all of the intra-articular pathoanatomy. We evaluate and re-establish the suprapatellar pouch followed by the medial and lateral gutters. Next, the anterior interval, infrapatellar fat pad, and pretibial recess should be re-established. The medial and lateral retinaculum are evaluated and releases performed if necessary. Electrocautery is essential to minimize bleeding. The intercondylar notch must be carefully evaluated because this is often a major site of pathology. Scar tissue, ACL nodules, bony nodules, or malpositioned grafts can all cause loss of motion problems.

The final two steps involve evaluation of the medial and lateral posterior capsule at both the tibial and femoral insertions. For those patients with persistent loss of extension after comprehensive arthroscopic treatment, limited open releases should be undertaken.

Open releases are reserved for severe cases in which patients have failed other treatments or the scarring is so complete that arthroscopy is technically impossible.

REFERENCES

1. Dandy DJ, Edwards DJ. Problems in regaining full extension of the knee after anterior cruciate ligament reconstruction: does arthrofibrosis exist? *Knee Surg Sports Traumatol Arthrosc* 1994;2: 76–79.
2. Irrgang JJ, Harner CD. Loss of motion following knee ligament reconstruction. *Sports Med* 1995;19:150–159.
3. Jackson DW, Schaefer RK. Cyclops syndrome: Loss of extension following intra-articular anterior cruciate ligament reconstruction. *Arthroscopy* 1990;6:171–178.
4. Cosgarea AJ, Sebastianelli WJ, DeHaven KE. Prevention of arthrofibrosis after anterior cruciate ligament reconstruction using the central third patellar tendon autograft. *Am J Sports Med* 1995;23:87–92.
5. Fried JA, Bergfeld JA, Weiker G, et al. Anterior cruciate reconstruction using the Jones-Ellison procedure. *J Bone Joint Surg Am* 1985;67:1029–1033.
6. Harner CD, Irrgang JJ, Paul J, et al. Loss of motion after anterior cruciate ligament reconstruction. *Am J Sports Med* 1992;20:499–506.
7. Johnson RJ, Eriksson E, Haggmark T, et al. Five- to 10-year follow-up evaluation after reconstruction of the anterior cruciate ligament. *Clin Orthop* 1984;183:122–140.

8. Kornblatt I, Warren RF, Wickiewicz TL. Long-term followup of anterior cruciate ligament reconstruction using the quadriceps tendon substitution for chronic anterior cruciate ligament insufficiency. *Am J Sports Med* 1988;16:444–448.

9. Plancher KD, Steadman JR, Briggs KK, et al. Reconstruction of the anterior cruciate ligament in patients who are at least forty years old. A long-term follow-up and outcome study. *J Bone Joint Surg Am* 1998;80:184–197.

10. Shelbourne KD, Wilckens JH, Mollabashy A, et al. Arthrofibrosis in acute anterior cruciate ligament reconstruction. The effect of timing of reconstruction and rehabilitation. *Am J Sports Med* 1991;19:332–336.

11. Zarins B, Rowe CR. Combined anterior cruciate-ligament reconstruction using semitendinosus tendon and iliotibial tract. *J Bone Joint Surg Am* 1986;68:160–177.

12. Millett PJ, Wickiewicz TL, Warren RF. Motion loss after ligament injuries to the knee. Part I: Causes. *Am J Sports Med* 2001;29:664–675.

13. Shelbourne KD, Rask BP. Controversies with anterior cruciate ligament surgery and rehabilitation. *Am J Knee Surg* 1998;11:136–143.

14. Fullerton LR Jr, Andrews JR. Mechanical block to extension following augmentation of the anterior cruciate ligament. A case report. *Am J Sports Med* 1984;12:166–168.

15. Recht MP, Piraino DW, Cohen MA, et al. Localized anterior arthrofibrosis (cyclops lesion) after reconstruction of the anterior cruciate ligament: MR imaging findings. *AJR Am J Roentgenol* 1995;165:383–385.

16. Fisher SE, Shelbourne KD. Arthroscopic treatment of symptomatic extension block complicating anterior cruciate ligament reconstruction. *Am J Sports Med* 1993;21:558–564.

17. Marzo JM, Bowen MK, Warren RF, et al. Intraarticular fibrous nodule as a cause of loss of extension following anterior cruciate ligament reconstruction. *Arthroscopy* 1992;8:10–18.

18. Sprague NF III: Motion-limiting arthrofibrosis of the knee: the role of arthroscopic management. *Clin Sports Med* 1987;6:537–549.

19. Sprague NF III, O'Connor RL, Fox JM. Arthroscopic treatment of postoperative knee fibroarthrosis. *Clin Orthop* 1982;166:165–172.

20. Petsche TS, Hutchinson MR. Loss of extension after reconstruction of the anterior cruciate ligament. *J Am Acad Orthop Surg* 1999;7:119–127.

21. Fu FH, Bennett CH, Ma CB, et al. Current trends in anterior cruciate ligament reconstruction. Part II. Operative procedures and clinical correlations. *Am J Sports Med* 2000;28:124–130.

22. Yaru NC, Daniel DM, Penner D. The effect of tibial attachment site on graft impingement in an anterior cruciate ligament reconstruction. *Am J Sports Med* 1992;20:217–220.

23. Melby A III, Noble JS, Askew MJ, et al. The effects of graft tensioning on the laxity and kinematics of the anterior cruciate ligament reconstructed knee. *Arthroscopy* 1991;7:257–266.

24. Enneking WF, Horowitz M. The intra-articular effects of immobilization on the human knee. *J Bone Joint Surg Am* 1972;54:973–985.

25. Paulos LE, Rosenberg TD, Drawbert J, et al. Infrapatellar contracture syndrome: an unrecognized cause of knee stiffness with patella entrapment and patella infera. *Am J Sports Med* 1987;15:331–341.

26. Sisto DJ, Warren RF. Complete knee dislocation. A follow-up study of operative treatment. *Clin Orthop* 1985;198:94–101.

27. Millett PJ, Wickiewicz TL, Warren RF. Motion loss after ligamentous injuries to the knee: Part II: Prevention and treatment. *Am J Sports Med* 2001;29:822–828.

28. Noyes FR, Barber-Westin SD. Reconstruction of the anterior and posterior cruciate ligaments after knee dislocation. Use of early protected postoperative motion to decrease arthrofibrosis. *Am J Sports Med* 1997;25:769–778.

29. Noyes FR, Mangine RE, Barber SD. The early treatment of motion complications after reconstruction of the anterior cruciate ligament. *Clin Orthop* 1992;277:217–228.

30. Shelbourne KD, Gray T. Anterior cruciate ligament reconstruction with autogenous patellar tendon graft followed by accelerated rehabilitation. A two- to nine-year followup. *Am J Sports Med* 1997;25:786–795.

31. Steadman JR, Burns TP, Peloza J. Surgical treatment of arthrofibrosis of the knee. *J Orthop Tech* 1993;1:119–127.

32. Montgomery JB, Steadman JR. Rehabilitation of the injured knee. *Clin Sports Med* 1985;4:333–343.

33. Paulos LE, Wnorowski DC, Greenwald AE. Infrapatellar contracture syndrome. Diagnosis, treatment, and long-term followup. *Am J Sports Med* 1994;22:440–449.

34. Delince P, Krallis P, Descamps PY, et al. Different aspects of the cyclops lesion following anterior cruciate ligament reconstruction: a multifactorial etiopathogenesis. *Arthroscopy* 1998;14:869–876.

35. Torry MR, Decker MJ, Viola RW, et al. Intra-articular knee joint effusion induces quadriceps avoidance gait patterns. *Clin Biomech (Bristol, Avon)* 2000;15:147–159.

36. Ahmad CS, Kwak SD, Ateshian GA, et al. Effects of patellar tendon adhesion to the anterior tibia on knee mechanics. *Am J Sports Med* 1998;26:715–724.

37. Patel D. Proximal approaches to arthroscopic surgery of the knee. *Am J Sports Med* 1981;9:296–303.

38. Windsor RE, Insall JN. Exposure in revision total knee arthroplasty: the femoral peel. *Tech Orthop* 1988;3:1–4.

39. Millett PJ, Williams RJ III, Wickiewicz TL. Open debridement and soft tissue release as a salvage procedure for the severely arthrofibrotic knee. *Am J Sports Med* 1999;27:552–561.

40. Millett PJ, Johnson B, Carson J, Krishnan S, Steadman JR. Rehabilitation of the arthrofibrotic knee. *Am J Orthop* 2003;32:531–538.

41. Marzo JM, Bowen MK, Warren RF, et al. Intraarticular fibrous nodule as a cause of loss of extension following anterior cruciate ligament reconstruction. *Arthroscopy* 1992;8:10–18.

42. Shelbourne KD, Johnson GE. Outpatient surgical management of arthrofibrosis after anterior cruciate ligament surgery. *Am J Sports Med* 1994;22:192–197.

43. Shelbourne KD, Patel DV, Martini DJ. Classification and management of arthrofibrosis of the knee after anterior cruciate ligament reconstruction. *Am J Sports Med* 1996;24:857–862.

44. Sterett WI, Hutton KS, Briggs KK, Steadman JR. Decreased range of motion following acute versus chronic anterior cruciate ligament reconstruction. *Orthopedics* 2003;26:151–154.

Lysis of Adhesions / Arthrofibrosis

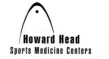

Howard Head
Sports Medicine Centers
A service of Vail Valley Medical Center

Name: _____

Dr. _____ Date: _____

● = Do exercise for that week

ROM RESTRICTIONS
(full prom)
_____
_____
_____
_____

BRACE SETTINGS
(no brace)

WEIGHT BEARING STATUS
Partial 30% WB
x 1-2 weeks

TIME LINES
Week 1 (1-7POD)
Week 2 (8-14POD)
Week 3 (15-21POD)
Week 4 (22-28POD)

Initial Exercises — WEEK	1	2	3	4	5	6	7	8	9	10	13	17	21	25
Extension/Flexion–wall slides	●	●	●	●	●	●	●	●	●	●				
Extension/Flexion–sitting	●	●	●	●	●	●	●	●	●	●				
Quad sets with straight leg raises	●	●	●	●	●	●								
Patellar mobilizations/quad-patellar tendon	●	●	●	●	●	●	●	●	●	●				
Hamstring sets	●	●	●	●	●	●								
Ankle pumps	●	●	●	●										
Sit and reach for hamstrings (towel)	●	●	●	●	●	●	●	●	●	●	●	●	●	●
Runners stretch for calf and achilles	●	●	●	●	●	●	●	●	●	●	●	●	●	●
Stork stand/quad stretching			●	●	●	●	●	●	●	●	●	●	●	●
Toe and heel raises		●	●	●	●	●								
1/3 knee bends						●	●							

Cardiovascular Exercises	1	2	3	4	5	6	7	8	9	10	13	17	21	25
Bike with single leg/single leg rowing	●	●	●	●	●	●								
Bike with both legs	●	●	●	●	●	●	●	●	●	●	●	●	●	●
Aquajogging			●	●	●	●	●	●	●	●	●	●	●	●
Treadmill–incline 7-12%							●	●	●	●	●	●	●	●
Swimming with fins							●	●	●	●	●	●	●	●
Elliptical trainer									●	●	●	●	●	●
Rowing									●	●	●	●	●	●
Stair stepper											●	●	●	●

Resisted Exercises	1	2	3	4	5	6	7	8	9	10	13	17	21	25
Double knee bends							●	●	●	●				
Carpet drags							●	●	●	●				
Gas pedal							●	●	●	●				
Leg press–double leg											●	●	●	●
Single knee bends											●	●	●	●
Balance squats											●	●	●	●
Forward/backward jogging											●	●	●	●
Side to side lateral agility											●	●	●	●

Agility Exercises	1	2	3	4	5	6	7	8	9	10	13	17	21	25
Running progression											●	●	●	●
Initial											●	●	●	●
Advanced												●	●	●
Functional Sports Test												●	●	●

High Level Activities	1	2	3	4	5	6	7	8	9	10	13	17	21	25
(After Cleared by Physician)														
Golf											●	●	●	●
Running												●	●	●
Skiing, basketball, tennis, football, soccer													●	●

181 West Meadow Drive
Vail, Colorado 81657
970-476-1225
Fax 970-479-7193

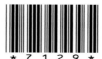

7129

_____
Therapist Name

Arthroscopic Treatment of the Degenerative Knee

12

J. Richard Steadman

■ INTRODUCTION 177

■ INITIAL EVALUATION 177

■ PATIENT SELECTION 178

■ TREATMENT PACKAGE 178

■ POSTOPERATIVE CARE 182

■ OUTCOMES 182

The usefulness of arthroscopic treatment of osteoarthritis of the knee was recently challenged after one article showed there was no benefit when it was compared with irrigation or placebo.[1] Although this article was statistically well constructed, it did fail to address several issues that, in my opinion, are crucial to the success of arthroscopic treatment of osteoarthritis of the knee. There are many characteristics in the degenerative knee that can produce pain. These include stiffness, synovitis, loose bodies, meniscus tears, and closed spaces due to compartmentalization, or old adhesions. Also, chondral defects or flaps can cause pain. In my experience, painful symptoms decrease about 70% of the time if these conditions are treated arthroscopically. Many of the studies have used arthroscopic techniques that include lavage, debridement, and abrasion arthroplasty.[2–14] However, these studies have not focused on increasing joint volume, treating capsular contracture,

and performing synovectomy. Furthermore, most of the studies have not emphasized the importance of the role of postoperative rehabilitation. *Correct rehabilitation is essential to address stiffness, maintain joint volume, and achieve maximum range of motion.* Strengthening exercises also protect the joint by improving concentric and eccentric muscle contraction. The goal of my arthroscopic treatment regimen is to allow patients to resume their active lifestyles, decrease their disability, and delay total knee arthroplasty.

INITIAL EVALUATION

Patients may present with a variety of conditions. Many patients have malalignment, joint stiffness, a prior meniscectomy, and/or instability with stiffness. Symptoms include pain, swelling, stiffness, and mechanical symptoms. In the degenerative knee, pain generators include stiffness, synovitis, loose bodies, meniscus tears, and stiffness due to closed spaces from compartmentalization or old adhesions. Loss of patellar mobility is common in the knee with degenerative joint disease. This is usually accompanied by diminished range of motion, particularly in extension. Loss of articular cartilage in the degenerative knee may not cause pain if these other conditions are corrected.

Radiographic evaluation includes standing anteroposterior, 45 degree flexion posteroanterior, long standing, and patellar views. The long standing view from hip to ankle allows for the evaluation of malalignment, and the 45 degree flexion view will show any diminished joint space posteriorly. Evaluating joint malalignment is discussed further in Chapter 13.

PATIENT SELECTION

This arthroscopic treatment protocol is appropriate for all age groups. It is usually considered after nonoperative measures such as weight loss, strengthening, medications, icing, and flexibility have not been successful in relieving pain. A knee sleeve can be helpful, but unloading braces are more effective if they are comfortable, well tolerated, and do not slip. Activity modification, such as changing from jogging to cycling or water exercise, is another option to consider. Additionally, injection with a cortisone preparation or viscosupplementation with a hyaluronic acid solution can be useful.

TREATMENT PACKAGE

My surgical treatment regimen for knees with severe osteoarthritis focuses on increasing joint volume with arthroscopy, and maintaining it with rehabilitation to provide symptomatic relief. This relief occurs when joint contact pressures are decreased, and correct rehabilitation keeps the joint spaces open. The comprehensive arthroscopic regimen consists of distinct procedures, which are performed after general anesthesia or spinal anesthetic is administered. A tourniquet is rarely used.

The first step in the procedure is to expand the joint space using insufflation. In the severely degenerative knee, the joint volume is contracted, with a volume of only 60 to 90 mL, whereas a normal knee has about 180 mL of volume. An 18-gauge needle and a 60-mL syringe are used to inflate the joint with a saline solution (Fig. 12.1).

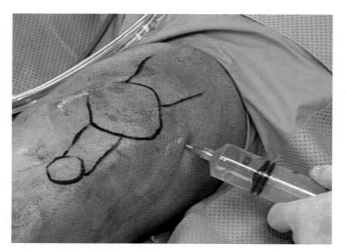

Figure 12.1 Needle placed in the suprapatellar pouch for the lateral side of the knee to inject fluid. A large needle is used to allow for tactile feedback to ensure that the fluid is flowing freely into the true joint space.

> **TIP:** It is important to make certain the needle is in the joint, and not in the subcutaneous tissue. Great care should be taken to avoid the back wall of the pouch. If the joint is entered superolateral to the patella and the needle is angled down, it is more likely to enter the joint and avoid injecting the back wall of the pouch. There should be an easy flow of solution into and out of the joint.

Fluid is inserted under manual pressure. As pressure increases, the outflow of fluid, when the syringe is removed from the needle, progresses from a drip to a steady flow, and then to a strong stream (Fig. 12.2). The joint is not like a balloon. If it is stretched, it will not just spring back. The degenerative joint has soft tissue contracture, and once it is stretched the resulting increased volume is maintained by fluid inflow during surgery, followed by mobilization and range of motion after surgery.

Following insufflation, a superomedial inflow portal is established followed by an anterolateral viewing portal and anteromedial working portal. The position of the viewing portal is more proximal than a standard lateral portal, permitting better visualization of the suprapatellar and infrapatellar areas. Unstable edges of the cartilage and loose bodies are removed, along with fragments and particulate in the joint. It is my impression that the particulate clogs the system. The body wants to get rid of the particulate, which gets in the joint lining and capsule and contributes to stiffness.

If the patient has never had an arthroscopic procedure, the meniscus may be causing pain, so I always trim a meniscus tear to a stable rim. Retaining volume of meniscus is important, even in chronic degenerative knees.[15]

Anterior osteophytes often block extension (Fig. 12.3). The quadriceps muscle can never relax when a flexion contracture is present. Standing on a normal bent knee is tiring, and to rest the muscle, the knee is straightened and locked, allowing the muscle to relax. *It is impossible for the knee with a flexion contracture to accomplish this relaxation of the quadriceps muscle.*

To improve extension, osteophytes are removed with a burr or shaver. In the process of removing osteophytes, inflammatory elements (bone marrow) enter the joint. Therefore, a drain is recommended for several hours after the surgery in order to remove the marrow elements released by the osteophytectomy.

The synovium is often inflamed and becomes hypertrophic (Fig. 12.4). Hypertrophic synovium is ablated using a thermal ablation device (Arthrocare; Arthrocare Corporation, Sunnyvale, CA). With the device on a low intensity (setting 5), I brush the surface to remove the inflamed portion of the synovium. If the synovium is dense, a higher intensity (setting 8) is used. The goal is to

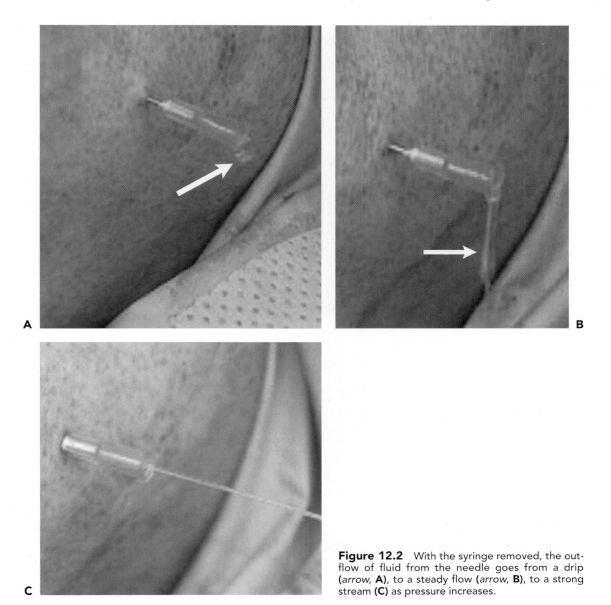

Figure 12.2 With the syringe removed, the outflow of fluid from the needle goes from a drip (*arrow*, **A**), to a steady flow (*arrow*, **B**), to a strong stream (**C**) as pressure increases.

remove the inflamed, hypertrophic synovium, which is a pain-generator. Emphasis should be placed on the area adjacent to chondral damage. Infrapatellar plica and suprapatellar plica are also removed (Fig. 12.5). Plica often contributes to tightness in the joint, which results in reduced joint volume. *It is important to achieve hemostasis when removing these tissues.*

TIP: The suprapatellar plica can compartmentalize the suprapatellar pouch, decreasing joint volume. If a compartmentalization is present, the quadriceps tendon is not visible in the pouch. If the compartmentalization is removed, increased joint volume results.

The anterior interval is the space between the infrapatellar fat pad and patellar tendon anteriorly, and the anterior border of the tibia and the transverse meniscal ligament (anterior intermeniscal ligament) posteriorly. No bridging scar tissue is normally present in this region; however, scarring in this region is commonly found in the degenerative knee or knees with prior surgery (Fig. 12.6). In order to have proper kinematics in the joint, the anterior interval needs to be open.[16] The infrapatellar fat pad is often scarred or overdeveloped (Fig. 12.7). In the normal knee, the interval between the patellar tendon and the tibia separates approximately 1.5 cm when the knee is moved in the range from 0 to 120 degrees. If there is scarring in this interval, the separation cannot occur, causing painful joint compression. This compression can also damage the cartilage.

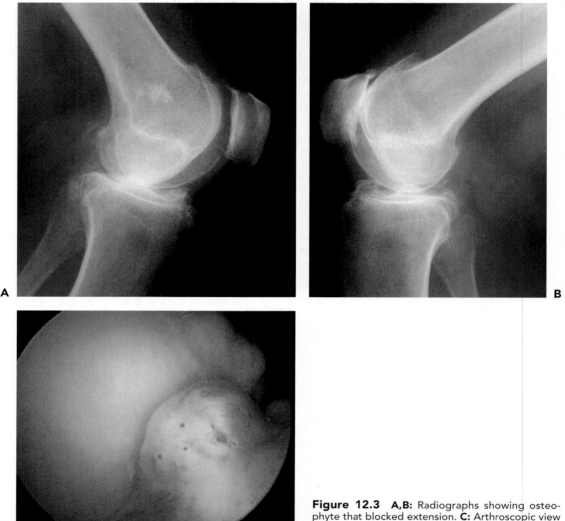

Figure 12.3 A,B: Radiographs showing osteophyte that blocked extension. **C:** Arthroscopic view of osteophyte in the notch.

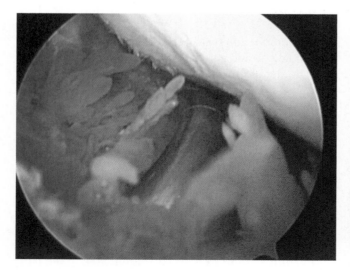

Figure 12.4   Hypertrophic synovium.

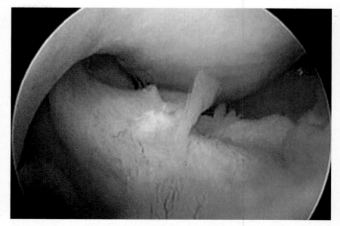

Figure 12.5   Infrapatellar plica in the knee can often cause loss of joint volume.

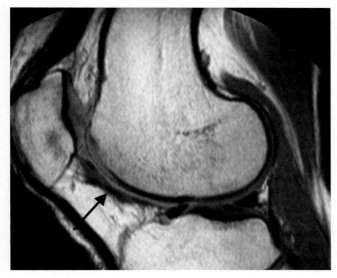

Figure 12.6 Magnetic resonance image demonstrating a scarred anterior interval. Scar tissue *(arrow)* bridges the gap between infrapatellar fat pad and patellar tendon.

The anterior interval is opened by releasing the area just anterior to the intermeniscal ligament (Fig. 12.8). This is done from medial to lateral, just anterior to the peripheral rim of the anterior horn of each meniscus. The release can be performed with either electrocautery or a thermal

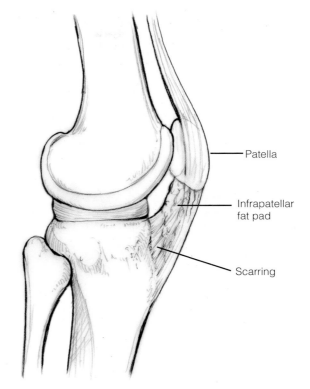

Figure 12.7 Illustration showing scarring of the infrapatellar fat pad, which results in reduced volume in the knee.

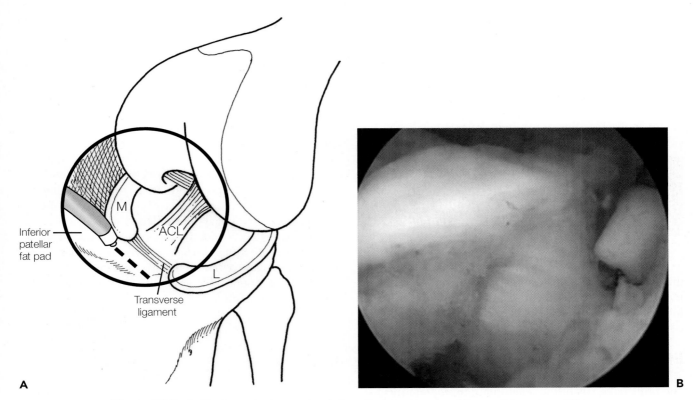

Figure 12.8 A: The interval release extends from the lateral border of the medial meniscus (M) to the medial border of the lateral meniscus (L), just anterior to the intermeniscal ligament. Care is taken to avoid injury to the anterior meniscal attachment during release. **B:** Arthroscopic view of anterior interval release. ACL, anterior cruciate ligament.

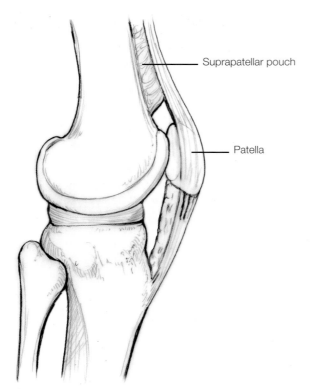

Suprapatellar pouch

Patella

Figure 12.9   Scarring of the suprapatellar pouch compartmentalizes the space, which reduces the volume of the knee.

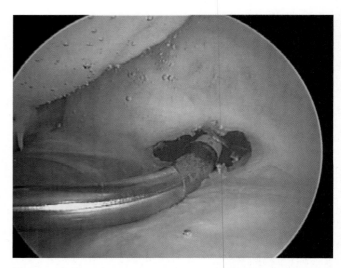

Figure 12.10   Release of the suprapatellar compartmentalization.

ablation device (Arthrocare). The release also should proceed from proximal (at the level of the meniscus) to approximately 1 cm distal along the anterior tibial cortex. Great care should be taken to avoid cauterizing or causing thermal necrosis to bone of the anterior tibia or the patellar tendon. Meticulous hemostasis should be obtained in the anterior interval and infrapatellar fat pad to prevent postoperative bleeding or recurrent scarring.

> **TIP: It is sometimes possible to release less-severe contractures just posterior to the intermeniscal ligament, but care must be taken to avoid the anterior meniscal attachments.**

In addition to the anterior interval, I also make sure that the suprapatellar pouch is not compartmentalized by scar tissue or plica (Fig. 12.9). The scar tissue or plica is released in a similar manner (Fig. 12.10).

POSTOPERATIVE CARE

The principal goals of the rehabilitation program include the maintenance of joint volume and the prevention of scar reformation, while preserving joint mobility.[17] Regaining strength is secondary to these goals. Throughout the rehabilitation program, exercises that elicit significant pain are strictly avoided. The postoperative regimens are specifically tailored to each patient.

The initial phase of rehabilitation focuses on passive and active-assisted range of motion exercises, patellar mobility, and stretching exercises. Patients are limited to touch-down weightbearing for the initial 1 to 2 weeks after surgery. Continuous passive motion machines are used during the first postoperative week. Extensor mechanism mobilization exercises include patellar and patellar tendon mobilization and are central to the rehabilitation protocol. Strength exercises include quadriceps and hamstring isometric sets, as well as heel and toe raises. Stationary bicycling, with no resistance, helps sustain flexibility while improving muscle tone. Patients proceed with stretching throughout rehabilitation.

After approximately 6 weeks, the next phase of rehabilitation begins, with the goal of achieving functional strength. To supplement the bicycle, treadmill walking, elastic resistance exercises, and one-third knee bends are begun, avoiding deeper bends more than 30 degrees. If pain is encountered during any of these exercises, the patient resumes training at a lower level that is pain-free. After approximately 3 months, the patient proceeds to advanced strengthening and return to sport. At 4 months, weight training exercises can begin if full range of motion is achieved. Outdoor biking and golf are also started at this point. After 5 months, patients can generally resume higher-level activities such as skiing and tennis.

OUTCOMES

In a recent study, we looked at patients who had undergone this treatment regimen for severe osteoarthritis of the knee.[17] All patients were considered candidates for knee replacement, but underwent this arthroscopic treatment instead. Thirteen

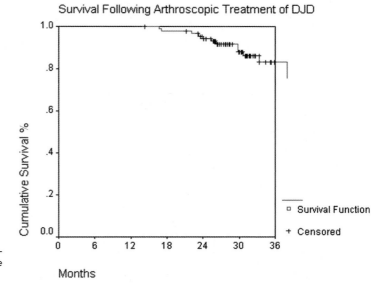

Figure 12.11 Survivorship curve of patients who underwent the arthroscopic treatment package. DJD, degenerative joint disease.

percent of the patients required total knee arthroplasty within the first 3 years following arthroscopy. Average survivorship (not requiring arthroplasty) at 1 year was 100%, 94% at 2 years, and 83% at 3 years (Fig. 12.11). Patients who required arthroplasty were older than those patients who did not. Of those patients whose treatment did not require arthroplasty, Lysholm scores improved from 49 preoperatively to 74 postoperatively. The average Tegner score postoperatively was 4, which is compatible with recreational sports participation. Patients were very satisfied with their outcomes. Knees with greater than 50% shift in their mechanical axis had lower postoperative Lysholm scores compared with knees with less than 50% shift in their mechanical axis. Patient satisfaction in patients with greater than 50% shift in mechanical axis was 7.6 (scale 1 to 10, with 10 being very satisfied), which was not statistically different from patients with less than 50% shift, whose average satisfaction was 8.3.

For patients who would like to delay joint replacement, arthroscopic surgery that addresses the pain generators in the joint is an option that can usually postpone replacement for several years. This approach can be incorporated with or without osteotomy. If osteotomy is performed, microfracture can be included as described in Chapter 13.

REFERENCES

1. Moseley JB, O'Malley K, Petersen NJ, et al. A controlled trial of arthroscopic surgery for osteoarthritis of the knee. *N Engl J Med* 2002;347:81–88.
2. Bert JM, Maschka K. The arthroscopic treatment of unicompartmental gonarthrosis: a five-year follow-up study of abrasion arthroplasty plus arthroscopic debridement and arthroscopic debridement alone. *Arthroscopy* 1989;5:25–32.
3. Harwin SF. Arthroscopic debridement for osteoarthritis of the knee: predictors of patient satisfaction. *Arthroscopy* 1999;15:142–146.
4. McGinley BJ, Cushner FD, Scott WN. Debridement arthroscopy. 10-year followup. *Clin Orthop* 1999;367:190–194.
5. Rand JA. Role of arthroscopy in osteoarthritis of the knee. *Arthroscopy* 1991;7:358–363.
6. Yang SS, Nisonson B. Arthroscopic surgery of the knee in the geriatric patient. *Clin Orthop* 1995;316:50–58.
7. Baumgaertner MR, Cannon WD Jr, Vittori JM, et al. Arthroscopic debridement of the arthritic knee. *Clin Orthop* 1990;253:197–202.
8. Dervin GF, Stiell IG, Rody K, et al. Effect of arthroscopic debridement for osteoarthritis of the knee on health-related quality of life. *J Bone Joint Surg Am* 2003;85:10–19.
9. Gibson JN, White MD, Chapman VM, et al. Arthroscopic lavage and debridement for osteoarthritis of the knee. *J Bone Joint Surg Br* 1992;74:534–537.
10. Edelson R, Burks RT, Bloebaum RD. Short-term effects of knee washout for osteoarthritis. *Am J Sports Med* 1995;23:345–349.
11. Friedman MJ, Berasi CC, Fox JM, et al. Preliminary results with abrasion arthroplasty in the osteoarthritic knee. *Clin Orthop* 1984;182:200–205.
12. Livesley PJ, Doherty M, Needoff M, et al. Arthroscopic lavage of osteoarthritic knees. *J Bone Joint Surg Br* 1991;73:922–926.
13. Ogilvie-Harris DJ, Fitsialos DP. Arthroscopic management of the degenerative knee. *Arthroscopy* 1991;7:151–157.
14. Salisbury RB, Nottage WM, Gardner V. The effect of alignment on results in arthroscopic debridement of the degenerative knee. *Clin Orthop* 1985;198:268–272.
15. Rodkey WG, Briggs KK, Steadman JR. Tissue loss at meniscectomy correlates with clinical symptoms, function and activity levels. *Arthroscopy* 2007;23:e16.
16. Ahmad CS, Kwak SD, Ateshian GA, et al. Effects of patellar tendon adhesion to the anterior tibia on knee mechanics. *Am J Sports Med* 1998;26:715–724.
17. Steadman JR, Ramappa AJ, Maxwell RB, et al. An arthroscopic treatment regimen for osteoarthritis of the knee. *Arthroscopy* 2007;23:948–955.

Debridement / Arthroscopy

Howard Head
Sports Medicine Centers
A service of Vail Valley Medical Center

Name: _____

Dr. _____   Date: _____

● = Do exercise for that week

ROM RESTRICTIONS
(full prom)
_____
_____
_____
_____

BRACE SETTINGS
(no brace)

WEIGHT BEARING STATUS
Partial 30% WB
x 1 weeks

TIME LINES
Week 1 (1-7POD)
Week 2 (8-14POD)
Week 3 (15-21POD)
Week 4 (22-28POD)

Initial Exercises — WEEK	1	2	3	4	5	6	7	8	9	10	13	17	21	25
Extension/Flexion–wall slides	●	●	●	●	●	●								
Extension/Flexion–sitting	●	●	●	●	●	●								
Quad sets with straight leg raises	●	●	●	●										
Patellar mobilizations/quad-patellar tendon	●	●	●	●	●	●								
Hamstring sets	●	●	●	●										
Ankle pumps	●	●	●	●										
Sit and reach for hamstrings (towel)	●	●	●	●	●	●	●	●	●	●	●	●	●	●
Runners stretch for calf and achilles	●	●	●	●	●	●	●	●	●	●	●	●	●	●
Stork stand/quad stretching			●	●	●	●	●	●	●	●	●	●	●	●
Toe and heel raises		●	●	●	●	●								
1/3 knee bends			●	●										
Cardiovascular Exercises	1	2	3	4	5	6	7	8	9	10	13	17	21	25
Bike with single leg/single leg rowing	●	●	●	●	●	●								
Bike with both legs	●	●	●	●	●	●	●	●	●	●	●	●	●	●
Aquajogging			●	●	●	●	●	●	●	●	●	●	●	●
Treadmill–incline 7-12%			●	●	●	●	●	●	●	●	●	●	●	●
Swimming with fins			●	●	●	●	●	●	●	●	●	●	●	●
Elliptical trainer			●	●	●	●	●	●	●	●	●	●	●	●
Rowing				●	●	●	●	●	●	●	●	●	●	●
Stair stepper				●	●	●	●	●	●	●	●	●	●	●
Resisted Exercises	1	2	3	4	5	6	7	8	9	10	13	17	21	25
Double knee bends			●	●	●	●	●	●	●	●				
Carpet drags			●	●	●	●	●	●	●	●				
Gas pedal			●	●	●	●	●	●	●	●				
Leg press–double leg					●	●	●	●	●	●	●	●	●	●
Single knee bends					●	●	●	●	●	●	●	●	●	●
Balance squats					●	●	●	●	●	●	●	●	●	●
Forward/backward jogging						●	●	●	●	●	●	●	●	●
Side to side lateral agility							●	●	●	●	●	●	●	●
Agility Exercises	1	2	3	4	5	6	7	8	9	10	13	17	21	25
Running progression							●	●	●	●	●	●	●	●
Initial							●	●	●	●	●	●	●	●
Advanced							●	●	●	●	●	●	●	●
Functional Sports Test							●	●	●	●	●	●	●	●
High Level Activities	1	2	3	4	5	6	7	8	9	10	13	17	21	25
(After Cleared by Physician)														
Golf							●	●	●	●	●	●	●	●
Running							●	●	●	●	●	●	●	●
Skiing, basketball, tennis, football, soccer							●	●	●	●	●	●	●	●

181 West Meadow Drive
Vail, Colorado 81657
970-476-1225
Fax 970-479-7193

* 7 1 2 7 *

Therapist Name

Joint Preservation: Care of the Older Athlete

William I. Sterett   Mark Adickes   Karen Briggs

■ **GOALS OF JOINT PRESERVATION 185**

■ **THE POSTMENISCECTOMY KNEE 186**

■ **ALIGNMENT 186**

■ **DESIRED VERSUS CURRENT ACTIVITY LEVELS 187**

■ **INTERVENTIONS 188**
Nonoperative 188
Operative 188
  Chondral Resurfacing 188
  Meniscal Replacement 189
High Tibial Osteotomy 189
High Tibial Osteotomy and Microfracture 189
  Templating 189
  Surgical Technique 190
Postoperative Management and Rehabilitation 192
Complications 193
Outcomes and Expectations 193

■ **SUMMARY 193**

GOALS OF JOINT PRESERVATION

Joint preservation in the older athlete has become more and more of an important tactic. Continued physical activity, longer life expectancies, and activity restrictions following arthroplasty have all led sports medicine physicians to get more creative about ways to preserve the native joint. Although arthroplasty components and techniques have seen recent dramatic improvements, these changes have not kept up with the increased longevity and activity levels of our maturing athletes. Joint preservation can actually be better interpreted as *activity preservation* techniques.

Preserving activity levels in our practice starts with understanding our patient's activity desires. All patients come to see us with both a chief complaint and a desired activity level. Two patients may present with a current level of activity involving discomfort while walking 18 holes on a golf course. The first patient really wants to get back to skiing more aggressively or playing better singles tennis, while the second patient simply wants a little less discomfort following a round of golf. Even before we see x-rays or examine the patient, we must be contemplating different treatment strategies in these two patients. Our advice will rarely involve counseling the patient to simply give up the activity for which he or she desires pain relief. Most patients realize that if they simply give up their desired activities, their knee will no longer hurt. Having said this, realistic counseling about interventions required to decrease, but possibly not eliminate, their pain should be undertaken with the patient.

In our patient population the chief complaint is usually one of pain. Considerable time should be spent clarifying the location and extent of their pain. Questions that should be asked of all patients with chronic pain include the following:

1. Location of the pain. We often ask the patient to point with one finger to the predominant location, if they can.
2. Quality of the pain. Specifically, we ask whether the pain is sharp, stabbing, and mechanical in nature, or more of a dull achy type of pain.
3. Severity of the pain. Use a visual analog scale to describe the pain at its worst and typical levels.
4. Duration of the pain. When did it start? How did it start? Was there an injury or an insidious onset?

5. What previous treatments have been attempted? Most patients in this category have had previous surgery. Identify all previous interventions and diagnostics, and have a good understanding of whether each intervention helped, helped briefly, or did not help.

6. Is the pain getting better, worse, or staying the same? Treatment recommendations are very different for severe pain that is getting rapidly better versus pain that has been slowly getting worse during the past year.

7. Finally, we always ask a question regarding relief of pain. "If we were able to relieve all of the pain today, what would you be doing differently in your life?" Treatment recommendations will again be very different depending on whether the answer is simply sleeping better or running the Boston Marathon.

The goal of joint preservation is really one of activity preservation and matching treatment plans with activity expectations and desires. As patients are maintaining higher activity levels for longer periods of time, traditional thoughts about age and arthroplasty no longer necessarily apply. Our treatment regimens are dictated much more strongly by the patients' desired activity level than by their age. The positive benefits of an ongoing exercise regimen to the overall health of an individual far outweigh any negative effects of joints "wearing down." From nutritional supplements, exercise regimens, and viscosupplementation, to arthroscopic and realignment techniques to preserve the native joints, we are requiring more and more novel ideas to preserve our patient's desired activity levels.

THE POSTMENISCECTOMY KNEE

Without question, the most common finding in a patient needing a joint preservation algorithm is the patient who has had a partial or complete meniscectomy in the distant past. This patient often has a pre-existing or congenital varus to the knee as evidenced by the bilateral nature of the alignment. Alternatively, this may be a developmental varus secondary to the meniscectomy. With normal alignment we should be putting roughly 50% of our weight during stance on the medial side of our knee and 50% on the lateral side. With less meniscal tissue we may shift this percentage very slightly toward the medial side. Over the years, this will cause further collapse of the medial plateau, which will further change the weightbearing percentages. Once we get into this cycle, it is very difficult to escape. Once more, without a sufficient meniscus, we are concentrating this higher percentage of our weight over a smaller surface area, again wearing down the native articular cartilage further.

On initial presentation, we have often seen the knee with medial compartment arthrosis, varus malalignment, and a limited amount of meniscal tissue to protect the joint further. We now classify this as the *hostile knee environment*, making our choice of intra-articular procedures much more limited. Meniscus replacement surgery is not an option in the varus, degenerative knee. Chondral resurfacing options are limited only to the marrow stimulation techniques and are destined to short-term successes because of the lack of meniscus to protect any "regenerate cartilage" that may be formed, and a higher percentage of body weight being placed on this area. Our algorithms for treating this knee will always take the surrounding environment into account in deciding the best short- and long-term recommendations.

ALIGNMENT

There is no single factor that affects nonoperative and surgical prognosis more than presenting alignment. Alignment appears to play a larger role than weight, body mass index, or previous surgeries in determining the rate of articular cartilage wear.[1]

There does not seem to be universal agreement about the effect of congenital varus on cartilage wear in the uninjured knee. The Framingham Osteoarthritis Study found that "baseline knee alignment is not associated with either incident radiographic or medial specific OA (osteoarthritis)".[2] Other magnetic resonance imaging studies have shown that baseline knee angle is associated with the rate of knee cartilage loss in patients with OA.[3] It appears from these studies that malalignment by itself will not wear down a knee. In OA, cartilage volume will decrease by an average of 5% per year, and this will decrease much more rapidly in the malaligned knee.[4]

Varus alignment will predispose the knee to meniscal tears from a combination of compression and shear (Fig. 13.1). Once the knee has less meniscus, the malalignment will

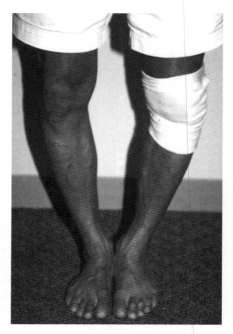

Figure 13.1 Patient with extreme varus deformity.

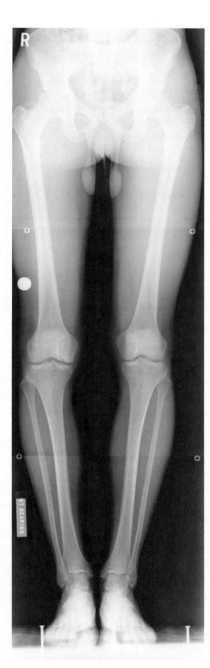

Figure 13.2 Long standing radiograph of hip, knee, and ankle joint.

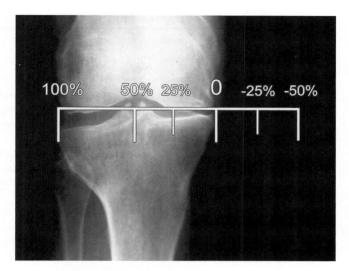

Figure 13.3 The weightbearing line crosses the tibia to calculate percent weightbearing.

more rapidly accelerate the cartilage loss than would have otherwise occurred. The malalignment itself will progress as the cartilage volume decreases and we come back to the hostile knee environment.

Alignment has been measured anatomically via the femorotibial angle. This may be a less exacting method for determining true weightbearing as it does not account for hip rotations, or femoral or tibial rotational or coronal malalignments. We believe that the most accurate method for determining the weightbearing characteristic at the level of the knee joint is the standing three-joint radiograph from hip to ankle (Fig. 13.2). Although variations exist, it is easiest for both surgeons and patients to understand that when a line connecting the center of the hip to the center of the ankle falls directly bicondylar in the center of the tibial plateau, we have a relatively equal weight distribution between our medial and lateral sides of the knee. As this weightbearing line (WBL) falls more medially (or possibly laterally), we are placing more and more of our weight on an isolated compartment of the knee. It is equally easy to visualize that if we are placing 70% of our weight on the portion of the knee that has less meniscus, more cartilage volume will be lost over a given time period. With articular cartilage wear, the bony hypertension that develops will create more concentrated pain and problems for the patient with a more difficult problem for the physician to solve.

The WBL can typically be reported as a percentage across the tibial plateau. When the WBL falls right in the middle, this can be reported as a WBL of 50% or 0.5. If the WBL actually falls medial to the medial plateau, this will be reported as a negative number. As the WBL falls lateral to the lateral aspect of the tibia, the WBL will be a number larger than 100% or 1.0 (Fig. 13.3).

DESIRED VERSUS CURRENT ACTIVITY LEVELS

When we initially see a patient, we like to know the disease (pain) severity and activity levels for both current and desired participation. Disease severity is most often described for us using the Lysholm subjective rating system, which can be completed by the patient prior to our initial introduction.[5] We use the Tegner Activity Scale to help decide treatment protocols (Fig. 13.4).[6] Most patients present with a current activity score around 3 (walking in forest, light labor). If they are looking to stay at 3 but simply with less pain, joint preservation techniques are probably not

Please choose one of the following which best describes your current activity level.

◯	Level 10	Competitive Sports(Soccer, Football, Rugby (national elite)
◯	Level 9	Competitive Sports(Soccer, Football, Rugby (lower divisions), hockey, wrestling, gymnastics)
◯	Level 8	Competitive Sports(Racquetball, Squash, Track and Field, Alpine Skiing)
◯	Level 7	Competitive Sports(Tennis, Athletics(Running), Handball, Basketball, Motorcross, Cross country track) Recreational Sports (Soccer, Football, Hockey, Squash, Athletics(jumping), Cross country track)
◯	Level 6	Recreational Sports (Tennis, Handball, Basketball, Alpine skiing, Jogging 5X/week)
◯	Level 5	Work (Heavy Labor) Competitive Sports (Cycling, X-country Skiing) Recreational (Jogging on uneven ground 2x/week)
◯	Level 4	Work (Moderately Heavy Labor (truck driving, etc) Recreational Sports (Cycling, Cross Country Skiing, Jogging on even ground 2X/week)
◯	Level 3	Work (Light Labor) Comp & Rec Sports (Swimming), Hiking, Backpacking
◯	Level 2	Work (Light Labor) Walking on uneven ground possible but impossible to backpack or hike
◯	Level 1	Work (Light Labor) Walking on even ground possible
◯	Level 0	Sick leave or disability pension because of knee problems

Figure 13.4   Tegner Activity Scale used to determine patients current activity level and desired activity level.

necessary. Often, more predictable outcomes with maintenance of the desired activity levels can occur with arthroplasty procedures. When the desired activity score of the patient is 6 or higher (alpine skiing, recreational tennis), it becomes more imperative to employ a joint preservation protocol. This is especially true when the patient is younger because of the high likelihood of revision arthroplasty, or even multiple revisions, being required during the lifespan of the young patient desiring higher activity scores.

Total knee arthroplasty (TKA) outcomes are predictable and result in satisfied patients.[7] Unfortunately, we need to treat patients, not x-rays. In the world's literature to date, there have been no published reports of long-term follow-up in patients undergoing TKA and returning Tegner Activity Scores above 4. We all have patients following arthroplasty who return to skiing or singles tennis, but this is rarely our counsel. When a postarthroplasty patient returns to these sports, we can no longer make accurate predictions about the longevity of these implants. There is risk of early polyethylene wear with these activities as well as risk of more catastrophic sequelae such as loosening or fracture. Rather than predicting a 15-year lifespan for the implant in these active patients, much more caution in the longevity should be expressed. Joint preservation is once again recommended for those not desiring to modify their activities to gain a more predictable outcome from their arthroplasty.

INTERVENTIONS

Nonoperative

From a nonoperative standpoint, quadriceps and hamstring muscle strengthening allows the knee to rely as much as possible on the musculature rather than the bony architecture for support. Providing a well-cushioned insole transfers some of that cushion at foot strike into the knee. Nutritional supplements such as glucosamine and chondroitin sulfate are becoming increasingly popular and seem to help a percentage of the population.[8-10]

Activities in an unloader brace often identify those patients who may benefit from an osteotomy. It is unclear, radiographically or mechanically, the extent to which these braces actually unload the knees.[11,12] Intermittent and judicious use of nonsteroidal anti-inflammatory medications can help break the cycle of inflammation that causes pain and more inflammation. The injectable viscosupplementations with hyaluronic acid have also become increasingly popular. It is unclear whether or not these provide benefits to the cartilage itself or have any actual long-term benefit.[13]

Operative

Chondral Resurfacing

It has become clear that acute chondral defects will predictably lead to further degenerative changes in the ensuing years. Therefore, even the asymptomatic chondral lesion should be treated surgically with attempts at repair or restoration. Acute chondral defects may be treated with a variety of techniques, including marrow stimulation techniques such as microfracture and auto- or allograft plugs such as mosaicplasty or osteochondral autologous transplantation.[14-16]

Finally, attempts at regeneration of true hyaline cartilage can be made with autologous chondrocyte transfer.[17] All of these have well-outlined benefits, as well as risks, with approximately an 85% rate of success in the athletic population. Further discussion about the treatment of the acute chondral defect can be found in other parts of this textbook and is beyond the scope of true joint preservation, which is typically a chronic problem.

Meniscal Replacement

Few aspects in sports medicine are undergoing as rapid a change as meniscal replacement. This calls for a heightened awareness of rapid degeneration following meniscectomy, particularly on the lateral side. Early-generation meniscal allograft replacements had significant problems. Studies were difficult to interpret as a variety of grafts and sizing techniques were being reported.[18] It is probably not feasible to make adequate comparisons between first-generation and more recent implants. First-generation implants were reported with freeze-dried grafts, cryopreserved grafts, and fresh-frozen grafts. The fresh-frozen grafts came highly irradiated to kill all virus particles; however, this denatured the graft. If limited irradiation was used, bacteria were killed, but not virus. Also, nonirradiated grafts, which were more like natural collagen, posed a significant safety risk.

Nevertheless, early reports were still fairly promising, with about 75% good or excellent results at 2-year follow-up.[19] In these patients, any remnant meniscus, functional or not, required removal prior to implantation; therefore, any failures were actually worse off, as they now had a failed meniscal allograft and less native meniscus than prior to surgery.

Newer sizing techniques are much more exacting, using a combination of computed tomography or magnetic resonance imaging for data.[20] Shrinkage can now be more predictably accounted for. With newer biological cleansing, less or no irradiation is required, which will lead to less stiffness and denaturing of the graft.

To date, there is evidence that good pain relief can be had in the 5- to 8-year period following meniscal transplantation. There is limited evidence that an allograft meniscus will be able to prevent further arthritic changes, despite having similar size and midbody motion as the native menisci with good vascular ingrowth.[21] Immediate meniscal transplantation in rabbits did not significantly reduce degenerative changes of articular cartilage when compared with meniscectomy.[22]

High Tibial Osteotomy

Since its description by Jackson and Waugh[23] in 1957, high tibial osteotomy (HTO) has become a widely accepted treatment for patients with moderately severe, primarily unicompartmental, varus degenerative arthritis of the knee. Tibial osteotomies can be performed using a medial opening or lateral closing wedge technique.[24] Advantages of the medial opening technique include accurate correction of deformity, avoidance of surgical insult to the peroneal nerve, and proximal tibia-fibula joint, lengthening an already shortened limb, and a near-midline incision that can be easily converted to a TKA. In a recently published series of lateral closing wedge osteotomies, the authors reported a 9.2% incidence of partial peroneal nerve palsy.[25] Less

than half of these injuries demonstrated complete recovery. This complication has not been reported in association with a medial opening technique.

Medial opening wedge HTO has gained popularity as a treatment option for the varus degenerative knee in the young, active patient.[26,27] The goal of HTO in this setting is correction of alignment deformity in the coronal plane; however, because of the triangular cross-sectional anatomy of the tibia, as well as technical challenges associated with this surgical procedure, the medial opening HTO may also alter alignment in the sagittal plane.

A review of the literature identifies several consistent contraindications to high tibial osteotomy. These include significant lateral compartment disease, markedly diminished range of motion, bone loss, ligamentous laxity, and excessive angular deformity.[14,28] The presence of preoperative patellofemoral arthrosis has raised some controversy. In our hands, the presence of patellofemoral arthrosis did not lead to worse outcomes when the chief complaint was medial-sided knee pain.

Case Study

A 62-year-old singles tennis player presents for treatment of medial knee pain. The patient has varus malalignment and moderate patellofemoral arthritis. The preoperative Lysholm score is 52 points with a current Tegner activity level of 3. The patient's desired activity level was a Tegner level 6. In the clinical decision-making scheme, this patient was not an appropriate candidate for unicompartmental knee arthroplasty (UKA) or total knee arthroplasty (TKA) based on their desired activity score. A microfracture and HTO were recommended for this patient.

High Tibial Osteotomy and Microfracture

Beginning in 1995, we began performing an opening wedge osteotomy on the medial side of the proximal tibia, in conjunction with a chondral resurfacing procedure, in the degenerative varus knee.[14] This combination produced more accurate realignment; extensile incisions that should not complicate TKA, if necessary, in the future; and restoration of the native height to the tibia. By avoiding the lateral side, complications with the proximal tibiofibular joint or the peroneal nerve have been essentially eliminated.

Templating

Long standing radiographs of the patient's knees are taken preoperatively. From these x-rays, a template is created. This is done by measuring the WBL and the mechanical axis deviation. From here, a paper cut-out of the actual tibia is created. Next, the paper cut-out is incised medially, and placed on top of the x-ray (Fig. 13.5). The cut-out is then opened to the appropriate width in millimeters, according to the precalculated correction (Fig. 13.6). This paper cut-out

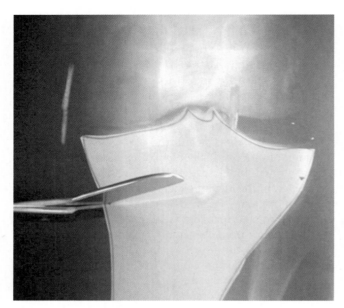

Figure 13.5 Preoperative preparation includes templating of the osteotomy. A paper template is made and then cut medially.

will then serve as the template for the HTO. The amount of millimeters is then recorded and an appropriate plate size is selected (Fig. 13.7).

Surgical Technique

The patient is placed supine on the operating room table. The head of the bed is reversed to aid in fluoroscopic visualization from the hip to the ankle. Diagnostic arthroscopy is performed viewing all compartments. If the lateral compartment has diffuse grade 4 change, an osteotomy is not performed. If less than 2 cm² of grade 4 changes are present in the lateral compartment, an osteotomy is still done, but overcorrection is no longer the goal. In this case, we correct only to neutral. We also visualize and document the condition of the medial and patellofemoral compartments. All pathology discovered during diagnostic arthroscopy is

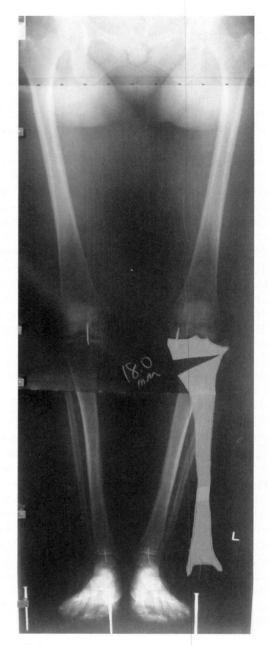

Figure 13.7 Paper template is laid over long standing radiograph to show change in alignment.

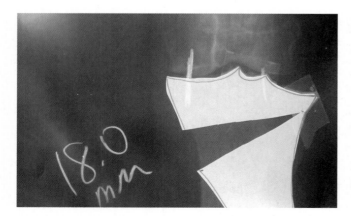

Figure 13.6 The paper template is opened and the millimeters of correction are measured.

addressed, including meniscal tears, synovitis, and adhesions.

With all intra-articular pathology addressed, chondral resurfacing is initiated. First, all loose flaps and unstable rim articular cartilage is debrided. Once a stable rim is established, the true size of the lesion is noted, and a rough shave is performed to create a bed with uniform punctuate bleeding. A 45-degree arthroscopic awl (Microfracture Awl; Linvatec, Largo, FL) is used to make multiple 2-mm holes in the subchondral bone. These holes are placed as close together as possible without breaking into one another. Fluid pressure is decreased to allow for visualization and

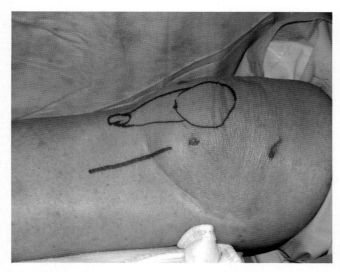

Figure 13.8 Preoperative markings to identify appropriate incision locations.

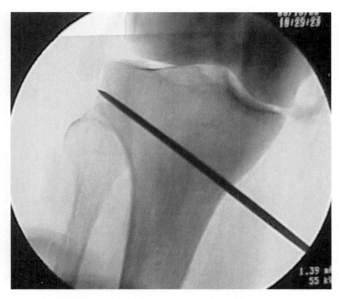

Figure 13.9 Kirschner wire placement, which serves as a template for oscillating saw.

documentation of good bleeding from the microfracture holes. The arthroscopy equipment is then removed from the knee and the portals closed with 4-0 Monocryl (Ethicon, Somerville, NJ) suture in a subcutaneous fashion.

An Esmark bandage is used to exsanguinate the limb, a tourniquet is elevated and the leg is prepared again with Betadine solution. Another extremity drape is then placed and a sterile pen is used to mark the incision site (Fig. 13.8). An incision is made centered on the tibial tubercle proximally and distally and placed one fingerbreadth medially. An inverted L-shaped incision is made and careful subperiosteal dissection is carried posteromedially to posterior cortex of the tibia. A formal anterior interval release is performed with a no. 10 blade by releasing the fat pad from the anterior tibia proximal to the patellar tendon insertion. A Z-retractor can then be placed anteriorly under the patellar tendon to protect this vital structure and posteriorly along the line of the osteotomy to protect the neurovascular bundle.

Two Kirschner wires are then placed to serve as a template for the oscillating saw. The first wire should be placed from the level of the tibial tubercle medially aiming to a point approximately 1.5 cm from the joint line laterally. Using fluoroscopy, the first wire should bisect the anterior and middle thirds of the tibia (Fig. 13.9). The second wire should be parallel to the first in the coronal plane and should bisect the middle and posterior thirds of the tibia. Both wires should contact but not penetrate the lateral cortex. A wide oscillating saw blade is then used to cut along the guide wires, staying in the center of the tibia and ending the cut, using fluoroscopy, 1 cm from the lateral cortex. Osteotomes are then used to complete the tibial cut anteriorly and posteriorly, taking care to leave intact bone laterally to provide crucial stability. Anteriorly, the cut in the cortical bone is made just beneath the patellar tendon attachment site, so careful technique must be used to avoid damaging this structure.

With the cut complete, the osteotomy site is checked for mobility and, if adequate, the EBI-articulated osteotome (EBI, Parsippany, NJ) is inserted to the desired depth and the osteotomy is opened to the predetermined amount per preoperative templating (Fig. 13.10). A long guide wire and fluoroscopy are then used to assess the weightbearing axis (Fig. 13.11). We site the wire in the center of the femoral head and, while holding this in place, move the distal guide wire to the center of the talus. While holding both ends of the wire still, the image is moved over the knee to assess the mechanical axis. If an acceptable amount of correction has been achieved based on templating and intraoperative arthroscopic findings, the plate of the correct size is inserted with the articulated osteotome remaining in place and fixed first distally and then proximally.

With the plate firmly held, the osteotome/distraction device is removed and all screw holes in the plate are filled (Fig. 13.12). Bone graft substitute mixed with autologous blood (Fig. 13.13) is tamped firmly in place, with care taken to fill the defect completely, particularly laterally (Fig. 13.14). Fluoroscopy should be used prior to definitively fixing the plate to assess the posterior slope of the tibia.

There is increasing evidence that release of the superficial medial collateral ligament (MCL) is required to effectively reduce contact pressures on the medial compartment following an opening wedge osteotomy.[29,30] At the time of surgical exposure we now routinely release the distal fibers of the MCL as we reflect both the MCL and pes tendons posteriorly during the osteotomy. We perform the osteotomy ar or below the level of the tibial tubercle. This requires careful attention to cut the bone behind the patellar tendon but leave the tendon alone. Because the tendon inserts over a 3.5 cm area, the tendon is allowed to "sleeve" over the osteotomy as it is distracted. A portion of the

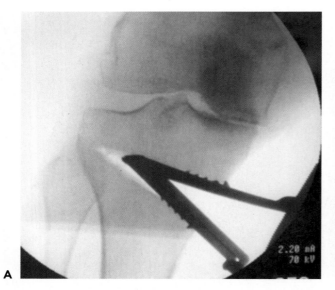
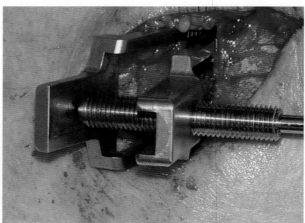

Figure 13.10   Osteotome inserted and opened to precalculated amount. **A:** Fluoroscopic view. **B:** External view.

tendon remains attached to the proximal fragment, while the majority routinely remains attached to the distal fragment. Utilizing this technique, and not distalizing the tubercle itself, we have been able to avoid any change in our Insall-Salvatti ratios.[31]

Postoperative Management and Rehabilitation

The rehabilitation protocol for osteotomy follows the rehabilitation program of the microfracture technique (see Chapter 9). If a microfracture is performed, the patient is placed in a continuous passive motion machine in the recovery room. The initial range of motion is typically 30 to 70 degrees, and it can be increased as tolerated by the patient. We push patients to gain full passive range of motion of the injured knee as soon as possible after surgery. We prescribe crutch-assisted touch-down weightbearing. Patients are touch-down weightbearing, placing 10% of their body weight on the injured leg during weightbearing. At 2 weeks, patients begin stationary biking without resistance, straight-leg raises, and a deep-water exercise program. The program is structured for 6 to 8 weeks. Terminal extension is the long-term focus. This is the one factor that seems to be most difficult for these patients to regain.

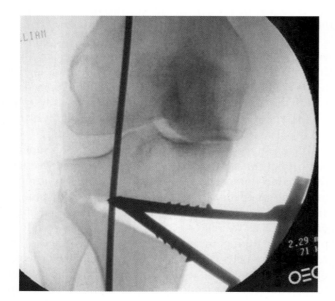

Figure 13.11   Osteotome being opened, with distal guide wire in place.

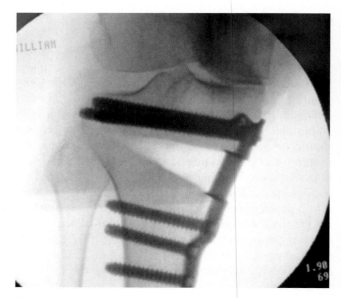

Figure 13.12   Plate fixation before wedge is packed with bone graft substitute.

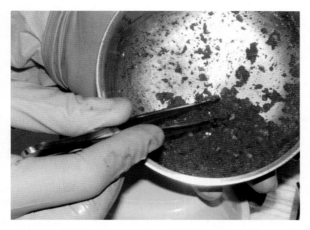

Figure 13.13 Mixture of bone graft substitute and autologous blood.

Complications

Reported complications include loss of correction,[32] delayed union,[33] nonunion,[33] peroneal nerve palsy,[28] vessel injuries and infection.[34] While complications were all initially high with first generation plates, newer instrumentation and implants have almost eliminated these complications.

Outcomes and Expectations

Outcomes following HTO have shown high patient satisfaction and return to function. One study determined the outcome of patients with varus malalignment who underwent both a chondral resurfacing procedure and an HTO.[14] Patients underwent an opening wedge HTO with microfracture if medial chondral degeneration was present, the

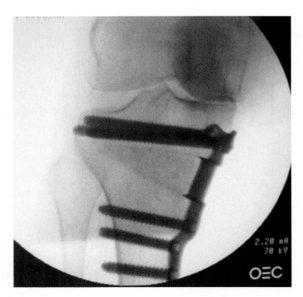

Figure 13.14 Plate fixation after opened wedge has been filled with bone graft substitute.

patient's weightbearing axis measured more than 5 degrees of varus or their WBL fell in the medial third of the tibial plateau, the chief complaint was medial sided knee pain, and the desired Tegner activity score was 4 or greater. All osteotomies in this study were done with an external fixator. Kaplan-Meir survivorship analysis showed a 96% survivorship at 3 years and an 84% survivorship at 5 years. The end point for survivorship analysis was defined as a revision HTO or total knee replacement following initial HTO. When these patients were compared with patients who underwent microfracture with joint-space narrowing and no osteotomy, greater improvement was seen. Postoperative Lysholm scores for the osteotomy/microfracture group had a mean of 81.0, which was significantly higher than the Lysholm score (73) in patients with microfracture only and joint-space narrowing ($p = 0.03$).

In the study by Miller et al.,[27] factors associated with patient satisfaction were determined in 30 patients who were treated with plate fixation and 31 treated with distraction osteogenesis and external fixation. The average magnitude of correction was 15.5 mm (range, 10 to 25 mm). Nineteen patients had degenerative changes in the patellofemoral compartment. At an average of 3 years postoperatively, the average Lysholm score was 75.4. The mean patient satisfaction score was 7.6 (range, 1 to 10). Patient satisfaction was not related to age, fixation technique, magnitude of corrections, or patellofemoral arthrosis. The independent predictor of patient satisfaction was postoperative Lysholm score.

In a recent study, we compared patient expectations in patients undergoing HTO compared with those patients undergoing TKA. The HTO patients had higher expectations for improvement in more athletic knee movements. These included squatting, kneeling, and running. HTO patients also had higher expectations for improvement in knee stiffness. For the TKA patients, confidence in their knee was the most important expectation.

SUMMARY

Joint preservation or "activity preservation" is an art and a science. Careful consideration of the patient and his or her needs are essential. We have outlined our approach to the patient, techniques for evaluation of pain, and current activity level, and placed emphasis on determining the desired activity level. Within these parameters a plan can be formulated to best fit the patient, which includes the desires and the pathoanatomic conditions present. We have had excellent results from opening wedge HTO in appropriately selected patients. Our technique is outlined in detail and includes attention to intra-articular pathology to include microfracture as necessary. We encourage the reader to think in terms of activity preservation, not just joint preservation, in the approach to older patients with limiting knee symptoms.

REFERENCES

1. Brouwer GM, van Tol AW, Bergink AP, et al. Association between valgus and varus alignment and the development and progression of radiographic osteoarthritis of the knee. *Arthritis Rheum* 2007; 56:1204–1211.

2. Hunter DJ, Niu J, Felson DT, et al. Knee alignment does not predict incident osteoarthritis: the Framingham osteoarthritis study. *Arthritis Rheum* 2007;56:1212–1218.

3. Cicuttini F, Wluka A, Hankin J, et al. Longitudinal study of the relationship between knee angle and tibiofemoral cartilage volume in subjects with knee osteoarthritis. *Rheumatology (Oxford)* 2004;43:321–324.

4. Wluka AE, Stuckey S, Snaddon J, et al. The determinants of change in tibial cartilage volume in osteoarthritic knees. *Arthritis Rheum* 2002;46:2065–2072.

5. Lysholm J, Gillquist J. Evaluation of knee ligament surgery with special emphasis on use of a scoring scale. *Am J Sports Med* 1982;10:150–154.

6. Tegner Y, Lysholm J. Rating systems in the evaluation of knee ligament injuries. *Clin Orthop Relat Res* 1985;198:43–49.

7. Kane RL, Saleh KJ, Wilt TJ, et al. The functional outcomes of total knee arthroplasty. *J Bone Joint Surg Am* 2005;87:1719–1724.

8. Bassleer C, Rovati L, Franchimont P. Stimulation of proteoglycan production by glucosamine sulfate in chondrocytes isolated from human osteoarthritic articular cartilage in vitro. *Osteoarthritis Cartilage* 1998;6:427–434.

9. Deal CL, Moskowitz RW. Nutraceuticals as therapeutic agents in osteoarthritis. The role of glucosamine, chondroitin sulfate, and collagen hydrolysate. *Rheum Dis Clin North Am* 1999;25:379–395.

10. Uebelhart D, Thonar EJ, Delmas PD, et al. Effects of oral chondroitin sulfate on the progression of knee osteoarthritis: a pilot study. *Osteoarthritis Cartilage* 1998;6(Suppl A):39–46.

11. Kirkley A, Webster-Bogaert S, Litchfield R, et al. The effect of bracing on varus gonarthrosis. *J Bone Joint Surg Am* 1999;81:539–548.

12. Lindenfeld TN, Hewett TE, Andriacchi TP. Joint loading with valgus bracing in patients with varus gonarthrosis. *Clin Orthop Relat Res* 1997;344:290–297.

13. Listrat V, Ayral X, Patarnello F, et al. Arthroscopic evaluation of potential structure modifying activity of hyaluronan (Hyalgan) in osteoarthritis of the knee. *Osteoarthritis Cartilage* 1997;5:153–160.

14. Sterett WI, Steadman JR. Chondral resurfacing and high tibial osteotomy in the varus knee. *Am J Sports Med* 2004;32:1243–1249.

15. Hangody L, Fules P. Autologous osteochondral mosaicplasty for the treatment of full-thickness defects of weight-bearing joints: ten years of experimental and clinical experience. *J Bone Joint Surg Am* 2003;85:25–32.

16. Lahav A, Burks RT, Greis PE, et al. Clinical outcomes following osteochondral autologous transplantation (OATS). *J Knee Surg* 2006;19:169–173.

17. Peterson L, Minas T, Brittberg M, et al. Two- to 9-year outcome after autologous chondrocyte transplantation of the knee. *Clin Orthop Relat Res* 2000;374:212–234.

18. Shaffer B, Kennedy S, Klimkiewicz J, et al. Preoperative sizing of meniscal allografts in meniscus transplantation. *Am J Sports Med* 2000;28:524–533.

19. Cole BJ, Dennis MG, Lee SJ, et al. Prospective evaluation of allograft meniscus transplantation: a minimum 2-year follow-up. *Am J Sports Med* 2006;34:919–927.

20. Donahue TL, Hull ML, Howell SM. New algorithm for selecting meniscal allografts that best match the size and shape of the damaged meniscus. *J Orthop Res* 2006;24:1535–1543.

21. Cole BJ, Carter TR, Rodeo SA. Allograft meniscal transplantation: background, techniques, and results. *Instr Course Lect* 2003;52: 383–396.

22. Rijk PC, Tigchelaar-Gutter W, Bernoski FP, et al. Histologic changes in articular cartilage after medial meniscus replacements in rabbits. *Arthroscopy* 2004;20:911–917.

23. Jackson J, Waugh W. Tibial osteotomy for osteoarthritis of the knee. *J Bone and Joint Surg Br* 1961;43:746–751.

24. Hoell S, Suttmoeller J, Stoll V, et al. The high tibial osteotomy, open versus closed wedge, a comparison of methods in 108 patients. *Arch Orthop Trauma Surg* 2005;125:638–643.

25. Sprenger TR, Doerzbacher JF. Tibial osteotomy for the treatment of varus gonarthrosis. Survival and failure analysis to twenty-two years. *J Bone Joint Surg Am* 2003;85:469–474.

26. Meding JB, Keating EM, Ritter MA, et al. Total knee arthroplasty after high tibial osteotomy. A comparison study in patients who had bilateral total knee replacement. *J Bone Joint Surg Am* 2000;82: 1252–1259.

27. Miller BS, Steadman JR, Briggs KK, et al. Patient satisfaction and outcome after microfracture of the degenerative knee. *J Knee Surg* 2004;17:13–77.

28. Naudie D, Bourne RB, Rorabeck CH, et al. The Install Award. Survivorship of the high tibial valgus osteotomy. A 10- to 22-year followup study. *Clin Orthop Relat Res* 1999;367:18–27.

29. Agneskirchner JD, Hurschler C, Wrann CD, et al. *Arthroscopy* 2007;23:852–861.

30. Pape D, Duchow J, Rupp S, et al. *Knee Surg Sport Traumatol Arthrosc* 2006;14:141–148.

31. Wright JM, Heavrin B, Begg M, et al. Observations on patellar height following opening wedge proximal tibial osteotomy. *Am J Knee Surg* 2001;14:163–173.

32. Myrnerts R. Failure of the correction of varus deformity obtained by high tibial osteotomy. *Acta Orthop Scand* 1980;51:569–573.

33. Coventry MB. Upper tibial osteotomy for osteoarthritis. *J Bone Joint Surg Am* 1985;67:1136–1140.

34. Coventry M. Upper tibial osteotomy for gonarthrosis. The evolution of the operation in the last 18 years and long term results. *Orthop Clin North Am* 1979;10:191–210.

HTO   Microfracture: Femoral Condyle / Tib Plateau

Howard Head
Sports Medicine Centers
A service of Vail Valley Medical Center

Name: _____

Dr. _____ Date: _____

● = Do exercise for that week

ROM
RESTRICTIONS
(full prom)
_____
_____
_____
_____

BRACE
SETTINGS

(no brace)

WEIGHT
BEARING
STATUS

Touch Down WB
x 6-8 weeks

TIME LINES
Week 1 (1-7POD)
Week 2 (8-14POD)
Week 3 (15-21POD)
Week 4 (22-28POD)

Initial Exercises	WEEK	1	2	3	4	5	6	7	8	9	10	13	17	21	25
Extension/Flexion–wall slides		●	●	●	●	●	●	●	●	●	●				
Extension/Flexion–sitting		●	●	●	●	●	●	●	●	●	●				
Quad sets with straight leg raises		●	●	●	●	●	●	●	●						
Patellar mobilizations/quad-patellar tendon		●	●	●	●	●	●	●	●	●	●				
Hamstring sets		●	●	●	●	●	●	●	●						
Ankle pumps		●	●	●	●										
Sit and reach for hamstrings (towel)		●	●	●	●	●	●	●	●	●	●	●	●	●	●
Runners stretch for calf and achilles										●	●	●	●	●	●
Stork stand/quad stretching										●	●	●	●	●	●
Toe and heel raises										●	●	●			
1/3 knee bends										●	●	●			
Cardiovascular Exercises		**1**	**2**	**3**	**4**	**5**	**6**	**7**	**8**	**9**	**10**	**13**	**17**	**21**	**25**
Bike with single leg/single leg rowing		●	●	●	●	●	●								
Bike with both legs				●	●	●	●	●	●	●	●	●	●	●	●
Aquajogging				●	●	●	●	●	●	●	●	●	●	●	●
Treadmill–incline 7-12%											●	●	●	●	●
Swimming with fins											●	●	●	●	●
Elliptical trainer												●	●	●	●
Rowing												●	●	●	●
Stair stepper													●	●	●
Resisted Exercises		**1**	**2**	**3**	**4**	**5**	**6**	**7**	**8**	**9**	**10**	**13**	**17**	**21**	**25**
Double knee bends												●	●		
Carpet drags										●	●	●			
Gas pedal										●	●	●			
Leg press–double leg												●	●	●	●
Single knee bends												●	●	●	●
Balance squats												●	●	●	●
Forward/backward jogging													●	●	●
Side to side lateral agility													●	●	●
Agility Exercises		**1**	**2**	**3**	**4**	**5**	**6**	**7**	**8**	**9**	**10**	**13**	**17**	**21**	**25**
Running progression													●	●	●
Initial													●	●	●
Advanced														●	●
Functional Sports Test														●	●
High Level Activities		**1**	**2**	**3**	**4**	**5**	**6**	**7**	**8**	**9**	**10**	**13**	**17**	**21**	**25**
(After Cleared by Physician)															
Golf													●	●	●
Running															●
Skiing, basketball, tennis, football, soccer															●

Copyright ©2006 Rehabilitation and Performance Center at Vail

181 West Meadow Drive
Vail, Colorado 81657
970-476-1225
Fax 970-479-7193

* 7 1 2 0 *

_____
Therapist Name

A Look Beyond the Horizon

14

William G. Rodkey

▬ **INTRODUCTION 197**

▬ **THE COLLAGEN MENISCUS IMPLANT 197**
Collagen Meniscus Implant Fabrication 198
Indications 198
Surgical Technique 198
Clinical Studies 199

DISCLAIMER: The Collagen Meniscus Implant (CMI) described in this presentation is not currently (2007) available for sale or distribution in the United States. Studies described in this presentation were performed under a U.S. Food and Drug Administration (FDA) Investigational Device Exemption (IDE). The FDA has classified the CMI as an investigational device, and it may be used in the United States only within the standards set forth in the IDE.

A roll of the dice? Picking the winning lottery numbers? Having a wild idea or just an intuitive hunch? What do these all have in common? They all deal with our curiosities and wondering what the future might hold. They are all beyond the horizon, but the horizon is always changing as long as we are moving, both physically and intellectually. Whether it takes only a "blink,"[1] or whether it takes 20 years of laboratory and clinical research, the future is suddenly on us. *The future is now!*

I have been fortunate enough to see a number of ideas that once lay beyond the horizon suddenly come into full view. Most were from great people; many were from the amazing people who conceived and have contributed to writing this book; a few were my own. Although we do not yet have all the answers to joint preservation and joint restoration, and perhaps our generation never will, our group is convinced that the future solutions are biological. We all look beyond metal and plastic; instead, we focus on orthobiologics, tissue engineering, gene therapy, scaffold and matrices, adult mesenchymal stem cells, biological modulators, and the likes. There are many examples that could be included in this section of the book, but I have chosen to focus on one that now is on "this side" of the horizon, and it may be nearing reality. More than 20 years ago, Dr. Steadman, I, and others started to seriously and scientifically pursue the idea of regrowing lost meniscus tissue. This chapter on the collagen meniscus implant (CMI) is evidence that no matter how long it takes, the future is now.

And so remember, "The real voyage of discovery consists not in finding new lands, but rather in seeing with new eyes."[2] Your "new eyes" will help you to look beyond the horizon.

THE COLLAGEN MENISCUS IMPLANT

Tissue engineering is a relatively new discipline that recently has received significant attention.[3] Tissue engineering has provided a fundamental understanding and technology that has permitted the development of structures derived from biological tissues. Bioresorbable collagen matrices are one important example of innovative new devices that resulted from the discipline of tissue engineering.[4–6] These collagen matrix materials have many positive features for use in preservation and restoration of meniscus tissue, including a controlled rate of resorption based on the degree of cross-linking. Most noteworthy, processing of the collagen can minimize any immune response, and the extremely complex biochemical composition of the normal meniscus might be recapitulated during the production process.[4-6] If such a material could serve successfully as a scaffold for regeneration of new tissue, then many of the previously noted negative effects of losing the meniscus cartilage might be prevented or at least minimized.[7]

We started development of this collagen scaffold, which we refer to as the *collagen meniscus implant* (CMI), with straightforward goals. We set out to generate or grow new meniscuslike tissue in an effort to restore or preserve the critical functions of the meniscus.[8-10] We also hoped to prevent further degenerative joint disease and osteoarthritis that likely would be progressive and lead to multiple surgeries, possibly including total knee replacement. Another goal for this regenerated tissue was to enhance joint stability. And finally, we wanted the implant and the new tissue to have the effect of providing pain relief and precluding the necessity for constant medication. We also focused on several criteria for design of the CMI.[8-10] We desired to have a material that would be resorbable over time so that as the collagen of the scaffold was metabolized, the regenerated tissue would have the opportunity to replace it. We also planned for the CMI to maintain its structural integrity in the intra-articular environment for a period that would be adequate to support the new matrix formation and maturation. It was essential that the material be nonimmunogenic to minimize reactions that might cause rejection or destruction of the implant. Consequently, biochemical techniques were developed as part of the processing procedures to minimize such reactions.[4-6] We designed the implant to be technically straightforward to implant surgically with a minimum of sizing considerations. We thought that the implant would have to be nonabrasive, not produce any wear particles, and not incite an excessive inflammatory response. And finally, it was extremely critical that the implant be nontoxic to the cells that invaded the scaffold and eventually produced the new matrix.[8-10]

Hence, it was our hypothesis that if we could provide such an environment, the meniscus fibrochondrocytes, or other progenitor cells as we would learn later, would migrate into the scaffold, divide and populate the scaffold, produce extracellular matrix, and finally lead to the generation of new meniscuslike tissue. This new tissue then would preserve and help restore the damaged meniscus cartilage and would function like the meniscus to be chondroprotective. We affirmed our hypothesis and confirmed that we had met our requirements in various animal studies.[6,8,11]

Collagen Meniscus Implant Fabrication

The CMI is fabricated from bovine Achilles tendons (Fig. 14.1). The tendon tissue is trimmed and minced and then washed copiously with tap water to remove blood residue and water-soluble materials. The Type I collagen fibers are purified using various chemical treatments such

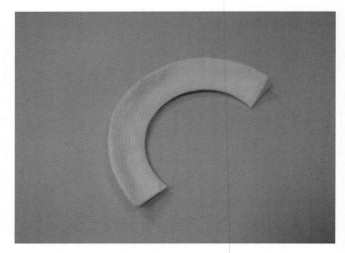

Figure 14.1   The collagen meniscus implant as it appears prior to implantation.

as acid, base, and enzymatic processes to remove noncollagenous materials and lipids. The isolated Type I collagen fibers then are analyzed for purity. After further processing, terminal sterilization is done by gamma irradiation.[4-6]

Indications

Initially, the CMI was designed for use only in the medial compartment of the knee. However, a lateral CMI has been developed and is in use outside the United States. The CMI is indicated for use in acute or chronic irreparable meniscus injuries or after previous partial meniscectomy. There must be enough remaining meniscus rim to which the CMI can be sutured. The CMI is contraindicated after total meniscectomy, if there is uncorrected ligamentous instability, if there is uncorrected axial malalignment, if there is untreated full-thickness loss of articular cartilage with exposed bone, or if there is documented evidence of allergy to collagen. Other systemic conditions may also preclude use of the CMI.

Surgical Technique

The CMI is placed using arthroscopic surgical procedures.[12-14] The damaged meniscus tissue is debrided minimally until healthy tissue is reached. If the debridement does not reach the red zone of the meniscus, a microfracture awl or similar instrument is used to perforate the host meniscus rim until a bleeding bed is assured.[13,14] A special malleable measuring device developed for this procedure is used to measure the exact size of the defect. The CMI is measured and trimmed to the correct size on the sterile field of the operating environment to fit the meniscus defect. If an inside-out suture technique is to be used, a posteromedial or posterolateral incision is made approximately 3 cm in length parallel and just posterior to the collateral ligament directly over the joint line so that the

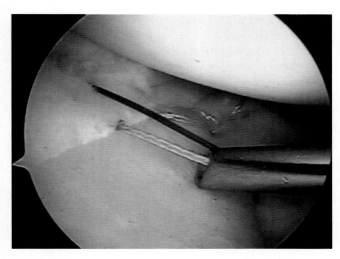

Figure 14.2 The collagen meniscus implant has been inserted into the lesion and is being sutured into place using an inside-out technique.

inside-out meniscus repair needles can be captured and the sutures tied over the capsule.[13,14] A specially designed introducer, which protects the rehydrated CMI, is inserted through the ipsilateral portal, and then a plunger pushes the implant out of the delivery device and into the joint. Alternatively, the CMI can be inserted into the joint dry with the aid of an atraumatic vascular clamp.

After satisfactory positioning, the implant is sutured to the host meniscus rim using standard inside-out techniques with zone-specific meniscus repair cannulae (Fig. 14.2).[13,14] We prefer to use a suture "gun," called the SharpShooter (ReGen Biologics, Franklin Lakes, NJ), to pass the sutures. Sutures are placed approximately 4 to 5 mm apart using size 2-0 nonabsorbable braided polyester suture material. Sutures are placed in a vertical mattress pattern around the rim of the meniscus remnant, and a horizontal pattern is used in the anterior and posterior horns.[13] Typically, eight to ten sutures are used to secure the implant in place. The sutures then are tied over the capsule in a standard manner.

Recently, we have gained positive experience with use of an all-inside fixation technique. For the all-inside technique, we prefer the FasT-Fix (Smith & Nephew, Andover, MA). However, additional care must be exercised to avoid damage to the CMI when using all-inside devices because they usually are larger and stiffer than needles and sutures.

Clinical Studies

In a phase II feasibility study, eight patients underwent arthroscopic placement of the CMI to reconstruct and restore the irreparably damaged medial meniscus of one knee during the first half of 1996.[13] Seven patients had one or more prior partial medial meniscectomies, and one patient had an acute irreparable medial meniscus injury. Patients were observed with frequent clinical, serologic, radiographic, and magnetic

resonance imaging (MRI) examinations for at least 24 months (range, 24 to 32 months) initially. As a part of the initial study, all patients underwent relook arthroscopy and biopsy of the CMI-regenerated tissue at either 6 or 12 months after implantation.[13] All patients improved clinically from preoperatively to 1 and 2 years postoperatively based on pain, Lysholm scores, Tegner activity scale, and self assessment. Relook arthroscopy revealed tissue regeneration in all patients with apparent preservation of the joint surfaces based on visual observations.

Based on measurements, the average amount of meniscus loss (defect) before placement of the CMI was 62%. That is, only 38% of the meniscus remained. At the initial relook surgery, the average filling of the meniscus defect was 77%, with a range of 40% to 100% based on actual measurements. Histologic analysis of the CMI-regenerated tissue confirmed new fibrocartilage matrix formation. Radiographs confirmed no progression of degenerative joint disease in the medial compartment.[13]

As a part of a long-term (5 to 6 years) follow-up study, all eight patients described previously returned for clinical, radiographic, and MRI examinations.[14] Clinical outcome measurements were virtually unchanged from the 2-year follow-up examination. Radiographs confirmed that the medial compartment chondral surfaces continued to be protected from further degeneration. MRI revealed that the CMI-regenerated tissue continued to mature, and it was often indistinguishable from the native meniscus tissue. All eight patients underwent relook arthroscopy to assess the status of the CMI-regenerated tissues as well as the condition of the chondral surfaces. The CMI-regenerated tissue appeared similar to the earlier relook arthroscopy, and its appearance was meniscuslike, both grossly and histologically (Fig. 14.3).[14]

At arthroscopy, the amount of the original meniscus defect remaining filled by newly generated meniscuslike tissue was determined with physical measurements and by comparison to video images of the index surgery and the

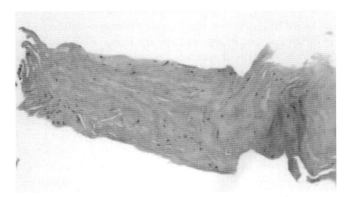

Figure 14.3 A biopsy obtained 6.3 years after placement of the collagen meniscus implant showing fibrocartilaginous tissue that is meniscuslike in appearance. The original magnification is ×25; the stain is hematoxylin and eosin.

first relook procedures. Physical measurements were made using the same arthroscopic measuring device that had been used during the index surgery. For example, if the original implant was 50 mm long and 7 mm wide, then it covered an area of 350 mm². If the newly generated tissue was measured and determined to cover 300 mm², then the original defect was calculated to remain 86% filled. The average amount of the original defect remaining filled at nearly 6 years after placement of the CMI was 69% (range, 50% to 95%).[14] That is, only a small loss of tissue had occurred since the initial relook about five years earlier when 77% of the defect was filled on average.[13] By adding the amount of filled defect to the amount of meniscus remaining at the time of index surgery, this group of eight patients had 81% of their normal meniscus (range, 66% to 98%) at about 6 years after placement of the CMI.[14] The percent of meniscus gain compared with the index remnant (the quotient of the percent of new tissue divided by the percent of remaining meniscus at index surgery) averaged 170% (range, 27% to 340%). No negative findings, such as damage to the chondral surfaces or exuberant tissue growth, attributable to the implant were observed.[14]

The positive results of this phase II feasibility study after 2 years[13] led to Food and Drug Administration approval of a large multicenter randomized (CMI versus meniscectomy alone) clinical trial of more than 300 patients in the United States. These patients were enrolled at 16 sites throughout the United States. Additionally, about 100 nonrandomized patients were enrolled at 10 sites in Europe and 2 sites in Japan. Patients who received the CMI had partial medial meniscus loss with an intact meniscus rim and no full-thickness chondral defects. Patients in the U.S. multicenter trial underwent frequent clinical examinations and relook arthroscopy with biopsy at 1 year postimplantation.

For patients enrolled in this multicenter study at our institution (n = 41), no serious or unanticipated complications have been attributed to the CMI. Patients routinely returned to daily activities by 3 months and most were fully active by 6 months, and then they continued to improve through at least 2 years, as evidenced by Tegner and Lysholm scores. Enzyme-linked immunosorbent assay testing failed to detect any increase in antibodies to the collagen material. No increased degenerative joint disease was observed, nor was there radiographic evidence of further joint-space narrowing. Sequential MRI examinations revealed progressive signal intensity changes indicating ongoing tissue ingrowth, regeneration, and maturation of the new tissue. At relook arthroscopy, gross appearance and shape of the regenerated tissue generally were similar to native meniscus cartilage with solid interface to the host meniscus rim in the majority of patients. The average amount of defect filled, calculated as previously described, was greater than 50%, with a range of 40 to 90%. Histologically, the collagen implant was progressively invaded and replaced by cells similar to meniscal fibrochondrocytes with production of new matrix. No inflammatory cells or histologic evidence of immunologic or allergic reactions were observed.

For all patients in the multicenter trial, we prospectively determined changes in Tegner activity levels from preoperative to 2 years postoperative in patients who received CMIs and were documented to have more than 50% total meniscus tissue at 1-year relook arthroscopy. One hundred thirty-eight patients, 18 to 60 years old, underwent partial medial meniscectomy and placement of a CMI to fill the meniscus defect. There were 64 acute (no prior meniscus surgery) and 74 chronic (1 to 3 prior partial meniscectomies on the involved meniscus) patients. At index surgery, meniscus defect size was measured with specially designed instruments, and the percent of meniscus loss was calculated based on these actual measurements. Relook arthroscopy was performed at 1 year on 124 patients (90% surgical follow-up), and percent total meniscus tissue (remnant plus new tissue) was determined by making these same measurements and calculations. Patients were followed clinically for a minimum of 2 years after CMI placement. At each follow-up, all patients completed questionnaires, including a Tegner score to assess activity. We then determined changes in Tegner score from the index surgery to 2 years status following CMI in these patients.

Of 124 relooks, 111 patients (90%) had more than 50% total meniscus tissue. In these patients, average Tegner activity scores improved by two levels, from 3 to 5 from preoperative to 2 years status following CMI. This increased change in activity level significantly correlated with total meniscus tissue more than 50% ($r = 0.21$, $p = 0.02$). These findings mirrored those we previously reported for partial meniscectomy patients in which more than 50% of the meniscus was maintained. Based on these observations, we conclude that there is a significant correlation between change (increase) in Tegner activity levels during 2 years and percent total meniscus tissue in patients who receive the CMI as treatment for meniscus loss and have more than 50% total meniscus tissue. This study confirms the importance of preserving as much meniscus tissue as possible at the time of repair or meniscectomy. It clearly supports the potential positive benefits of regrowing or regenerating lost meniscus tissue to assist patients in regaining their activity.

In the control group of this same randomized study, we prospectively determined the amount of tissue loss at time of partial medial meniscectomy and then correlated the extent of meniscus loss with clinical symptoms, function, and activity levels 2 years following the index meniscectomy. One hundred forty-nine patients, 18 to 60 years old, underwent partial medial meniscectomy and served as controls. There were 81 acute (no prior meniscus surgery) and 68 chronic (1 to 3 prior partial meniscectomies on the involved meniscus) patients. At index surgery, size of the meniscus defect was measured using specially designed instruments, and percent of meniscus loss was calculated based on actual measurements. Patients were followed clinically for a minimum of 2 years following meniscectomy. At each follow-up, every patient completed questionnaires, including Lysholm and Tegner scores, to assess function and activity. Amount of meniscus tissue at index surgery was correlated with the individual domains of the Lysholm scale. Tegner index was calculated to determine the amount of lost activity regained 2 years after surgical intervention.

Two-year data were available for 127 patients (85% follow-up). There was a significant correlation between the amount of meniscus tissue remaining following the index meniscectomy and 2-year Lysholm domains of squatting ($r = 0.28$, $p = 0.001$), stair-climbing ($r = 0.25$, $p = 0.004$), and swelling ($r = 0.26$, $p = 0.003$). In particular, it is noteworthy that patients who had more than 50% of their meniscus remaining had significantly better function than patients who had less than 50% meniscus remaining. Patients who had worse or no improvement in pain symptoms at 2 years averaged 42% meniscus remaining, while patients who had improved pain scores had on average 51% meniscus remaining. Tegner index for patients with less than 50% meniscus remaining averaged 24%, and for patients with more than 50% meniscus remaining averaged 52% ($p = 0.02$); hence, a greater amount of meniscus tissue remaining allowed patients to regain significantly more of their lost activity.

Based on these findings, we concluded that there is a significant correlation between the amount of meniscus tissue removed at meniscectomy and symptoms, function, and activity 2 years after surgery. This study confirms the importance of preserving as much meniscus tissue as possible at the time of meniscus repair or meniscectomy as well as the potential positive benefits of regrowing or replacing lost meniscus tissue in order to minimize clinical symptoms that may be suggestive of early degenerative changes.

Early in 2006, the lateral CMI received approval and the CE (Conformité Européene) mark in Europe. A limited release of that device is underway as of late 2006. No clinical data are yet available.

Based on our personal experiences with the limited long-term feasibility study and the randomized multicenter clinical trial, we conclude that the CMI is implantable, biocompatible, and bioresorbable. It supports new tissue regeneration as it is resorbed, and the new tissue appears to function similar to normal meniscus tissue. The advantage of the CMI, as opposed to partial meniscectomy alone, in limiting the progression of degenerative joint disease over the long term has not been definitely proven yet, but the results of the studies described here provide evidence that a CMI-based, tissue-engineered meniscus structure can survive within the joint.

Based on the relook procedures, the chondral surfaces are protected by the CMI-regenerated tissue. No serious or unanticipated complications directly related to the CMI have thus far been observed, and most patients have functioned well based on clinical examination and outcomes assessment. Relook arthroscopy results are positive and encouraging. These findings lend strong support to the concept that a CMI can be used to replace irreparable or removed meniscus tissue. Similar positive European observations resulted in obtaining the European Union CE mark for the CMI in 2000. Regulatory approval was obtained in Australia and Chile in 2002. Approval is pending in other non-U.S. countries at this time.

REFERENCES

1. Gladwell M. *Blink. The Power of Thinking Without Thinking.* New York: Little, Brown and Company; 2005.
2. Proust M. In: Jackson GS, ed. *Never Scratch a Tiger with a Short Stick.* Colorado Springs, CO: NavPress; 2003.
3. Vunjak-Novakovic G, Goldstein SA. Biomechanical principles of cartilage and bone tissue engineering. In: Mow VC, Huiskes R, eds. *Basic Orthopaedic Biomechanics and Mechano-Biology.* Philadelphia: Lippincott William & Wilkins; 2005:343–407.
4. Li S-T. Biologic biomaterials: tissue-derived biomaterials (collagen). In: Bronzino J, ed. *The Biomedical Engineering Handbook.* Boca Raton, FL: CRC Press; 1995:627–647.
5. Li S-T, Yuen D, Li PC, Rodkey WG, Stone KR. Collagen as a biomaterial: an application in knee meniscal fibrocartilage regeneration. *Materials Research Society Symposium Proceedings* 1994;331: 25–32.
6. Li S-T, Rodkey WG, Yuen D, Hansen P, Steadman JR. Type I collagen-based template for meniscus regeneration. In: Lewandrowski K-U, Wise DL, Trantolo DJ, et al., eds. *Tissue Engineering and Biodegradable Equivalents. Scientific and Clinical Applications.* New York: Marcel Dekker, Inc.; 2002:237–266.
7. Arnoczky SP. Building a meniscus. Biologic considerations. *Clin Orthop* 1999;367:S244–S253.
8. Stone KR, Rodkey WG, Webber RJ, McKinney LA, Steadman JR. Future directions: collagen-based prosthesis for meniscal regeneration. *Clin Orthop* 1990;252:129–135.
9. Rodkey WG, Stone KR, Steadman JR. Prosthetic meniscal replacement. In: Finerman GAM, Noyes FR, eds. *Biology and Biomechanics of the Traumatized Synovial Joint: The Knee as a Model.* Rosemont, IL: American Academy of Orthopaedic Surgeons; 1992:222–231.
10. Stone KR, Rodkey WG, Webber RJ, McKinney LA, Steadman JR. Development of a prosthetic meniscal replacement. In: Mow VC, Arnoczky SP, Jackson DJ, eds. *Knee Meniscus: Basic and Clinical Foundation.* New York: Raven Press, 1992;165–173.
11. Stone KR, Rodkey WG, Webber RJ, McKinney LA, Steadman JR. Meniscal regeneration with copolymeric collagen scaffolds: in vitro and in vivo studies evaluated clinically, histologically, biochemically. *Am J Sports Med* 1992;20:104–111.
12. Stone KR, Steadman JR, Rodkey WG, Li S-T. Regeneration of meniscal cartilage with use of a collagen scaffold: analysis of preliminary data. *J Bone Joint Surg Am* 1997;79A:1770–1777.
13. Rodkey WG, Steadman JR, Li S-T. A clinical study of collagen meniscus implants to restore the injured meniscus. *Clin Orthop* 1999; 367S:S281–S292.
14. Steadman JR, Rodkey WG. Tissue-engineered collagen meniscus implants: 5 to 6-year feasibility study results. *Arthroscopy* 2005; 21:515–525.

Rehabilitation Principles

15

Steve Stalzer   John Atkins   Gene Hagerman

■ INTRODUCTION 203

■ THE CRUCIAL PRINCIPLES OF
REHABILITATION 204
Teamwork 204
  Goals 205
  Communication 205
  Motivation 205
  Compliance 205
  Reinforcement 205
  Managing Complications 205
  Optimizing Results 205

■ REHABILITATION PROTOCOLS 206

■ HEALING TISSUE SHOULD NEVER BE
OVERSTRESSED 206

■ PREVENTING THE DETRIMENTAL EFFECTS OF
IMMOBILIZATION 206
Cardiopulmonary Conditioning 207

■ THE REHABILITATION PROGRAM MUST BE
BASED ON CURRENT RESEARCH 207
Options for Rehabilitation 207
  Home Versus Supervised Therapy 208
  Home Exercise Versus Weight Machines 208
  Aquatic Therapy 208
  Open Versus Closed Chain Exercise 208

■ PROGRESSION OF REHABILITATION MUST BE
BASED ON OBJECTIVE CRITERIA 208
Phase I: Immediate Rehabilitation 208
  Goals 208
Phase II: Intermediate Rehabilitation 209
  Goals 209

Phase III: Advanced 210
  Goals 210
Phase IV: Sport-Specific Training 211
  Goals 211

■ CASE STUDY 1: FEMORAL CONDYLE
MICROFRACTURE 216

■ CASE STUDY 2: ANTERIOR CRUCIATE
LIGAMENT RECONSTRUCTION
(BONE-TENDON-BONE GRAFT) 217

■ CASE STUDY 3: LYSIS OF ADHESIONS/ANTERIOR
INTERVAL RELEASE 217

■ THE FUTURE TRENDS IN REHABILITATION 218
The Facility 218
Influence of Technology 218

■ SUMMARY 218

In 1977 Dr. Steadman enlightened us (John Atkins and Gene "Topper" Hagerman) with his vision of rehabilitation. This vision has formed the basis of our rehabilitation philosophy—principles and practices—in the care of athletes and others who come to our clinic. As one of the inventors of modern rehabilitation, Dr. Steadman recognized the importance of progressing rehabilitation objectively and preventing the detrimental effects of immobilization, but also protecting the integrity of healing tissue. Dr. Steadman also values teamwork, research-based rehabilitation, and using rehabilitation guidelines that assure consistency in patient care and outcomes.

While we were working with the U.S. Alpine Ski Team in Squaw Valley, California, Dr. Steadman was practicing orthopaedics in South Lake Tahoe. If an athlete needed rehabilitation, Dr. Steadman would initiate the rehabilitation in his home, monitor and progress the rehabilitation, and analyze the outcomes.

When we were traveling with the ski teams, he was just a phone call away for advice. This communication sealed our bond as a team. In 1984, after the most successful Winter Olympics in Alpine history, we joined Dr. Steadman in South Lake Tahoe, where he invited us to work with all of his patients, including the athletes, no matter what the sport. We joined Dr. Steadman at local and national orthopaedic meetings and the trainers' conferences. We shared his vision and described our rehabilitation program. We met other orthopaedic surgeons. One orthopaedic surgeon, John A. Feagin, MD, in particular, was as enthusiastic as we were about Dr. Steadman's rehabilitation practices and philosophy. We were propelled by teamwork, passion, and knowledge. This combination has helped us create one of the most successful rehabilitation programs in the country.

Our rehabilitation team moved together with Dr. Steadman from South Lake Tahoe to Vail, Colorado, in 1990. As the number of patients grew, communication between physician, patient, and therapist became even more important. We designed clear and concise protocols to enable patients to follow our rehabilitation program even if they returned home to continue their rehabilitation. For those patients, we emphasized the importance of keeping in contact by phone calls. We wanted them to know that although we may not be physically involved in their rehabilitation, we were only a phone call away. That was important to us. Keeping in touch with patients, particularly returning their calls, is one practice that shows we care. Everyone associated with Dr. Steadman cares about the patient and the quality of care for each patient.

The rehabilitation team has grown from the 2 of us to almost 50 employees today (2006). Two leaders, Sean McEnroe and Steve Stalzer, joined the team in 1996 and 2001, respectively. They both share our values and work ethic. Together, Sean and Steve have started an extensive mentoring system for our therapists and have expanded our vision. The key to our growth is the wisdom of Dr. Steadman, who continues to guides us, the quality of the new therapists we hire, and always looking ahead and trying to get that much better in the arena of physical therapy, physical fitness, and health.

How do we know we are succeeding? After surgery, the Steadman Hawkins Research Foundation tracks patients and their outcomes. The Foundation has an extensive database on patient satisfaction, return to work, return to sports, and longevity of their lifestyles.

We still keep in touch with a remarkable number of patients and continue to tell each patient that we are a lifelong resource for them.

In the following pages, we share the principles of our rehabilitation program and conclude with our vision of the future. What new technology will arrive on the scene? How much of new technology will we incorporate into our program? We will adapt to the technology that is compatible with our philosophy so long as the technology does not eliminate the hands-on approach and the therapist-patient relationship. Our goals and values will never change. We will continue to be the best that we can be and we will aim to become better.

John and Topper

THE CRUCIAL PRINCIPLES OF REHABILITATION

A strong rehabilitation team is an essential part of the successful sports medicine clinic. It is important that the physician and rehabilitation team share common goals, mutual respect, and effective communication. Within the rehabilitation team, the following principles are vital to achieving consistently successful outcomes in rehabilitation.

- Teamwork with the physician, therapist, and patient, working toward a common goal, is essential.
- The rehabilitation protocol is not a cookbook, but a set of guidelines that assure consistency in patient care, compliance, and outcomes.
- The rehabilitation program must be based on current research and evidence-based practice.
- Healing tissue should never be overstressed.
- The detrimental effects of immobilization must be prevented.
- Progression through each stage of rehabilitation must be based on objective criteria.

Teamwork

An emphasis on teamwork is the foundation for the successful sports medicine program. The team must share a common goal, mutual respect, and attention to communication. The successful therapist also fulfills the roles of motivating the patient, assuring patient compliance, re-enforcing the physician's instructions, and managing complications to optimize results.

In 1989, before Dr. Steadman moved to Vail, he asked four individuals (John Atkins, Topper Hagerman, Crystal Adams, and Shirley Carlson) if they would move with him and continue to work as part of his team. To this day, Dr. Steadman insists that he would not have moved if any one member of the team had not been willing to relocate.

Each of these individuals has been a part of his team for more than 20 years.

Goals

The goals of rehabilitation are to return the patient to his or her desired level of activity as quickly and safely as possible. To achieve these goals, the physician, therapist, and patient must work together to determine the best rehabilitation course following injury or surgery. Often, success is measured by how quickly an athlete returns to competition. Although quick return is important, it is vital that the patient's safety not be compromised as a result. It is equally important that the patient has a long-term successful outcome that includes avoidance of additional injury. Longevity of patient satisfaction and overall health should never be compromised in the return to athletic competition.

Communication

Effective communication among the rehabilitation team members generates and perpetuates successful patient outcomes. The physician and rehabilitation team must communicate clearly about general rehabilitation principles as well as each patient's plan. We develop postoperative protocols that are fundamental for physician/therapist/patient communication. These protocols are developed through extensive collaboration of all team members including the patient. To assure clear communication, each physician starts his or her day with rounds to see postoperative patients in the rehabilitation clinic with the rehabilitation team. This time is dedicated to establishing each patient's postoperative rehabilitation course and to clarify individual protocol adjustments. Surgical findings are discussed with the therapist and patient as well as how these findings affect the rehabilitation program. Dedication to communication assures that the patient receives a consistent message from the physician and therapist. Close communication also allows us to respond quickly to any patient problems that arise during rehabilitation.

For the patient who does not live locally, communication is especially important. The patient must clearly understand his or her postoperative rehabilitation program following surgery. A clearly outlined protocol assists in guiding the patient through each phase of rehabilitation. The therapist must maintain adequate contact with the patient to assure that he or she stays on track with the rehabilitation program. Frequent communication allows the therapist to manage complications early and alter the rehabilitation program if needed. It is important to remember that communication does not happen automatically and cannot be taken for granted.

Motivation

Motivation is vital for individuals recovering from an injury, just as it is for optimal athletic performance. Each person is motivated in different ways. Understanding how to motivate each individual is essential for optimizing effectiveness as a rehabilitation provider. The first step in motivating a patient is to establish trust and make a personal connection with each patient.

- Take time to get to know patients beyond their current injury.
- Find out their interest, activities, sports, and where they are from.
- Find out their rehabilitation goals as well personal goals that relate to their health and fitness.

Compliance

Motivation is one key factor in patient compliance, but a well-designed rehabilitation program and the therapist's professional knowledge are also important. Proper motivation by the therapist leads the patient to be accountable to the rehabilitation program as well as his or her overall health. The patient must understand that his or her role is essential to the success of the rehabilitation program. In addition, a well-designed exercise program is important in achieving patient compliance. The program must be comprehensive, but not overwhelming. Patient compliance improves when the rehabilitation program is limited to the smallest number of exercises that adequately meet the needs of the patient. Patient understanding and knowledge of the rehabilitation program is the final element of compliance. The better the patient understands why each exercise is important, the more likely he or she is to be compliant with the exercise program.

Reinforcement

Because the therapist has the opportunity to see the patient weekly or even daily, it is important that the therapist reinforce key messages to the patient. Reinforcement is unique to each patient and may include weightbearing restriction, bracing, or specific exercises. Compliance must be continually reinforced for optimal patient outcomes.

Managing Complications

An awareness and proper management of potential complications is essential for consistently successful outcomes. Attention to joint effusion, joint pain, and tendonitis are all elements the therapist and the patient watch for during the rehabilitation program. Early treatment of complications can be the difference between a minor adjustment to the rehabilitation program and a major setback. The patient should also be properly instructed to watch for swelling and pain, particularly when advancements are made in the rehabilitation program. Close communication between the therapist and physician allows for expedited treatment of complications.

Optimizing Results

Optimal results are achieved when effective teamwork, communication, and patient compliance are combined with a sound rehabilitation program. Several key elements exist in optimizing the results of rehabilitation. The first key is to understand and follow the fundamental principles of rehabilitation. The second element is the "art" of progressing each patient appropriately through the rehabilitation program. It is equally important that the therapist understand when to accelerate and when to decelerate the patient's rehabilitation. Focusing on overall fitness is another key element of optimizing results. Working on cardiovascular fitness, core strength, and upper body strength all aid in improved fitness. The last element in optimizing results is accomplished by working on performance enhancement during the final stage of rehabilitation.

By initially building endurance, strength, and then power, the athlete has built a solid foundation for advanced sport specific training and plyometrics. Form running, speed training, and agility drills can push the athlete to be quicker, faster, and stronger than before injury.

Finally, accountability leads to improved compliance with the rehabilitation program and thus leads to improved outcomes and optimal results. Compliance also improves when the patient understands the rationale for the rehabilitation program. It is the role of the therapist to reinforce patient compliance and to keep the patients motivated as they progress through each phase of rehabilitation. The successful therapist understands that motivation is essential for consistently successful outcomes.

REHABILITATION PROTOCOLS

The rehabilitation protocol is not a cookbook, but a set of guidelines that assure consistent patient care, improved compliance, and improved outcomes. Consistent patient care is achieved when all patients follow a consistent rehabilitation philosophy. The rehabilitation protocol assures that the nonlocal patient will continue to follow the same philosophy after returning home. Improved compliance is achieved by providing the patient with a comprehensive protocol that provides the patient with knowledge of the rehabilitation program. The combination of consistent patient care and improved compliance results in improved outcomes and allows for analysis of outcomes. An additional benefit of protocols is that they provide an avenue for communication with other rehabilitation providers. The rehabilitation program or protocol should be based on fundamental rehabilitation principles. The protocol should be comprehensive yet simple enough to enhance patient compliance. It is a key element for patient, therapist, and physician communication and has allowed us to maintain consistent care with patients who complete their therapy in all parts of the world.

HEALING TISSUE SHOULD NEVER BE OVERSTRESSED

The management of knee injuries has evolved significantly in recent years with the advancement of arthroscopic techniques and rehabilitation knowledge. The application of minimally invasive surgical techniques has facilitated rela-

tively rapid returns to sporting activity in both recreational and elite athletes.[1] The dilemma in rehabilitation is that the rates of healing must be balanced with rehabilitation that stresses these injured, repaired, or reconstructed elements of the knee.[2] Rehabilitation involves restoration of normal range of motion, gait, proprioception, and strength to allow return to functional activity. In the recreational or professional athlete, the rehabilitation program must also focus on restoration of power, speed, and agility for optimal return to competition.

The need for return to activity as quickly as possible is clear, but the time at which safe return is possible is less clear.[3,4] If neuromuscular coordination, strength, or endurance is inadequate, static elements of joint stability share greater loads and the normal bone, cartilage, or ligaments may fail putting the repair or reconstruction at risk.[2,5,6] The dilemma in rehabilitation is that rates of healing must be balanced with coordination that stresses injured, repaired, or reconstructed elements of the knee. Delay in initiating physical conditioning lengthens the time for return to preinjury activity level and may encourage some patients to resume activity when healing is maximized, but conditioning is not optimal.[2] We do understand that healing tissue should not be overstressed.

Communication among the physician, therapist, and patient is essential in understanding the constraints of tissue healing related to the patient's injury, repair, or reconstruction. The physician and therapist must also stay abreast of current research related to time constraints of tissue healing. We have seen a trend for success to be measured by how fast a patient returns to sports. Although the time for return to competition is important, it is equally important that safety is not compromised. A truly successful outcome is measured by longevity of patient satisfaction and a long-term healthy, asymptomatic knee.

Knee joint effusion and the subsequent capsular distention can cause major alterations in the normal gait cycle and can be considered a causative factor promoting the acquisition of quadriceps avoidance gait patterns.[7] Weight-bearing restrictions are surgery-specific, but crutches should not be discontinued until the patient is able to demonstrate a pain-free, normal gait pattern. We typically instruct patients in partial weightbearing with crutches for a minimum of 1 week to assist in decreased knee stress and joint effusion.

PREVENTING THE DETRIMENTAL EFFECTS OF IMMOBILIZATION

The effects of joint immobilization are dramatic and include muscle atrophy, articular cartilage degeneration, ligament strength loss, and excessive adverse collagen formation.[1,8–17] Experimental studies in cat and rabbit knees show that the earliest changes with immobilization take place at about 15 days and include subsynovial intracapsular connective tissue proliferation in the infrapatellar and intercondylar regions. By 30 days, fibrofatty tissue enveloping the cruciate ligaments completely filled the notch, extending from the patellar tendon posteriorly to articular surfaces not in contact. The tissue density increased daily and was mature within 1 month. Adhesions forming over articular cartilage were present at 15 days and the cartilage surface was noted to lose definition with progressive loss of the tangential cell layer.[18]

Biochemically, the intra-articular and periarticular connective tissue shows a steady decrease in glycosaminoglycans and water. Collagen remains more stable with a half-life of 300 to 500 days and as a result forms random cross links. New, altered collagen is deposited in small amounts in a nonaligned fashion.[1] Immobility inevitably results in localized areas of articular cartilage that are subject to compression during a sustained period. Decreased cellular activity, loss of chondrocytes, and neovascularization results. Loss of chondroitin sulfate rapidly accelerates with time and the immobilized joint begins to resemble a degenerative joint by 4 weeks.[16] Clinically, the patellofemoral joint is at great risk.[2] Scarring of the anterior interval, the interval between the patellar tendon fat pad and the tibia, is a common reason for stiffness in the anterior cruciate ligament (ACL) reconstruction patient.[19] These adhesions can cause significant alterations in patellofemoral and tibiofemoral kinematics and contact, and reduce the knee extension force.[20]

Avoiding adhesion formation is accomplished by joint motion and preventing localized compressive forces. Joint motion is accomplished with the use of a continuous passive motion machine, passive range of motion (ROM) exercise, and patellar mobilization. The primary effects of continuous passive motion are increased synovial fluid movement, intermittent compression, and soft tissue tension in the knee. This results in more rapid clearing of hemarthroses, prevention of adhesion formation, and stress-induced connective tissue healing.[11] Passive ROM exercise and patellar mobilization exercises are performed three to four times daily. We instruct each patient to perform a total of 10 to 15 minutes of inferior-superior and medial-lateral patella glides as well as medial-lateral patellar tendon glides three times each day for up to 6 weeks following surgery.

Immobilization can also have detrimental effects on joint proprioception. It has been demonstrated that proprioceptive afferents conduct more rapidly than A-delta and C fibers. Thus, the proprioceptive afferents allow immediate reflex control of joint position.[21-24] Lack of tonic input through functional stimulation at the spinal level may act to imbalance the normal spinal tonic efferent output completely.[25] Alterations in tonic stimulus by immobilization and nonweightbearing may uncouple "learned" reflexes and require relearning to achieve preinjury levels of activity.[26] This first link of the kinetic chain is extremely important in achieving a high degree of coordination, agility, and dynamic joint stability.[2] Salter et al.[11] have shown that

early rehabilitation with continuous passive motion may, in fact, alter perception of pain by proprioceptive input using these reflex arcs, and this may ultimately help to keep these arcs functional.

The sequence of injury, pain, and immobilization inevitably results in muscle atrophy and loss of strength.[2] To achieve the goal of returning the athlete to sport as quickly and safely as possible, prevention of atrophy is as important as reconditioning.

Haggmark et al.[27] have demonstrated that pain and immobilization result in selective atrophy of type I (slow twitch or red muscle) fibers, which are most numerous in extensor or more tonic postural muscles. Type II fibers show resistance to change in fiber size and decreased glycolytic activity. It is also evident that muscle fiber type composition can change.

Immobilization has been shown to influence both the muscle itself and its innervation resulting in a significant decrease in percentage of type I muscle fibers.[7] Quadriceps and hamstring stretching has been postulated as decreasing atrophy from studies demonstrating diminished atrophy and type I fiber loss for muscles in tension[2] (secondary to monosynaptic extrafusal stimulation by muscle spindles). Passive range of motion and cocontraction may adequately reproduce this tension. Electrical stimulation to facilitate muscle contraction has been shown to prevent type I muscle atrophy and muscle inhibition due to pain and swelling.[28-31]

Cardiopulmonary Conditioning

The loss of aerobic conditioning following 7 weeks of immobility has been demonstrated by Costill et al.[32] Well-leg rowing and upper extremity ergometers are effective ways to prevent aerobic deconditioning. In addition, cross-extremity training has been demonstrated as a useful adjunct to muscle conditioning.[33] Upper body and core training are other methods used to provide vigorous exercise and thus a sense of well-being.

THE REHABILITATION PROGRAM MUST BE BASED ON CURRENT RESEARCH

The rehabilitation program must be based on current research and evidence-based practice. Many options exist in rehabilitation programs. Open versus closed chain exercise is one example of the options. It is important that the therapist continue to evaluate both current research and clinical results in developing and improving rehabilitation programs.

Options for Rehabilitation

Several options exist in accomplishing the goals of rehabilitation. These include home versus supervised therapy, home exercise or weight machines, and open versus closed chain exercise.

Home Versus Supervised Therapy

The decision for the patient to do home versus supervised therapy is as individualized as the program itself. Research completed by Beard and Dodd[34] has shown that structured supervised instruction by a trained therapist in combination with a home exercise program is more effective than a home program alone in the restoration of muscle strength, function, and ROM following knee surgery. For patients who will not attend supervised therapy, it is vital that they receive a comprehensive rehabilitation program and have a sufficient understanding of the key elements of their rehabilitation program.

Home Exercise Versus Weight Machines

All types of resistance training are beneficial for strengthening. Finding the type of program with which the patient is more likely to be compliant with is the most important factor for making the decision of home exercise versus free weights or machines. Because many of our patients prefer a home-based program that they can also perform while traveling, we often use Sport Cords (Topper Sports Medicine, Vail, CO) as a key element in our rehabilitation programs.

Aquatic Therapy

The use of aquatic therapy is beneficial for many patients with knee injuries.[35,36] Aquatic therapy is particularly beneficial for gait training, increasing ROM, decreasing joint compression stress during strengthening, providing cardiovascular exercise in a deweighted condition, and for low-impact agility drills.

Open Versus Closed Chain Exercise

An area of recent attention in rehabilitation is whether to strengthen through the use of open or closed kinetic chain exercises. Open kinetic chain exercises are described as those exercises in which the foot is not in contact with a solid surface or the ground (e.g., leg extensions). The resistive loads are applied to the tibia and are transferred directly to the knee. Only the muscles immediately surrounding the knee are required to perform the exercise, which allows for specific strengthening but which also can place increased forces directly through the knee joint. Open kinetic chain exercises include leg extensions. Closed kinetic chain exercises are defined as exercises in which the foot is in contact with the ground or another solid surface (e.g., squats, leg press). The foot is opposed by a ground-reaction force, which is transmitted through all of the joints in the lower extremity.

Intersegmental forces at the knee indicate that closed kinetic chain exercises produce lower anterior shear load on the tibia, increase tibiofemoral compressive forces, enhance muscle contraction, and decrease patellofemoral compressive forces near extension. These factors are thought to protect the ACL graft and better restore knee function.[37,38] A recent comparison of exercises found that an increase in resistance during open kinetic chain extension exercise produced increased ACL strain that did not occur during closed kinetic chain exercise.[38] Increased ACL strain has also been noted with open kinetic chain quadriceps contraction at 30 and 15 degrees of flexion compared with no ACL strain noted at 60 and 90 degrees.[38] In contrast, hamstring dominated open kinetic chain flexion appears to pose little risk to the ACL throughout the entire flexion arc. If open kinetic chain extension strengthening is used following ACL injury, care must be taken to avoid the ranges of 0 to 30 degrees of knee motion.

A thorough understanding of joint kinematics as well as open kinetic chain and closed kinetic chain exercises must be attained before deciding which should be used for each patient. In addition to anterior and posterior tibial translation, patellofemoral joint stresses must be considered as contact stresses through the patella change as the knee moves through a full arc of motion. Although it is important to consider each patient's needs individually, our rehabilitation programs have primarily focused on closed chain exercises performed within pain-free ranges of motion.

PROGRESSION OF REHABILITATION MUST BE BASED ON OBJECTIVE CRITERIA

Progression through each phase is based on clinical criteria and time frames as appropriate. It is important that the physician and therapist communicate clearly about criteria for progression of the rehabilitation program.

Phase I: Immediate Rehabilitation

Goals
- Protect integrity of repaired tissue
- Diminish pain and inflammation
- Restore ROM within restrictions
- Prevent muscular inhibition
- Maintain cardiovascular fitness

The initial phase of rehabilitation starts immediately following surgery and in general lasts until injured or repaired tissue can accept the stress of full weightbearing and full ROM. The goals during this phase are to protect the integrity of repaired tissue, diminish pain and inflammation, restore ROM within restrictions, prevent muscular inhibition, and maintain cardiovascular fitness.

To protect repaired tissue and limit joint stress, weightbearing and ROM are restricted for 1 to 8 weeks, depending on the surgical procedure. All postsurgical patients remain on partial weightbearing for at least 1 week or until they can ambulate with a normal gait pattern. By restricting weightbearing for at least 1 postoperative week, joint stress is decreased in the swollen knee, as is the potential for arthrofibrosis. A brace is used when limiting ROM or further protection is required to avoid tissue stress. We commonly use a postoperative brace to protect the knee following ACL reconstruction/repair, meniscus repairs, trochlear groove microfracture, and patellar tendon fenestrations and repairs.

Inflammation and pain are controlled through the use of ice, compression, elevation, nonsteroidal anti-inflammatory medications, and early ROM exercises. An early emphasis on reduction of swelling is important in achieving full ROM, preventing muscular inhibition, and reducing the potential for joint contractures and scar tissue formation. Effusion is monitored closely as we have found that unresolved swelling can be problematic for achieving the phase I goals of rehabilitation. Early ROM is started the day of surgery using a continuous passive motion machine, and passive ROM exercises to restore joint motion and decrease the potential for scaring in the joint. Stationary bicycling is added as soon as is safely allowed after the patient is able to achieve 110 degrees of knee flexion.

Early passive ROM and patellar mobility are emphasized starting the day of surgery. Early ROM exercises are performed through full ROM unless the range is limited to protect repaired tissue. Prone passive ROM and manual calf support are used to avoid posterior tibia translation following posterior cruciate ligament reconstruction or repair. Achieving full flexion and extension are both equally important and ROM is monitored daily during phase I. Much of the patient's time during this phase is spent focusing on ROM and patellar mobility as full ROM is required for normal joint mechanics and to avoid unnecessary joint stress that leads to future problems.

Along with early passive ROM, emphasis is placed on patella and patellar tendon mobility to prevent the formation of adhesions in the patellofemoral joint. Each patient is instructed to perform manual patella and patellar tendon mobility for 10 to 15 minutes two to three times each day. For most patients, patellar mobility is best achieved with a therapist or partner performing the mobility. This avoids hamstring tension and allows for muscular relaxation, which is ideal for patellar mobilization. Patients are instructed to perform medial/lateral and superior/inferior movement of the patella and medial/lateral movement of the patellar tendon (Figs. 15.1 and 15.2). Flexing the knee to 20 degrees allows the patient to more easily palpate the patellar tendon. However, this position may decrease mobility from increased patellar tendon tension.

The prevention of muscular inhibition is achieved through early strength exercises that limit joint stress while providing the appropriate load through the knee and lower extremity muscles. Isometric strengthening is typically initiated immediately following surgery for the quadriceps, hamstrings, and gluteal muscles. Hamstring isometrics are delayed for 6 weeks for patients with posterior cruciate ligament injury.

Maintaining cardiovascular fitness is important in maintaining overall fitness, to increase blood flow and tissue healing, and for psychological benefit. Single-leg rowing, aerodyne bicycling, and upper body exercises are the most

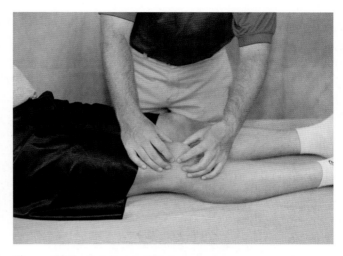

Figure 15.1 Patellar mobilization.

common exercises used at our clinic. Single-leg rowing is performed with the involved leg sliding passively on plexiglas placed next to the rower. For aerodyne bicycling, the involved leg is placed on a foot peg and only the upper body and uninvolved leg perform the exercise. Once the goals for phase I have been met and full weightbearing is allowed, patients are progressed to the intermediate phase of rehabilitation.

Phase II: Intermediate Rehabilitation

Goals
- Protect integrity of repaired tissue
- Restore full ROM
- Restore normal gait pattern
- Progressively increase muscle endurance/strength
- Restore and improve balance and proprioception
- Maintain and improve cardiovascular fitness

The intermediate phase of rehabilitation is typically started between 2 and 8 weeks postoperatively, depending

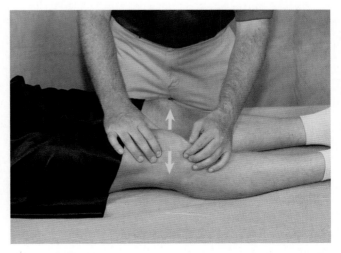

Figure 15.2 Medial/lateral movement (*arrows*) of the patellar tendon.

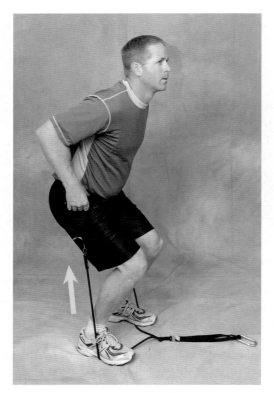

Figure 15.3 One-third knee bends using the Sport Cord. Arrow indicates direction of movement.

on the surgical procedure and weightbearing restrictions. The second phase of rehabilitation includes a progression of ROM/stretching, gait training, and strengthening. Passive ROM and stretching exercises should be continued as needed to maintain full ROM.

Gait training should take place both in the pool and on land as the patient is progressed off of crutches. Patients are instructed to wean off of crutches as tolerated and to avoid joint pain and swelling as they increase their time off crutches. Patients progress by increasing their weightbearing percentage before discontinuing one crutch then discontinuing both crutches. Patients are also instructed to progress through this phase without limping and are instructed to continue with the use of one or both crutches until they can ambulate without a limp. Once the patient can demonstrate a normal gait pattern, he or she is allowed to progress with weightbearing strength exercises.

Intermediate strength exercises include double one-third knee bends (Fig. 15.3), carpet drags (Fig. 15.4), and gas pedals (Fig. 15.5) using a Sport Cord. The use of a Sport Cord at this phase of rehabilitation allows for low-load endurance strengthening that also challenges the patient's proprioceptive system. These exercises are performed with a low load and high repetitions while focusing on proprioceptive control. Stationary biking with resistance, swimming with fins, and walking on an inclined treadmill are additional low-stress exercises used to work on cardiovascular fitness and muscular endurance. Once the goals of phase II have been met, patients are progressed to the advanced phase of rehabilitation.

Phase III: Advanced

Goals
- Restoration of muscular strength
- Improve cardiovascular fitness
- Optimize neuromuscular control/balance/proprioception

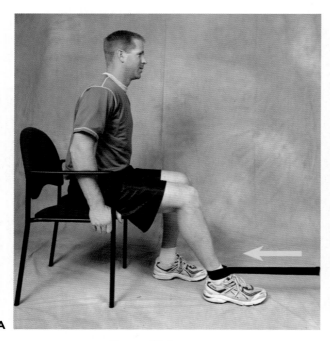
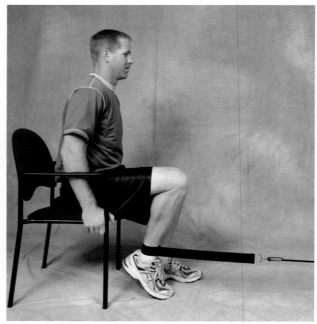

Figure 15.4 Carpet drags using the Sport Cord. Arrow indicates direction of movement.

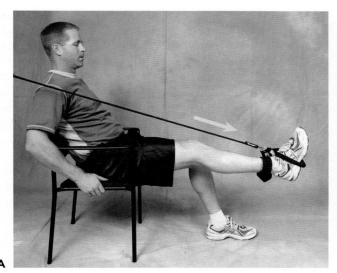
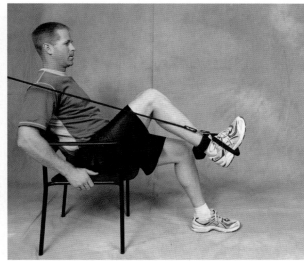

A   B

Figure 15.5   Gas pedals using the Sport Cord. Arrow indicates direction of movement.

The advanced phase of rehabilitation is started between 4 and 16 weeks postoperatively depending on the surgical procedure. During this phase, patients focus on restoration of muscular strength, improvement of cardiovascular fitness, and neuromuscular control.

Advanced strength and neuromuscular control exercises use a Sport Cord for forward (Fig. 15.6) and backward (Fig. 15.7) running, single-knee bends (Fig. 15.8), and side-to-side lateral agility (Fig. 15.9). Cardiovascular training should continue with progressive biking, inclined treadmill,

elliptical trainer, stair climber, and swimming. Once the goals of phase III have been met, patients are allowed to begin sport-specific training.

Phase IV: Sport-Specific Training

Goals
- Strengthen more than 85% of the uninvolved side
- Completion of functional sports test
- Completion of a return-to-sports program

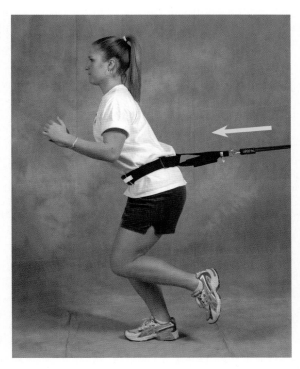
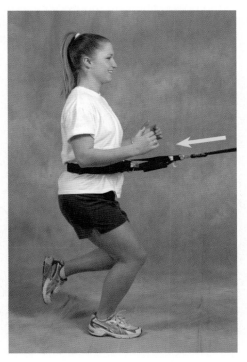

Figure 15.6   Forward running using the Sport Cord. Arrow indicates direction of movement.

Figure 15.7   Backward running using the Sport Cord. Arrow indicates direction of movement.

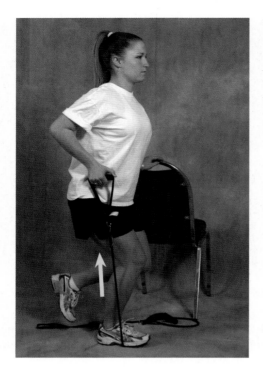

Figure 15.8 Single-knee bend using the Sport Cord. Arrow indicates direction of movement.

Sport-specific training is initiated between 6 and 24 weeks postoperatively. The goals of this phase are 85% strength compared with the uninvolved extremity, completion of a functional sports test, and completion of a return-to-sports program. Any deficits in ROM, strength, power, balance, and proprioception are addressed as needed.

Little has been published on functional sport testing. Although hop tests and isokinetic strength testing were pop-

ularized in the 1990s, no research has been published on reinjury rates following successful completion of these tests. Wilk et al.[39] established a correlation between the single-leg hop and isokinetic testing at 160 deg/sec, but no reinjury rates following successful completion of either test have been published. Although hop tests allow for easy comparison to the contralateral extremity, they are only good tests for the patient capable of passing the test. For the patient who is not ready to pass the test, the landing can place unnecessary stress on the ACL.

Our return-to-sports test was established in 1980 to test endurance, strength, power, agility, and the ability to accept a load through the hip, knee, and ankle. The test is safe for patients who fail testing, and in 25 years of testing, no patient has damaged his or her knee from testing. The test is also ideal because the test exercises are used as part of the patient's home program to work on continued endurance, strength, and agility. Because of our close interaction and communication with each physician, we have been able to successfully use this test within our clinic. Each physician has a good understanding of the test and its scoring system. In addition to the score, the therapist communicates the reason for lost points, which are from pain, lack of form, or endurance.

The test is used for assessment of knee pain as well as tested prior to return to participation in sporting events. The test is a valuable indicator of whether the patient with knee pain will be able to rehabilitate successfully without pain restricting his or her success. The test is also used for assessing the ability to return to sporting activities. The test consists of four exercises: single-leg squatting with resistance, lateral agility, forward jogging, and backward jogging, with a Sport Cord being used for each exercise. Figure 15.10 presents a complete description of the Howard Head Sports Medicine Return-to-Sport Test.

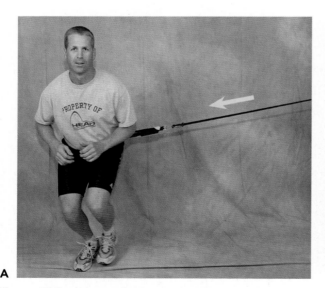
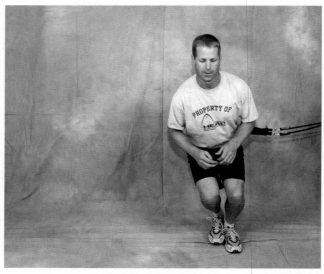

Figure 15.9 Side-to-side lateral agility using the Sport Cord. (**A**) Start position (lean against cord); (**B**) End cycle (weight transfer). Arrow indicates direction of movement.

Howard Head Sports Medicine
181 W. Meadow Dr., Vail, CO 81657
Phone: (970)476-1225 FAX: (970)479-7193

RETURN-TO-SPORT TEST

Name: _____   **Date:** _____

M.D. _____   **Dx** _____ **Mo.s/p** _____

Single Knee Dips (goal: 3 min). Time: _____
1 point for each 30 seconds (____/6)
Circle deductions: form pain endurance   Score _____/6

Lateral Agility (goal: 80 seconds) Time: _____
1 point for each 20 seconds (1 2 3 4)
1 point for 30° of knee flexion excursion (5)
Circle deductions: form pain endurance   Score _____/5

Forward Running (goal: 2 min) Time: _____
1 point for each 30 seconds (1 2 3 4)
1 point for 30° of knee flexion excursion (5)
Circle deductions: form pain endurance   Score _____/5

Backward Running (goal: 2 min) Time: _____
1 point for each 30 seconds (1 2 3 4)
1 point for 30° of knee flexion excursion (5)
Circle deductions: form pain endurance   Score _____/5

Score: _____/21
(18 pass)

Future Program Instructions:

Figure 15.10 Return-to-sport test. (Copyright © 2006, Rehabilitation and Performance Center, LLC. Reprinted with permission from Howard Head Sports Medicine, Vail, CO.)

Single Knee Bend

Purpose:	To test single leg strength/endurance and evaluate patellar tracking.
Supplies:	Sport Cord (Topper Sports Medicine, black cord)
	Goniometer
	Stopwatch
Description:	Cord setup: 1. The athlete places the heel of the foot on the cord. 2. The D ring of the handle is aligned with the knee joint line to remove slack from the cord. 3. Tension is set by pulling the cord handle to the waste line. 4. Having the athlete hook their thumb around their pant line is helpful in maintaining tension on the cord.

The Movement is a 1/3 single knee bend between 30°–60° of flexion. A chair can be utilized to mark 60° for the athlete prior to starting – the athlete's buttocks should lightly touch the chair at 60° of knee flexion.

The Athlete will perform knee bends to 60 degrees at a cadence of 1 second up and 1 second down for a goal of 3 minutes. Two fingers are allowed for balance on a chair back.

Technique:	The athlete must perform each repetition <u>without</u> a Trendelenburg sign, the knee locking in full extension, or the patella extending past the toe.
Scoring:	1 point is earned for each 30-second increment completed with proper form.

Testing is stopped if the subject is unable to complete with the above form on 5 consecutive repetitions or 10 nonconsecutive repetitions.

Testing is stopped if the patient has pain >3/10 for 30 seconds.

Lateral Agility

Purpose:	To test the ability of the knee/leg to accept load and push off in a lateral direction.
Supplies:	Sport Cord (Topper Sports Medicine, black cord)
	Goniometer
	Stopwatch
Description:	Cord setup: 1. Place waist belt through the handles; attach sport cord end to the door jam or secure post. 2. Attach waist belt. Stand with the involved leg toward the cord attachment. 3. Step away until tension is reached where the athlete compensates with leaning. 4. Tape a line on the lateral aspect of the involved foot. 5. Measure the distance from the greater trochanter to the floor. 6. Use this measured distance to place a second tape line parallel to the first.
Technique:	The athlete must land on/inside the first tape line with the <u>involved</u> foot and on/outside the second tape line with the <u>uninvolved</u> foot.

The athlete is to hop from one leg to the other; absorbing energy as he/she lands by bending at the knee (primary) and the hip (secondary). Instruct the athlete that one point is earned for achieving 30° of knee flexion excursion throughout the test. Excursion is defined as the amount of absorption from knee flexion at landing to max knee flexion.

Each repetition should take 1 second. Explain to the athlete that he/she must explode laterally, land, absorb, and maintain control for a goal of 80 seconds. Only one foot should be on the ground at any time.

Figure 15.10   *(continued)*

Scoring: 1 point is earned for every 20 seconds completed with proper form.

Testing is stopped if the subject is unable to complete with the form on 5 consecutive repetitions or 10 nonconsecutive repetitions.

Testing is stopped if the patient has pain >3/10 for 30 seconds.

1 point is given for good form/absorption if 30° of knee flexion excursion is achieved throughout the entire 80 seconds.

Forward Run

Purpose: To test lower extremity strength, endurance, and absorption.
Supplies: Sport Cord (Topper Sports Medicine, black cord)
Goniometer
Stopwatch
Description: Cord setup: 1. Place waist belt through handles, attach the sport cord end to a door jam or secure post. 2. Attach waist belt. Stand facing away from the wall. 3. The athlete is to maintain a distance in front of the proximal tape line set for the lateral agility test; keeping constant cord tension. 4. A second tape line may be placed at the toes for a visual cue.
Technique: The activity is a forward jog in place. The athlete must hop from one leg to the other using proper form; absorbing energy with each landing by bending at the knee (primary) and the hip (secondary). Instruct the athlete that one point is earned for achieving 30° of knee flexion excursion throughout the test.

Each repetition should take 0.5 seconds per foot. Correct performance of this activity is through proper absorption with knee flexion as the athlete transfers weight onto that extremity. Explain to the athlete that he/she must land, absorb, and maintain control for a goal of 2 minutes. Only one foot should be on the ground at any time.

Scoring: 1 point is earned for every 30 seconds completed with proper form.

Testing is stopped if the subject is unable to complete with the above form on 5 consecutive repetitions or 10 nonconsecutive repetitions.

Testing is stopped if the patient has pain >3/10 for 30 seconds.

1 point is added for good form/absorption if 30° of knee flexion excursion is achieved throughout the entire 2 minutes.

Backward Run

Purpose: To test lower extremity strength, endurance, and absorption.
Supplies: Sport Cord (Topper Sports Medicine, black cord)
Goniometer
Stopwatch
Description: Cord setup: 1. Place waist belt through handles, attach the sport cord end to a door jam or secure post. 2. Attach waist belt. Stand facing toward the wall. 3. The athlete is to maintain a distance in front of the proximal tape line set for the lateral agility test; keeping constant cord tension. 4. A second tape line may be placed at the toes for a visual cue.

Figure 15.10   (continued)

Technique:	The activity is a backward jog in place. The athlete must hop from one leg to the other through proper form; absorbing energy with each landing by bending at the knee (primary) and hip (secondary). Instruct the athlete that one point is earned for maintaining 30° of knee flexion excursion throughout the test.
	Each repetition should take 0.5 seconds per foot. Correct performance of this activity is through proper absorption with knee flexion as the athlete transfers weight onto that extremity. Explain to the athlete that he/she must land, absorb, and maintain control for a goal of 2 minutes. Only one foot should be on the ground at any time.
Scoring:	1 point is earned for every 30 seconds completed with proper form.
	Testing is stopped if the subject is unable to complete with the above form on 5 consecutive repetitions or 10 nonconsecutive repetitions.
	Testing is stopped if the patient has pain >3/10 for 30 seconds.
	1 point is added for good form/absorption if 30° of knee flexion excursion is achieved throughout the entire 2 minutes.

Figure 15.10   (*continued*)

CASE STUDY 1

Femoral Condyle Microfracture

A 21-year-old college football player presents with acute knee pain that has worsened during a period of 4 weeks. His pain was worse with weightbearing and impact activities. Pain is preventing participation in football practice and weight lifting. On physical examination, the patient had full ROM, ligament stability, and thigh girth. Magnetic resonance imaging revealed a 2 × 2 cm grade IV lesion of the medial chondral surface of the femur. After discussion between the patient and physician, the decision was made to have a microfracture surgical procedure.

The patient was referred to therapy immediately following surgery with the following instructions: nonweight-bearing for 8 weeks, no brace, full passive ROM. The first 8 weeks of rehabilitation included ROM exercises with a goal of full extension and flexion, edema control, quadriceps sets and leg raises, hamstring sets, hamstring stretching, and patella and patellar tendon mobility. A continuous passive motion machine was used 8 hours per day for the first 8 weeks. At week 3, spinning on a bike without resistance and aqua jogging in a deep pool were initiated.

At week 9 pregait activities began and the patient was weaned off crutches during a period of 7 days. Additional exercises included toe and heel raises, and one-third knee bends, hamstring curls, and leg press with a Sport Cord. The patient also began stationary biking with resistance, swimming with fins, and walking on the treadmill. All exercises were performed in a pain-free range.

At week 13 the elliptical trainer, rowing machine, and double-knee bends with a Sport Cord were added. At week 17 single-knee bends, lateral agility, and forward/backward jogging with a Sport Cord were added. These exercises were used to progress the patient's endurance, strength, and power and to work on his ability to accept a load with his knee. Initial agility drills began at week 17. Advanced agility drills and field work began at week 21.

At week 25 the patient had full ROM, equal thigh girth and strength bilaterally, and was able to pass a sport test with a 20/21. The physician cleared the patient to return to preseason conditioning and practice without activity restrictions.

CASE STUDY 2

Anterior Cruciate Ligament Reconstruction (Bone-Tendon-Bone Graft)

A 32-year-old male ski instructor presents following an acute grade III ACL tear. The patient's primary complaint is instability with athletic movements. On physical examination he lacks 2 degrees of extension and 8 degrees of flexion. Quadriceps and hamstring strength are rated 4/5 and 5/5, respectively. Thigh girth is equal bilaterally. After consulting with his physician, he scheduled ACL reconstruction with a bone-tendon-bone autograft.

The patient was referred to therapy preoperatively to decrease swelling, establish 0 to 120 degrees of ROM, and restore good quadriceps function. He attended therapy three times during a period of 1 week, during which he was treated with ROM exercises, patella and patellar tendon mobility, quadriceps sets and straight-leg raises, stationary biking, and modalities for edema control.

Following surgery, the patient was instructed to maintain partial weightbearing for 1 week, then to wean off crutches as tolerated. A postoperative knee brace was set at 0 to 90 degrees and was used at all times except for physical therapy. Full passive ROM was allowed and therapy was initiated the day of surgery.

The first week of rehabilitation included ROM exercises with a goal of achieving full passive flexion and extension, quadriceps sets and straight-leg raises, hamstring sets, hamstring stretching, and patella and patellar tendon mobility. Modalities were used for edema management and for facilitation of normal quadriceps function. At week 2 the patient began weaning off crutches and was able to ambulate with no limp and no assistive device by the end of the second postoperative week. Stationary biking with no resistance and toe and heel raises were added as well. Aqua jogging and one-third knee bends were added at week 3.

At week 7 the patient had full ROM, ambulated with no limp, and had good quadriceps function. There was no evidence of swelling and mild atrophy of the vastus medialis muscle. The patient was allowed to begin walking on an inclined treadmill, swimming with fins, and double-knee bends, hamstring curls, and leg press using a Sport Cord. At week 9 the elliptical trainer was added to the rehabilitation program. At week 10 single-knee bends and forward and backward jogging in place with a Sport Cord were added.

At week 12 the patient added the stair stepper, lateral agilities, and initial agility drills. The patient progressed from building endurance, strength, and then power. At 16 weeks the athlete had a 1-cm difference in quadriceps girth and scored a 16/21 on a functional sports test. The patient had restored preinjury endurance and cardiovascular fitness but lacked strength and power as well as the ability to fully accept an eccentric load during agility drills. At 20 weeks quadriceps girth was equal bilaterally and the patient passed the functional sport test with a score of 19/21. A postoperative brace was used as the patient returned to recreational skiing before returning to ski instructing full time at week 22.

CASE STUDY 3

Lysis of Adhesions/Anterior Interval Release

A 29-year-old female nurse presents with right anterior knee pain and tightness in the patellar tendon region with running, skiing, and hiking. She is 2 years status following right ACL reconstruction with a hamstring autograft. The first year and a half following ACL reconstruction she was able to resume full function, including trail running, skiing, hiking, and mountain biking. The patient had failed an 8-week course of physical therapy including modalities, patellar mobility, stretching, and quadriceps, hamstring, and gluteal muscle strengthening. On physical examination the patient lacked 2 degrees of hyperextension and 1 cm of thigh girth with comparison to the contralateral leg. Patella and patellar tendon mobility were decreased as well. After discussion between the patient and physician, the decision was made to have an arthroscopic lysis of adhesion and anterior interval release procedure.

The patient was referred to therapy immediately following surgery with the following orders: partial weightbearing for 2 weeks, full passive ROM, and emphasis on patella and patellar tendon mobility. The first week of rehabilitation included ROM exercises including manual hamstring and posterior capsule stretching and prone hangs to achieve full passive extension. Manual patella and patellar tendon mobility was performed for 15 minutes three times per day. Additional exercises included spinning on a stationary bike with no resistance, quadriceps sets and straight-leg raises, and hamstring sets. The patient was weaned off crutches following 2 weeks of partial weightbearing.

At week 3 the patient demonstrated a normal pain-free gait pattern, full flexion and extension ROM, and no edema. At week 3 aqua jogging was added 3 days per week. No additional strengthening was added to avoid joint stress that might cause adhesion formation.

At week 7 the patient began closed chain exercises including biking with resistance, inclined treadmill, swimming with fins, and one-third knee bends, hamstring curls, and leg press with a Sport Cord. At week 10 the patient initiated advanced Sport Cord exercises including single-leg squats and forward and backward jogging in place. Lateral agility exercises were added at week 11.

At week 12 the patient demonstrated full ROM and patellar mobility, no edema, no pain with exercise, and equal thigh girth. The patient passed a functional sport test with an 18/21 and was cleared to return to skiing, yoga, Pilates, and trail running.

THE FUTURE TRENDS IN REHABILITATION

The Facility

Our facility has been successful in creating the culture we want. There are times when privacy is desirable, and even necessary. However, our gymnasium environment has been appreciated by many of our patients. Patients are motivated by seeing others who are a month ahead of them postoperatively. Those patients get to know one another and develop a camaraderie that helps in attaining successful outcomes. Having such a facility that allows privacy when appropriate but also allows a motivating environment is compatible with our philosophy and principles. Being as close to the physicians as possible is key for teamwork and communication. There is nothing special about our rehabilitation equipment. A million-dollar facility is not worth anything until you have quality staff who relate to patients and a systematic program.

Influence of Technology

As time goes on, technological advances continue to play a role in our rehabilitation programs. We have found visual feedback provided by equipment such as Monitored Rehabilitation Systems (Haarlem, The Netherlands) to be very beneficial for our patients. We expect this technology to continue to assist patients in the development of neuromuscular control, proprioception, and even motivation. Computer modeling in biomechanics is another way that the science behind rehabilitation will continue to improve. There are also places for monitoring equipment that technology could enhance, such as ROM and strength data collection. We must keep our eyes and ears open to technology and keep exploring advances in rehabilitation technology.

One area that we hope future technology does not take away is the "hands-on" interaction between the therapist and patient. We will lose the culture, the touch, and the trust that develops between that of a patient and a therapist if rehabilitation becomes automated. To make everything easier by treating patients with impersonal machines would be a detriment.

SUMMARY

Rehabilitation guidelines and protocols following knee arthroscopy or injury must be followed to assure consistent rehabilitation and patient outcomes and to return the patient to full functional activities as quickly and safely as possible. While surgical procedures continue to advance, athletes are already pushing the limits to return to competition as quickly as possible. As postoperative protocols evolve, it is essential to follow the basic guidelines of rehabilitation. Initially, soft tissue healing constraints must be considered while focusing on controlling inflammation and pain, restoring full ROM, and preventing muscle atrophy. As physiological healing occurs, rehabilitation must address progressive lower extremity strengthening, proprioceptive retraining, and sport-specific training. In our opinion, a functional return to sports test is the best way to assess readiness to return to sports activities.

ACKNOWLEDGMENTS

We would like to thank Molly Scanlan, MPT, OCS, and Dirk Kokemeyer, MPT, COMT, for case study contributions, and Meredith Mueller, PT, and Sean McEnroe, PT, MBA, for text editing.

REFERENCES

1. Akeson WH, Woo SL-Y, Amiel D, et al. The connective tissue response to immobility: biochemical changes in periarticular connective tissue of the immobilized rabbit knee. *Clin Orthop* 1973;93:356–362.
2. Steadman, JR, Forster RS, Silferskiöld, JP. Rehabilitation of the knee. *Clin Sports Med* 1989;8:605–627.
3. Higgins RW, Steadman JR. Anterior cruciate ligament repair in world class skiers. *Am J Sports Med* 1987;15:439–447.
4. Paulos L, Noyes FR, Grood E. et al. Knee rehabilitation after ACL reconstruction and repair. *Am J Sports Med* 1981;9:140–149.
5. Noyes FR, Mooar PA, Matthews DS, et al. The symptomatic anterior cruciate-deficient knee. Part I. The long term functional disability in the athletically active individuals. *J Bone Joint Surg Am* 1983;65:154–162.
6. Noyes FR, Torvik PJ, Hyde WB, et al. Biomechanics of ligament failure. II. An analysis of immobilization, exercise, and re-conditioning effects in primates. *J Bone Joint Surg Am* 1974;56:1406–1418.
7. Torry MR, Decker MJ, Viola RW, et al. Intra-articular knee joint effusion induces quadriceps avoidance gait patterns. *Clin Biomech* 2000;15:147–159.
8. Dehne E, Tory R. Treatment of joint injuries by immediate mobilization, based upon the spinal adaptation concept. *Clin Orthop* 1971;77:218–232.
9. Haggmark T, Erikson E. Cylinder or mobile cast brace after knee ligament surgery: a clinical analysis and morphologic and enzymatic

study of changes of the quadriceps muscle. *Am J Sports Med* 1979;7: 48–56.

10. Noyes FR, Mangine RE, Barber S. Early knee motion after open and arthroscopic anterior cruciate ligament reconstruction. *Am J Sports Med* 1987;15:149–160.

11. Salter RB, Simmonds DF, Malcolm BW, et al. The biological effects of continuous passive motion on the healing of full thickness defects of articular cartilage. An experimental investigation in the rabbit. *J Bone Joint Surg Am* 1980;62:1232–1251.

12. Salter RB, Bell RS, Kealey F. The protective effect of continuous passive motion on living articular cartilage in acute septic arthritis: an experimental investigation in the rabbit. *Clin Orthop* 1981;159:223–247.

13. Woo SL-Y, Mathews SU, Akeson WH. Connective tissue response to immobility. *Arthritis Rheum* 1975;18:257–264.

14. Wilk KE, Andrews JR. Current concepts in the treatment of anterior cruciate ligament disruption. *J Orthop Sports Phys Ther* 1992;15:279–293.

15. Baber YF, Robinson AH, Villar RN. Is diagnostic arthroscopy of the hip worthwhile? A prospective review of 328 adults investigated for hip pain. *J Bone Joint Surg Br* 1999;81:600–603.

16. Ginsberg JM, Eyring EJ, Curtiss PH, Jr. Continuous compression of rabbit articular cartilage producing loss of hydroxyproline before loss of hexosamine. *J Bone Joint Surg Am* 1969;51:467–474.

17. Troyer H. The effect of short term immobilization on the rabbit knee joint cartilage: A histochemical study. *Clin Orthop* 1975;107: 249–257.

18. Evans EB, Eggers GWN, Butler JK, et al. Experimental immobilization and remobilization of rat knee joints. *J Bone Joint Surg Am* 1960;42:737–758.

19. Steadman JR, Bollum TS. Principles of ACL revision surgery and rehabilitation. *Sports Med Arthrosc Rev* 2005;13:53–58.

20. Ahmad CS, Kwak SD, Ateshian GA, et al. Effects of patellar tendon adhesions to the anterior tibia on knee mechanics. *Am J Sports Med* 1998;26:715–724.

21. Kennedy JC, Alexander IJ, Hayes KC. Nerve supply of the human knee and its functional importance. *Am J Sports Med* 1982;10: 329–335.

22. Limbird TJ, Shiavi R, Frazer M, et al. EMG profiles of knee joint musculature during walking: changes induced by anterior cruciate ligament deficiency. *J Orthop Res* 1988;6:630–638.

23. Slocum DB, Larson RL. Rotary instability of the knee: Its pathogenesis and a clinical test to demonstrate its presence. *J Bone Joint Surg Am* 1968;50:211–225.

24. Walla DJ, Albright JP, McAuley E, et al. Hamstring control and the unstable anterior cruciate ligament-deficient knee. *Am J Sports Med* 1985;13:34–39.

25. Dehne E. Treatment of fractures of the tibial shaft. *Clin Orthop* 1969;66:159–173.

26. Basmajian JV. *Muscles Alive* 3rd ed. Baltimore: Williams & Wilkins, 1974:1–139.

27. Häggmark T, Jansson E, Eriksson E, et al: Fiber-type area and metabolic potential of the thigh muscle in man after surgery and immobilization. *Int J Sports Med* 1981;2:12–17.

28. Delitto A, Rose SJ, McKowen JM. Electrical stimulation versus voluntary exercise in strengthening thigh musculature after anterior cruciate ligament surgery. *Phys Ther* 1988;68:660–663.

29. Eriksson E, Haggmark T. Comparison of isometric muscle training and electrical stimulation supplementing isometric muscle training in the recovery after major knee ligament surgery. *Am J Sports Med* 1979;7:169–171.

30. Lossing I, Grinby G, Johnson T. Effects of electrical muscle stimulation combined with voluntary contractions after knee ligament surgery. *Med Sci Sports Exerc* 1988;20:93–98.

31. Morissey MC, Brewster CE, Shields CL. The effects of electrical stimulation on the quadriceps during post-operative knee immobilization. *Am J Sports Med* 1985;13:40–44.

32. Costill DL, Fink WJ, Habansky AJ, et al. Muscle rehabilitation after knee surgery. *Phys Sports Med* 1971;5:71.

33. Hellebrandt FA, Waterland JC, et al. Indirect learning: The influence of unimanual exercise on related muscle groups of the same and opposite side. *Am J Phys Med* 1962;41:45–55.

34. Beard DJ, Dodd CA. Home or supervised rehabilitation following anterior cruciate ligament reconstruction: a randomized controlled trial. *J Orthop Sports Phys Ther* 1998;27:134–143.

35. Suomi R, Collier D. Effects of arthritis exercise programs on functional fitness and perceived activities of daily measures in older adults with arthritis. *Arch Phys Med Rehabil* 2003;84: 1589–1594.

36. Wyatt FB, Milam S, Manske RC, et al. The effects of aquatic and traditional exercise programs on persons with knee osteoarthritis. *J Strength Cond Res* 2001;15:337–340.

37. Brotzman SB, Wilk KE. *Clinical Orthopaedic Rehabilitation.* 2nd ed. Philadelphia: Mosby, 2003:267–270.

38. Fleming BC, Oksendahl H, Beynnon BD. Open- or closed-kinetic chain exercises after anterior cruciate ligament reconstruction. *Exerc Sport Sci Rev* 2005;33:134–140.

39. Wilk KE, Romaniello ET, Soscia SM, et al. The relationship between subjective knee scores, isokinetic testing, and functional testing in the ACL-reconstructed knee. *J Orthop Sports Phys Ther* 1994;20:60–73.

ADDITIONAL SUGGESTED READING

Dorfman H, Boyer T. Arthroscopy of the hip: 12 years of experience. *Arthroscopy* 1999;15:67–72.

Hagerman GR, Atkins JA, Dillman C. Rehabilitation of chondral injuries and chronic degenerative arthritis of the knee in the athlete. *Oper Tech Sports Med* 1995;3:127–135.

Haggmark T, Eriksson E, Jansson E. Muscle fiber type changes in human skeletal muscle after injuries and immobilization. *Orthopedics* 1986;9:181–185.

Irrgang JJ, Pezzullo D. Rehabilitation following surgical procedures to address articular cartilage lesions of the knee. *J Orthop Sports Phys Ther* 1998;28:232–240.

Steadman JR, Rodkey WG, Rodrigo JJ. Microfracture: surgical technique and rehabilitation to treat chondral defects. *Clin Orthop* 2001;391(Suppl):362–369.

Steadman JR, Rodkey WG, Singleton SB, et al. Microfracture technique for full-thickness chondral defects: technique and clinical results. *Oper Tech Orthop* 1997;7:300–304.

The Horse-Human Relationship: Research and the Future

16

C. Wayne McIlwraith   William G. Rodkey

■ INTRODUCTION 221

■ THE HORSE AS A MODEL FOR ARTICULAR DEFECTS IN THE HUMAN KNEE 222

■ EARLY STUDIES OF MICROFRACTURE IN THE HORSE 222

■ OTHER LESSONS LEARNED FROM THE HORSE: IMPORTANCE OF REMOVAL OF CALCIFIED CARTILAGE 223

■ FURTHER ATTEMPTS TO AUGMENT THE ENDOGENOUS REPAIR FROM MICROFRACTURE USING GENE THERAPY 224

■ EVALUATION OF CHONDROCYTE TRANSPLANTATION TECHNIQUES IN AN EQUINE MODEL 224

■ THE FUTURE 226

The horse is a magnificent athlete. The athletic pursuits include racing, show jumping, eventing (combined training), dressage, cutting, reining, and the rodeo events of roping, team roping, steer wrestling, and barrel racing. Elite equine athletes, like elite human athletes, suffer trauma to the limbs in general and joints in particular. They also suffer a similar range of diseases as occur in the elite human athlete. Like human patients, arthroscopic surgery revolutionized our ability to treat these athletes. Arthroscopic techniques were developed for the horse closely behind those developed for humans. Their ability to return a horse to racing at the same level was exemplified by "Spend A Buck" winning the Kentucky Derby in the first weekend of May 1985, after having arthroscopic surgery for carpal chip removal by the first author in December 1984. However, osteoarthritis often accompanies acute trauma and also develops with repeated injury. The cartilage defects that limit the human's ability to compete are similar to those that limit the horse. Osteoarthritis has been estimated to cause the retirement of 60% of athletic horses.[1]

In 1992 the second author introduced the first author to J. Richard Steadman, MD. Dr. Steadman had developed the straightforward, but brilliant, idea of microfracture to facilitate access to healing elements in the bone marrow underneath cartilage defects. At this time the first author had become frustrated with previous methods of bone marrow access and attempts to heal articular cartilage defects in the horse. After some preliminary work evaluating the value of the horse as a model of cartilage healing in the human knee, a collaborative research project was initiated to do a controlled study evaluating microfracture in cartilage healing and this was funded by both the Steadman-Hawkins Research Foundation and the Orthopaedic Research Center at Colorado State University, where the first author is the director.

THE HORSE AS A MODEL FOR ARTICULAR DEFECTS IN THE HUMAN KNEE

From a clinical point of view, there are two distinct goals for cartilage repair: (a) restoration of joint function, which includes pain relief, and (b) prevention of, or at least delay of, the onset of osteoarthritis.[2] These goals can potentially be achieved through replacement of damaged or lost articular cartilage with a substance capable of functioning under normal physiologic environments for an extended period. Screening of potential procedures for human clinical use had been done by preclinical studies. Restoration of a joint surface is assessed by its appearance anatomically, histologically, biologically, and mechanically relative to the original tissue, hyaline cartilage. Preclinical studies use animal models. The choice of animal models is one of the most frequently discussed and controversial issues in biomedical research, especially in orthopaedics. It has been stated that the key issue in the selection of the appropriate model is to match the model to the question being investigated and the hypothesis being tested.[3]

In 1929, August Krogh, a Danish physiologist, wrote, "for a large number of problems there will be some animals of choice, or a few such animals, in which it [the problem] can be most conveniently studied."[4] However, it has also been pointed out that the uncritical application of this principle could lead to inaccurate generalizations, because extrapolating findings from one species to another is not without flaws.[5] The researcher must consider which animal model(s) most accurately represent(s) the human condition being investigated and to what extent the results obtained from these models might be extrapolated to humans.[6] The obvious critical questions with regard to joint defect repair are (a) which animal model(s) most accurately represents the critical chondral defect in humans and (b) to what extent can preclinical research results in this model be extrapolated to humans.[2] The equine stifle (femoropatellar and femorotibial articulations) are comparable to the human knee, and this joint also suffers considerable naturally occurring clinical disease. Osteoarthritis with erosion of articular cartilage occurs naturally on the medial condyle of the femur. In addition, the femoral trochlear ridges are commonly affected with osteochondritis dissecans.

A study was done in the first author's laboratory where histologic measurements of the thickness of noncalcified and calcified cartilage, as well as the subchondral bone plate in five locations on the femoral trochlea and medial femoral condyles of species used in preclinical studies of human articular cartilage were made and compared with those of the human knee.[7] Cadaveric specimens were obtained of six human knees, as well as six equine, six goat, six dog, six sheep, and six rabbit stifle joints (the animal equivalent to the human knee). Specimens were taken from the lateral trochlear ridge, medial trochlear ridge, and medial femoral condyle of the femur. After histopathologic

processing, the thickness of noncalcified and calcified cartilage layers, as well as the subchondral bone plate, was measured. Average articular cartilage thickness over five locations was 0.2 to 0.3 mm for the rabbit, 0.5 to 0.7 mm for the sheep, 0.5 to 0.8 mm for the dog, 0.6 to 1.5 mm for the goat, 1.8 to 2.2 mm for the horse; human femurs showed a range of 2.4 to 2.9 mm. It was concluded that the horse provided the closest approximation to humans in terms of articular cartilage thickness, and this approximation is considered relevant in preclinical studies of cartilage defects.[7]

The typical human lesion is a defect on the medial femoral condyles and the defect is limited to the articular cartilage. Hunziker[8] has given an example of the difficulty of creating an articular cartilage defect only in such species as the rabbit. If one created a 3-mm deep lesion in rabbit articular cartilage (the majority of which would be in the bone), 93% to 95% of the volume of this defect would be ensheathed by bone, bone marrow space, and vasculature (yielding an abundance of different cell types, growth factors, and signaling substances) and only 5% to 7% of the defect volume would abut on cartilage. Because of the thickness of articular cartilage on the medial condyle of the femur of the horse, experimental defects can be made without compromising the subchondral bone plate, but at the same time, removal of the calcified cartilage layer can be assured. In addition, these defects can be made arthroscopically, and after surgery the horses can be exercised at an increasingly athletic level on a high-speed treadmill.

EARLY STUDIES OF MICROFRACTURE IN THE HORSE

The use of microfracture, or *micropicking*, as it has been referred to in equine arthroscopy, has many of the advantages associated with subchondral drilling, including focal penetration of the dense subchondral plate to expose cartilage defects to the benefits of cellular and growth factor influx, as well as improving anchorage of the new tissue to the underlying subchondral bone, and to some extent, surrounding cartilage.[9–11] However, microfracture has the advantages over drilling in that there is no thermal necrosis, and the holes have rough edges, which seems to enhance clot adhesion. Additionally, the microfracture awls allow access to all areas of the joint, whereas some areas cannot be reached with drills. The simplicity of microfracture comes from the use of a tapered awl (Linvatec, Largo, FL; Arthrex, Naples, FL) that eliminates the need for powered instrumentation and gives accurate control. A tapered entry into the subchondral marrow space is achieved.

The first experimental study in the horse documented improvement in the quantity of tissue and the type II collagen content at 4 and 12 months after microfracture of full-thickness defects[12] (Fig. 16.1). The testing model was a 1-cm^2 defect made arthroscopically on the medial condyle of the femur. The medial femoral tibial joint is a separate

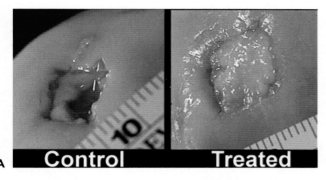

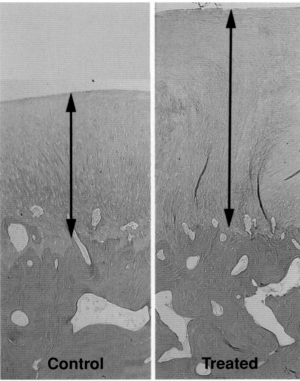

Figure 16.1 From the first experimental study in the horse, improvement was shown in the amount of tissue on **(A)** gross examination and **(B)** histologic examination 12 months after microfracture of full-thickness defects. Both images are at the same magnification and the arrows define the depth of repair tissue. (Reprinted with permission from Frisbie DD, Trotter GW, Powers BE, et al. Arthroscopic subchondral bone plate microfracture augments healing of large osteochondral defects in the radial carpal bone in medial femoral condyles of horses. *Vet Surg* 1999:28; 242–255.)

joint compartment. The arthroscope was placed into the joint from the lateral aspect. The anterior instrument portal allowed a curette to be used to debride the cartilage down to the subchondral bone plate. Evaluations were made at 4 and 12 months.

A second study at the Orthopaedic Research Center evaluated early events in cartilage repair after subchondral bone microfracture. The initial idea of this study (also funded by the Steadman-Hawkins Research Foundation) was to see if there was a "marker" signifying positive cartilage healing and also to see if microfracture affected the

early events in healing. Between 2, 4, 6, and 8 weeks, gene expression (using real-time polymerase chain reaction) showed an increase in mRNA expression for both type II collagen and aggrecan (Fig. 16.2). There was significant improvement in gene expression for type II collagen at 8 weeks.[13] Aggrecan increased but it was not significantly enhanced by microfracture.

These two studies in the horse confirmed that microfracture did have a significant effect on articular cartilage healing. It also initiated its use in our clinical practice patients in the horse, where it is used in a number of joints at arthroscopy if there is cartilage erosion with the subchondral plate still intact and/or sclerotic.

OTHER LESSONS LEARNED FROM THE HORSE: IMPORTANCE OF REMOVAL OF CALCIFIED CARTILAGE

During the previously mentioned equine studies looking at microfracture, it was noted that if there was retention of any calcified cartilage, inferior healing was obtained. This finding has also been reported in the dog, as well as in earlier equine studies from the Orthopaedic Research Center at Colorado State University, but no controlled work had been done to define the actual difference. Hence, a third study was done with the hypothesis that removal of the calcified cartilage with retention of subchondral bone enhances the amount of attachment of the repair tissue compared with retention of the calcified cartilage layer. This was a randomized, blocked experimental study, again involving 1-cm^2 articular cartilage defects made in 12 skeletal mature horses on the axial weightbearing portions of both medial femoral condyles. Using a custom measuring device and direct arthroscopic observation of the subchondral bone beneath the calcified cartilage layer, we either removed or retained the calcified cartilage layer in one defect of each horse.[14] The repair was assessed with arthroscopy, clinical examination, radiographic and magnetic resonance imaging examinations, biopsy at 4 months, gross and histopathologic examinations at 12 months, as well as small mRNA and immunohistochemical evaluations.

The results of the study described in the preceding paragraph showed that removal of calcified cartilage with retention of the subchondral bone plate increased the overall repair tissue, improved attachment to surrounding articular cartilage and underlying subchondral bone, as well as firmness on palpation (Fig. 16.3 and Fig. 16.4). The clinical pain, radiographic and magnetic resonance imaging evaluations, histologic character, matrix proteins, or mRNA expression did not appear to differ based on the level of defect debridement. It was concluded that removal of the calcified cartilage layer appears to provide optimal amount and attachment of repair tissue and that close arthroscopic visualization is recommended for the debridement of clinical lesions to ensure removal of the calcified cartilage layer.

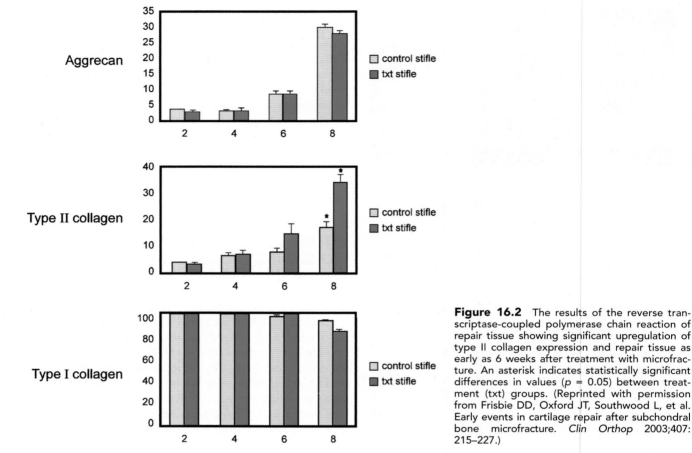

Figure 16.2 The results of the reverse transcriptase-coupled polymerase chain reaction of repair tissue showing significant upregulation of type II collagen expression and repair tissue as early as 6 weeks after treatment with microfracture. An asterisk indicates statistically significant differences in values ($p = 0.05$) between treatment (txt) groups. (Reprinted with permission from Frisbie DD, Oxford JT, Southwood L, et al. Early events in cartilage repair after subchondral bone microfracture. *Clin Orthop* 2003;407: 215–227.)

FURTHER ATTEMPTS TO AUGMENT THE ENDOGENOUS REPAIR FROM MICROFRACTURE USING GENE THERAPY

The most recent study done in horses has been evaluating the use of gene therapy in addition to subchondral microfracture using the same femoral condyle defects. As a collaborative effort between four universities—the Orthopaedic Research Center at Colorado State University, Cornell University, University of Pittsburgh, and Harvard—we were able to evaluate the usefulness of a combined gene therapy protocol using the interleukin-1 (IL-1) receptor antagonist to decrease the effects of IL-1 on cartilage repair, as well as insulinlike growth factor-1, which has been previously shown to enhance cartilage healing in an equine model, as well as to reduce the deleterious effects of IL-1.[6,15] Using an osteoarthritic IL-1 coculture (synovial membrane and articular cartilage), system gene transduction of insulinlike growth factor-1 and IL-1ra proteins was demonstrated using an adenoviral vector with protection of proteoglycan loss in the cartilage.[6] There was also restoration of cartilage

matrix without IL-1 present using the same *in vitro* system.[15] This combination gene therapy protocol was then evaluated using full-thickness articular chondral defects treated with microfracture in the horse.[16] The protocol enhanced the quality of the repair tissue in full-thickness equine chondral defects compared with microfracture alone in that there was increased type II collagen as well as aggrecan content in the defects.

EVALUATION OF CHONDROCYTE TRANSPLANTATION TECHNIQUES IN AN EQUINE MODEL

Autogenous chondrocyte transplantation is one of the few Food and Drug Administration (FDA)-approved tissue engineering techniques to treat articular cartilage injury in humans (Carticel; Genzyme, Cambridge, MA). It is a two-stage procedure in which articular cartilage biopsies are harvested arthroscopically from minimally weightbearing regions of the injured knee, propagated *ex vivo* in cell culture, and later implanted under an autoge-

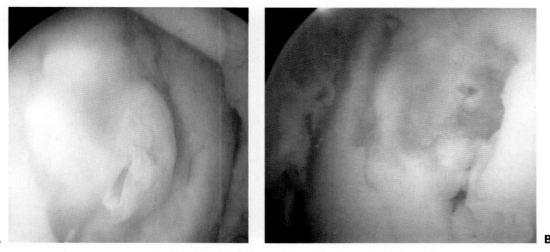

Figure 16.3 Arthroscopic comparison of microfractured defects with calcified cartilage removed **(A)** and calcified cartilage retained **(B)**. Reprinted with permission from Frisbie DD, Morisett S, Ho CP. et al. Effects of calcified cartilage on healing of chondral defects treated with microfracture. *Am J Sports Med* 2006;11:1824–1831.

nous periosteal tissue flap.[17] The delivery of cells requires an arthrotomy and the harvest and suture attachment of a periosteal flap, which is tedious and technically demanding. In Europe, other methods of autologous chondrocyte transplantation are used. Verigen in Germany (recently acquired by Genzyme) has developed a technique of autologous chondrocyte implantation that does not require harvesting or suturing on autologous periosteal flap, nor are the cells delivered in a liquid suspension. The technique uses a resorbable porcine collagen I/III membrane, and autologous chondrocytes are harvested, cultured, and expanded for a period of 3 to 4 weeks prior to seeding on the collagen

membrane. The collagen membrane is then attached into the defect with the cells toward the inside. This technique has been registered as matrix-induced autologous chondrocyte implantation (MACI, Genzyme Biosurgery, Cambridge, MA). Fibrin sealant is applied to the subchondral bone and the debrided defect and the MACI membrane is sealed into position using gentle pressure. A second "solid" form of autologous chondrocyte implantation has been developed by serum-free cultivation of cells combined with the use of another collagen type I/III membrane called Chondro-Gide (Geistlich Biomaterials, Wolhusen, Switzerland) and a third is an autologous bioengineered graft based on hyaluronan called

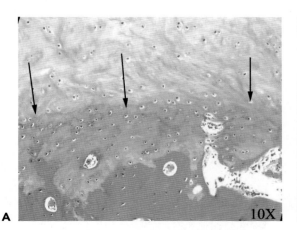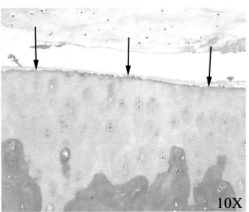

Figure 16.4 Histologic comparison of microfractured defect where calcified cartilage was removed **(A)** and calcified cartilage was retained **(B)**. Reprinted with permission from Frisbie DD, Morisett S, Ho CP. et al. Effects of calcified cartilage on healing of chondral defects treated with microfracture. *Am J Sports Med* 2006;11:1824–1831.

Hyalograft C (Fidia Advanced Biopolymers, Abano Terme, Italy).

Using two 15-mm defects on the medial trochlear ridge of the femur, we have evaluated the usefulness of cultured autologous chondrocytes, cultured expanded and seeded on a collagen membrane (small intestinal submucosa), and then reimplanted into the defects.[18] The use of this technique was compared with collagen scaffold alone and empty defects (CMA and ECD, respectively). Analysis of pathologic and histologic parameters demonstrated a significant improvement with autologous chondrocyte transplantation compared with either CMA- or ECD-treated defects (Fig. 16.5). The nature of the repair tissue was graded as being more hyalinelike in the autologous chondrocyte transplantation-treated defects compared with the CMA- and ECD-treated defects. This study was part of a Good Laboratory Practice study for FDA licensing, but the company is not moving the study further because of a one-step procedure that is now described.

Further work in our laboratory has tested a one-stage technique in 15-mm defects on the medial trochlear ridge of the femur in the horse, and the success of this technique has caused it to now go into human clinical trials.[19] Briefly, an articular cartilage biopsy of 300 mg is taken from the lateral trochlear ridge of the femur (follow-up at 12 months reveals no apparent morbidity associated with the cartilage biopsy). The cartilage is morselized into approximately 1 mm^3 and suspended in fibrin on a membrane (various membranes were tested, but the one that gave the best results was a polydioxanone [PDS]-reinforced foam). This morselized cartilage-fibrin-PDS membrane combination was then placed into the defect with the membrane uppermost and fixed with three specially developed PDS-PGA (polyglycolic acid) staples

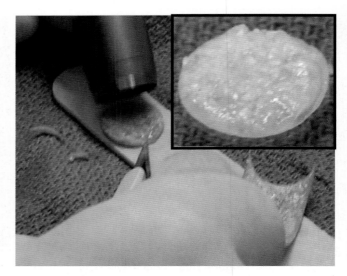

Figure 16.6 Morselized cartilage in fibrin and on a polydioxanone (PDS) membrane (*inset*) prior to being placed into a defect.

(Figs. 16.6 and 16.7). The follow-up results at 12 months were excellent (Fig. 16.8).

THE FUTURE

Following an FDA panel on optimal models for articular cartilage healing conducted in May 2005, there are conclusions that preclinical studies for cartilage healing in humans should involve the use of the goat or horse. It is envisaged that projects will continue and that the extrapolation from horse to human will increase. It is particularly exciting that important clinical answers can be obtained for both humans and horses using these equine models.

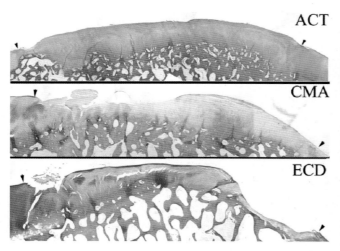

Figure 16.5 Histopathologic comparison of defects treated with autologous chondrocyte transplantation (ACT) compared with collagen membrane alone (CMA) and empty defects (ECD). The arrowheads delineate the extent of the experimental lesions.

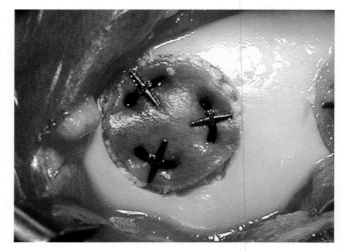

Figure 16.7 The construct with the polydioxanone (PDS) membrane uppermost is fixed with three specially developed PDS-polyglycolic acid staples.

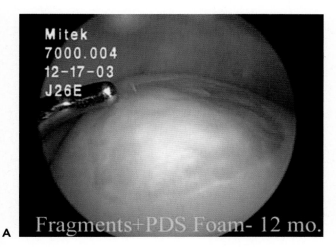

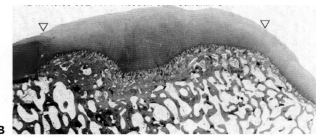

Figure 16.8 Arthroscopic view **(A)** and histologic appearance **(B)** 1 year following treatment with the morselized cartilage-fibrin-polydioxanone membrane technique.

REFERENCES

1. Caron JP, Genovese RL. Principles and practices of joint disease treatment. In: Ross MW, Dyson SJ, eds. *Diagnostics and Management of Lameness in Horse*. 1st ed. Philadelphia: Elsevier Science; 2003:746–763.
2. O'Driscoll SW. Preclinical cartilage repair: current status and future perspectives. *Clin Orthop* 2001;(391 Suppl):S397–401.
3. Arnoczky S. Animal models for knee ligament research. In: Daniel DM, ed. *Knee Ligaments: Structure, Function, Injury and Repair*. New York: Raven Press; 1990:401–417.
4. Krogh A. Progress of physiology. *Am J Physiol* 1929;90:243–251.
5. Krebs A, Krebs JR. The August Krogh principle. *Comp Biochem F Physiol* 1980;67B:379–380.
6. Houpt JL, Frisbie DD, McIlwraith CW, et al. Duel transduction of insulin-like growth factor-1 and interleukin receptor protein controls cartilage degradation in an osteoarthritic culture model. *J Orthop Res* 2005;23:118–126.
7. Frisbie DD, Cross M, McIlwraith CW. Articular cartilage thickness in the stifle of animal species used in human preclinical studies compared to the human knee. *Vet Comp Orth Traum* 2006;19:142–146.
8. Hunziker EB. Biologic repair of articular cartilage. Defect models in experimental animals and matrix requirements. *Clin Orthop* 1999;(367 Suppl):S135–146.
9. Rodrigo JJ, Steadman JR, Silliman JF, Fulstone HA. Improvement of full-thickness chondral defect healing in the human knee after debridement and microfracture using continuous passive motion. *Am J Knee Surg* 1994;7:109–116.
10. Steadman JR, Rodkey WG, Rodrigo JJ. Microfracture: surgical technique and rehabilitation to treat chondral defects. *Clin Orthop* 2001;391(Suppl):S362–S369.
11. Steadman JR, Rodkey WG, Briggs KK. Microfracture to treat full thickness chondral defects. Surgical techniques, rehabilitation, and outcomes. *J Knee Surg* 2002;15:170–176.
12. Frisbie DD, Trotter GW, Powers BE, et al. Arthroscopic subchondral bone plate microfracture augments healing of large osteochondral defects in the radial carpal bone in medial femoral condyles of horses. *Vet Surg* 1999;28:242–255.
13. Frisbie DD, Oxford JT, Southwood L, et al. Early events in cartilage repair after subchondral bone microfracture. *Clin Orthop* 2003;407:215–227.
14. Frisbie DD, Morisett S, Ho CP, et al. Effects of calcified cartilage on healing of chondral defects treated with microfracture in horses. *Am J Sports Med* 2006;34:1824–1831.
15. Nixon AJ, Houpt JL, Frisbie DD, et al. Gene mediated restoration of cartilage matrix by combination insulin-like growth factor-1/interleukin receptor-1 antagonist. *Gene Ther* 2005;12:177–186.
16. Morisset S, Frisbie DD, Robbins PD, et al. Healing of full-thickness chondral defects treated with arthroscopic subchondral bone plate microfracture and IL-1ra/IGF-1 delivered through gene transfer. *Clin Orthop* 2007;462:221–228.
17. Brittberg M, Lindhal A, Nilsson A, et al. Treatment of deep cartilage defects in the knee with autologous chondrocyte transplantation. *New Engl J Med* 1994;331:889–895.
18. Frisbie DD, Colhoun HA, Bowman S, McIlwraith CW. PDS/PGA staples compared to suture fixation of autologous chondrocyte constructs. In: Proceedings from the 49th Annual Meeting of the Orthopaedic Research Society; New Orleans, Louisiana, February 2003;28.
19. Frisbie DD, Lu Y, Colhoun HA, et al. *In vivo* evaluation of autologous cartilage resurfacing techniques in a long-term equine model. In: Proceedings from the 51st Annual Meeting of the Orthopaedic Research Society; Washington, DC, February 2005;30:1355.

17

Functional Biomechanics of Healthy, Anterior Cruciate Ligament-Deficient and -Reconstructed Knees

Kevin B Shelburne   *Marcus G. Pandy*   *Michael R. Torry*

◼ **PRELUDE 229**

◼ **BACKGROUND: COMPUTER SIMULATION AND *IN VIVO* MEASUREMENT OF HUMAN MOTION 230**

◼ **KNEE FUNCTION AND LOADS DURING ACTIVITIES OF DAILY LIVING 230**
Knee Flexion and Extension 231
Knee Bends and Squatting 233
Walking 233
　Ligament Loads During Walking 233
　Functional Adaptations in the Anterior Cruciate
　　Ligament-Deficient Knee 236
　Summary of Normal versus Anterior Cruciate
　　Ligament-Deficient Gait Adaptations 240
　Functional Adaptations in the Anterior Cruciate
　　Ligament-Reconstructed Knee 240
Landing 241
　Landing from a Drop Jump 241
　Landing Performance with Muscular Fatigue 243

◼ **SUMMARY AND CONCLUSION 244**

PRELUDE

Musculoskeletal biomechanics has the potential to make significant contributions to medicine, ergonomics, and sports performance. The study of human motion (kinesiology) is especially relevant, as it is segment motions and the interaction of the muscles and external forces that can cause the acute and/or chronic breakdown of physiologic tissue. Moreover, it is the extraordinary adaptability of the body that allows for continued activity, even in the presence of an injury or pathology. In the anterior cruciate ligament (ACL)-deficient knee, for instance, many individuals suffer through instability and episodes of giving way in an effort to remain physically active, only to be faced later on with meniscal damage and the development and progression of osteoarthritis. Equally, some individuals appear to compensate very well with an ACL deficient knee, as they appear to effectively utilize muscular strategies to stabilize the knee during activities.

This chapter focuses on the understanding of normal knee function and the biomechanics of the ACL-deficient and ACL-reconstructed knee during activities of daily living. Basic experiments concerning the performance adaptations in the ACL-deficient and ACL-reconstructed knee will be reviewed, and the biomechanics of the normal, ACL-deficient, and ACL-reconstructed knee under more strenuous activities, such as landing from a jump, will also be provided. By combining information obtained from two distinct but related scientific disciplines (*in vivo* experimentation and computer modeling), much of our work in recent years has focused on describing and explaining the intra-articular loads that occur at the knee.

BACKGROUND: COMPUTER SIMULATION AND *IN VIVO* MEASUREMENT OF HUMAN MOTION

The lower extremity musculoskeletal system is composed of a series of jointed links (segments) that can be approximated as rigid bodies. Six independent parameters (the degrees of freedom) are required to describe the location and orientation of each of the lower extremity body segments in three-dimensional (3D) space. *In vivo* measurements quantitatively describe the spatial motion of these segments and the movements of the joints connecting these segments over time and during dynamic motions. Historically, *in vivo* measurements of lower extremity mechanics for dynamic activities have been acquired with optical capture, accelerometer, or goniometric methods. The most common of these are the optical systems that employ high-speed cameras to capture the 3D motion of reflective markers that are placed on the limb segments and pertinent bony landmarks of the subjects. These systems produce 3D trajectories of the markers, which are used to estimate the position, velocity, and acceleration of the body segments during the activity. These kinematic parameters are then combined (in a process termed the *inverse dynamic solution*) with a subject's anthropometric measurements and external forces (commonly measured with a force-plate mounted in floor) to yield external reaction forces and net moments at the joints. The internal muscle contraction, passive soft tissues, and joint-reaction forces must generate equal and opposite forces to the externally measured moments and forces. These methods have been applied to a myriad of sporting motions and pathologic diseases. Yet, despite their widespread use in orthopaedic research, this technology cannot determine muscle forces and/or forces borne by the individual ligaments and other tissues. Without this information, specific conclusions regarding tissue loads are not possible.

To remove this limitation, scientists have developed sophisticated computer simulation techniques that estimate loads in the muscles and on specific tissues and intra-articular structures. Quite simply, computer simulation allows for the estimation of forces in specific tissues that cannot otherwise be measured *in vivo*. A computer simulation is based on a mathematical model of a biological system that represents the geometry, anthropometry, and mechanical

material properties of the tissues. Put simply, a *musculoskeletal model* of the body represents the bones, joints, muscles, and ligaments of the body. With today's computing technology, these models can often be visualized in 3D with moderately powered computer workstations. Because all models are simplifications of reality, there is always a trade-off between level of detail and computational complexity. Although models represent the physical properties of a system, *a simulation* applies conditions (such as the joint motion and external loads from walking) to the model and calculates the resultant motion and loads. Thus, a simulation generally refers to a computerized version of the model, which is used to study the muscle, ligament, and joint loads of a defined motion.

In vivo measurements and computer simulations form a continuous cycle of investigation (Fig. 17.1). Most often, investigation of a particular activity, condition, or pathology begins with laboratory measurements. In application to the knee and its function during activities of daily living and sporting motions, this means measurement of body segment kinematics, joint moments, external forces, and appropriate muscle electromyography (EMG) activations in subjects. Then, in order to understand the loads inside the body, the experimental data are used to develop a computer simulation. The outputs of the simulation are often the muscle forces, joint loads, and ligament loads during the measured activity. In many cases, the computer simulation yields results that lead to additional focused laboratory experiments. This process continues with refinement of the experimental and simulation methods until an adequate level of understanding is developed. In this way, experiments and simulation coexist as disciplines for developing a level of understanding of the interaction of all the individual parts of a system, and of the system as a whole.

In the following review of knee function, much of the scientific detail regarding the *in vivo* experimental methodology as well as the construction and performance of the computer simulations are omitted but are adequately referenced so that the reader may refer to the peer-reviewed articles for a detailed description of the specific methods.

KNEE FUNCTION AND LOADS DURING ACTIVITIES OF DAILY LIVING

Quantifying ligament loads at the knee during activity is motivated by the high incidence of knee ligament injuries, the frequency of their surgical treatment, and the subsequent rehabilitation protocols. In addition, onset and progression of knee osteoarthritis is often attributed to an injury or pathology that alters the way the knee carries force. Little is known about the way muscles, ligaments, and external forces contribute to loading of the knee joint during activities of daily living. Forces in the ligaments and between the bones are determined mainly by the forces in the muscles and the external loads on the

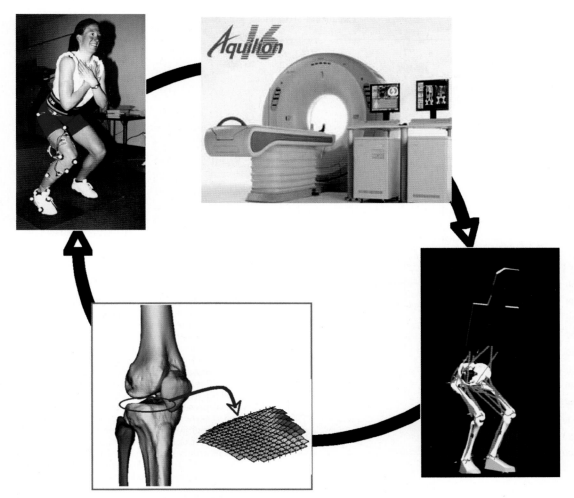

Figure 17.1 *In vivo* experiments conducted in the laboratory can provide a wealth of information on how a person performs a motion, but these methods cannot provide information about intra-articular loads. Computer modeling can predict these loads. These two disciplines work in continuity as computer models require *in vivo* data such as kinematics, ground-reaction force, and kinetics for comparison and model validity. This is illustrated above in which experimental data (upper left figure) is collected, then subject specific joint geometry is collected (upper right picture) using MRI and/or CT. These techniques provide modelers with the basic data to create realistic models and foward dynamic simulations (bottom right picture) by which intra-articular loads can be estimated (bottom left picture). Together, these techniques provide a very powerful tool in the understanding of human function and its consequences on tissue structure. (All photos contained in this figure are courtesy of Marcus G. Pandy, University of Melbourne, Melbourne, Australia; and Michael R. Torry and Kevin B. Shelburne, Steadman Hawkins Research Foundation, Vail, CO).

lower limb that accompany activity. Because these loads are large and specific to each activity, *in vitro* simulation of knee loading with cadaveric limbs is often insufficient to represent the *in vivo* loading environment of the knee. The following sections describe knee mechanics for a variety of activities of daily living and sport. Each activity is treated separately because the forces borne by the knee cannot be generalized from one activity to another.

Knee Flexion and Extension

Much attention has been given to understanding ligament function during flexion/extension of the knee. The reasons for this are that these can be well-controlled experiments and often form part of the rehabilitation protocol following knee injury. Knee flexion/extension with and without resistance forms part of many rehabilitation protocols following ligament injury or repair, and although conceptually simple, understanding the behavior of the knee during knee flexion and extension can enlighten the function of the knee ligaments during more demanding activities of daily living and sport. Shelburne and Pandy[1] used a computer simulation of knee flexion/extension to study ligament forces induced by isolated contractions of the extensor and flexor muscles with the specific goals of predicting the forces induced in the ACL and posterior cruciate ligament (PCL) and to explain how these forces were influenced by knee angle and the geometry of the knee tissues.

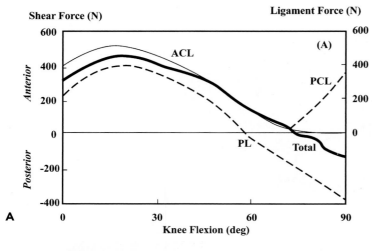

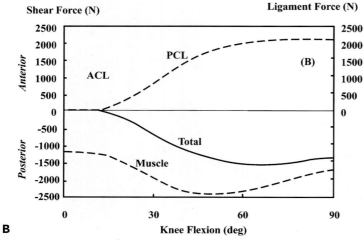

Figure 17.2 **A:** Anterior-posterior shear forces applied to the tibia *(thick line)* and resultant cruciate ligament forces *(thin line)* for a maximum isometric knee extension. Total shear force *(thick solid line)* represents the resultant shear force applied to the tibia and is equal and opposite to the net shear force supplied by all ligaments and capsular structures. **B:** Anterior-posterior shear forces applied to the tibia *(thick line)* and the resultant cruciate ligament forces *(thin line)* for maximum isometric knee extension. Muscle *(thick line)* represents the total shear supplied by the hamstrings and gastrocnemius. Hamstrings dominate the curve, with gastrocnemius only contributing less then 10% at all angles of knee flexion. ACL, anterior cruciate ligament; PCL, posterior cruciate ligament; PL, patellar ligament/tendon. (Reproduced with permission from Shelburne KB, Pandy MG. A musculoskeletal model of the knee for evaluating ligament forces during isometric contractions. *J Biomech* 1997;30:163–176.)

Results indicated that the ACL is loaded from full extension to approximately 80 degrees of flexion during maximum, isolated contractions of the quadriceps (Fig. 17.2A,B). This suggests that quadriceps exercises should be limited in this region if the ACL is to be protected from load. In contrast, isolated hamstring and gastrocnemius muscle contractions will protect the healing ACL graft throughout the entire range of knee flexion. The study also showed that the ACL cannot be protected from all load in the 0- to 10-degree range irrespective of any combination of hamstring, gastrocnemius, and quadriceps muscle activations as the ACL load in this range is determined mainly by the line of action of the ACL in relation to the shapes of the articulating surfaces of the medial and lateral compartments. As the knee flexes beyond 10 degrees, ACL load can be lowered by decreasing quadriceps activation or by increasing hamstrings activation. This is because the pattern of ACL loading in this range is governed by the geometry of the patellofemoral joint and the mechanical properties of the hamstrings. As the knee flexes, the angle between the patellar tendon and the long axis of the tibia also decreases. As this angle decreases, so does the shear force

supplied by the patellar tendon. ACL force decreases in proportion to the decrease in patellar tendon shear force because the ACL is the primary restraint to this force. In addition, the angle between the hamstrings and the tibia increases. Thus, the amount of shear force provided by the hamstrings increases because of geometry alone. In short, for a constant quadriceps and hamstrings force contraction, ACL force decreases monotonically as the knee flexes.

Rehabilitation following ACL injury or repair is often associated with knee extension exercises that also employ external loads (isometric, isokinetic, and isotonic knee extensions). Pandy and Shelburne[2] evaluated the influence of muscle activity in conjunction with an external restraining force (i.e., a tibial push pad as used in Cybex [Cybex, Inc, Ronkonkoma, NY] testing) on the forces induced in the knee ligaments during isometric knee extension exercises. Moving the tibial restraint closer to the flexion axis decreases the ACL load because it increases the amount of posterior shear force applied to the tibia by the pad. The study found that the ACL force is practically independent of the orientation of the restraining force. This means, at all angles of isometric loading, that decreasing the angle between the line of action of the restraining force and the long axis of the tibia has only a small effect on ACL loading.

Several studies have documented an increase in anterior tibial translation in the ACL-deficient knee during knee extensions. However, the numerous *in vitro* studies conducted in this area may be limited as ligament function in cadavers may be different compared with that of *in vivo* ligaments and because the muscle loads applied to cadavers are often much less than the muscle loads used during ordinary activities. Pandy and Shelburne[2] showed that anterior laxity in the intact knee is greatest between 20 and 30 degrees and the primary restraint to anterior tibial translation is the ACL, which provides 85% to 95% of the total restraining force. Anterior laxity increases when the ACL is removed. The greatest increase occurs between 15 and 30 degrees relative to the intact condition. The deep fibers of the MCL become more loaded during an anterior drawer providing up to 80% resistance to anterior tibial translation and this remains consistent throughout all flexion angles.

Even though anterior tibial translation increases in ACL-deficient knee extension, the extensor torque remains more or less the same relative to the intact knee. This is because the patellar tendon force and the moment arm of the patellar tendon do not change when the ACL is torn. In general, this analysis suggests that the knee extensor mechanism does not change much in the absence of the ACL as the force transmitted to the patellar tendon, the location of the flexion axis, the moment arm of the extensor mechanism, and the torque developed by the quadriceps are all nearly the same as compared to the intact knee. This is because the change in line-of-action of the patellar tendon relative to the rotational center of the knee changes little with increased anterior tibial translation. However, the decrease in patellar tendon angle relative to the long axis of the tibia reduces the anterior shear force applied to the shank. For this reason, although MCL force increases, MCL force in the ACL-deficient knee remains much lower than that found in the ACL in the intact knee under identical external and muscle loads. This is an important factor in the later description of ACL-deficient walking.[3]

Collectively, these data suggest that the performance differences often observed in ACL-deficient knees are a result of quadriceps strength deficits and not from an increase in anterior tibial translation. In addition, although function of the knee extensor mechanisms is not altered by loss of the ACL, the load sharing amongst the ligaments is substantially different; the deep fibers of the medial collateral ligament (MCL) bear nearly all the resistance to anterior tibial translation and the tibiofemoral joint load is carried farther posterior on the tibial plateau. These findings support the clinical observations of increased MCL and medial meniscal injuries in the ACL-deficient knee.

Knee Bends and Squatting

The previous discussion has focused on nonweightbearing knee extension exercises. However, weightbearing exercises such as squatting or "knee dips" are most often prescribed for post-ACL repairs. As with the knee extension exercise, very little experimental data are available because it is difficult to measure ACL loads *in vivo*; although these loads have been estimated using cadaveric specimens and are thought to be low, the muscles forces that are used in those studies are much lower (five to eight times lower) than what are actually occurring during the exercise.

In 2002, Shelburne and Pandy[4] investigated the squatting motion using a forward dynamic model based on optimization theory. In this simulation, the ACL was loaded from 15 to 40 degrees of knee flexion but the peak force in the ACL only reached a maximum of 20 N. The PCL was loaded at flexion angles greater than 30 degrees and reached a maximum value of 66 N at 81 degrees. Peak MCL force reached 40 N, which is roughly the same loads as reported during passive knee extension movements. The quadriceps developed nearly 3,000 N of force as the knee approached 80 degrees; compared to the maximum hamstring forces, which reached 500 N. The pattern of muscles forces created a similar pattern of tibiofemoral and patellofemoral loading and is representative of the acceleration of the body up from its squat position. The tibiofemoral and patellofemoral loads during squatting are much less than those occurring at the knee during active knee extension exercises. For comparison, during isometric, maximal contractions, tibiofemoral and patellofemoral loads are estimated at 6,000 and 10,000 N, and for the sit-to-stand motion these were estimated at 2,800 and 3,200 N, respectively. The results of Shelburne and Pandy[4] generally support the view that weightbearing, squatting exercises can be a relatively safe exercise following ACL repair.

Walking

Ligament Loads During Walking

Walking is one of the most common and basic of human movements. Although we usually take this motion for granted, it is one of the most complex and integrated motions all able-bodied persons do on a daily basis. It has been well described and scientifically analyzed in hundreds of laboratories throughout the world. This is important because a large body of data now exists by which standards and norms can be compared with pathologic conditions with ease. This allows for even the smallest deviations from normal gait patterns to be informative to the knowledgeable and discerning clinician.

A number of studies have inferred ACL loading from *in vivo* measurements of bony motion at the knee,[5-7] but very few studies have calculated knee-ligament forces in gait. Of those that have, there appears to be some disparity in the results. Morrison[8] used an inverse dynamics approach to estimate muscle, ligament, and joint contact forces at the knee during normal, level walking. His calculations showed that the ACL was loaded throughout the stance phase of walking, and that peak ACL force was 156 N

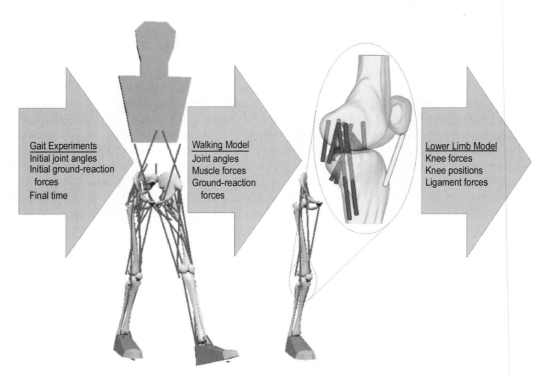

Figure 17.3 Schematic of the forward dynamic walking model used to determine individual muscles forces during the gait cycle. Muscle forces, ground-reaction forces, and lower limb motions obtained from the walking simulation matched experimental measures in the laboratory. These parameters were then input into a lower limb model. Ligament forces and joint contacts loads were then estimated using the three-dimensional model of the knee joint. (Reproduced with permission from Shelburne KB, Torry, MR, Pandy MG. Muscle, ligament, and joint-contact forces at the knee during walking. *Med Sci Sports Exerc* 2005;37:1948–1956.)

(approximately one-fourth body weight [BW]). Using a similar approach, Harrington[9] also found that the ACL was loaded throughout stance, but the peak force transmitted to the ligament was estimated to be much higher (approximately one-half BW).

In 2004, Shelburne et al.[3] using a 3D model of the lower limb (Fig. 17.3) and knee, described cruciate ligament forces during walking in terms of the shear force applied to

the knee. The ACL was loaded throughout the stance phase of gait (Fig. 17.4). Peak ACL force occurred at contralateral toe-off and was estimated to be 303 N, which is about 13% of the reported failure strength of the ligament[10] and is similar to the levels of ACL loading predicted for isokinetic knee-extension exercise at fast speeds.[11,12] The force induced in the ACL was explained by the balance of muscle forces, joint contact forces, and the ground-reaction force

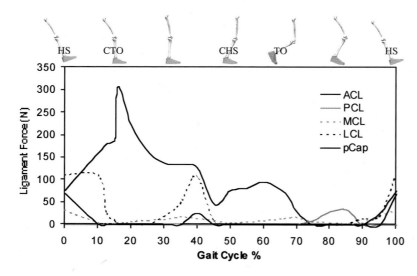

Figure 17.4 Forces in the cruciate ligaments (ACL, anterior cruciate ligament; PCL, posterior cruciate ligament), collateral ligaments (MCL, medial collateral ligament; LCL, lateral collateral ligament), and the posterior capsule (pCap) of the knee during one complete gait cycle. HS, heel strike; CTO, contralateral toe-off; CHS, contralateral heel strike; TO, toe-off. Peak force in the ACL coincided with peak knee extensor torque and quadriceps muscle forces. (Reproduced with permission from Shelburne KB, Pandy MG, Anderson FC, et al. Pattern of anterior cruciate ligament force in normal walking. *J Biomech* 2004;37:797–805.)

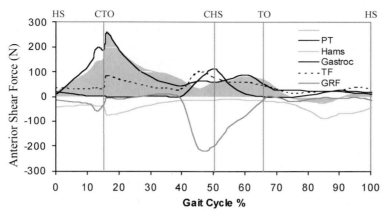

Figure 17.5 Shear forces acting on the leg (shank + foot) during the simulated gait cycle. The shaded region shows the total shear force borne by the knee ligaments in the model. Total shear force is the shear force due to the muscle forces, ground-reaction forces, and joint contact forces. Anterior shear forces (+ values) tended to translate the leg anteriorly; posterior shear forces (− values) tended to translate the leg posteriorly. Hamstrings always applied a posterior shear force. The ground-reaction force applied a posterior shear force to the leg because the line of action of the resultant ground force passed behind the knee. HS, heel strike; CTO, contralateral toe-off; CHS, contralateral heel strike; TO, toe-off; PT, patellar tendon; Hams, hamstrings; Gastroc, gastrocnemius muscle; TF, tibiofemoral contact force; GRF, ground-reaction force.). (Reproduced with permission from Shelburne KB, Pandy MG, Anderson FC, et al. Pattern of anterior cruciate ligament force in normal walking. *J Biomech* 2004;37:797–805.)

applied to the leg; each of these forces contributed to the resultant shear force acting at the knee. The patellar tendon, gastrocnemius muscle, and tibiofemoral contact force all applied anterior shear forces to the leg, while hamstrings and the resultant ground-reaction force applied posterior shear forces (Fig. 17.5).

In early stance, the shear force from the patellar tendon dominated the resultant shear force applied to the leg, and so maximum force was transmitted to the ACL at this time (Fig. 17.5). Patellar tendon shear force was large in early stance because quadriceps force was large and also because the line of action of the patellar tendon was inclined anteriorly relative to the long axis of the tibia.[1,11] ACL force was relatively small in late stance because the posterior component of the ground-reaction force was nearly equal to the sum of the anterior shear forces supplied by the patellar tendon, gastrocnemius muscle, and the tibiofemoral contact force at that time (Fig. 17.5). Gastrocnemius applied an anterior shear force to the shank because the knee was nearly fully extended just before contralateral heel strike, and at small flexion angles the gastrocnemius wraps around the back of the tibia.[1,11–13] Tibiofemoral contact force applied an anterior shear force to the leg because of the posterior slope of the tibial plateau.[2,11,14] The ground-reaction force applied a posterior shear force to the leg because the line of action of the resultant ground force passed behind the knee. The posterior shear force caused by the ground reaction increased prior to contralateral heel strike because the angle between the shank and the ground increased at this time.

The model PCL was unloaded during stance because the resultant shear force at the knee pointed anteriorly at this

time (Fig. 17.5, shaded region). This result of the model correlates with the clinical observation that the knee often responds adequately to conservative treatment after isolated rupture of the PCL, without the need for reconstruction.[15,16]

Peak force borne by the MCL was less than 20 N during stance (Fig. 17.4). The model MCL was not loaded much for two reasons: first, the ACL provided the primary restraint to anterior tibial translation in the intact knee; and second, the ground-reaction force applied an adductor moment to the leg, which could only be resisted by the structures on the lateral side of the knee. The study by Shelburne et al.[3] showed that the muscles that applied the largest forces at the knee during walking were the vasti and gastrocnemius. Peak force in vasti was 1,188 N, which occurred at contralateral toe-off. Peak force in gastrocnemius was lower at 849 N, and it occurred at contralateral heel strike. The hamstrings developed much lower forces during stance; peak force predicted for hamstrings was 495 N, which occurred at heel strike.

The model calculations showed a bimodal pattern for patellofemoral and tibiofemoral contact force (Fig. 17.6A,B), with the first and second peaks of tibiofemoral load aligning with peak forces developed by the quadriceps and gastrocnemius muscles. The calculations also showed that the center of pressure at the knee was concentrated on the medial side. Compressive force acting between the femur and tibia was much greater in the medial compartment than in the lateral compartment throughout the stance phase of gait. The compressive force was much greater on the medial side because the resultant ground-reaction force passed medial to the knee at all times during

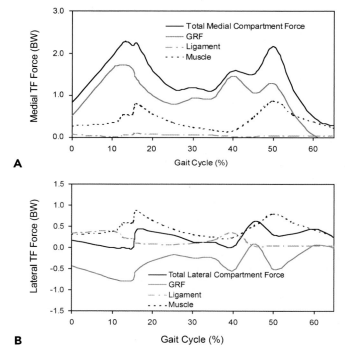

Figure 17.6   A: Components contributing to the composition of the medial tibiofemoral (TF) compartment joint reaction force. **B:** Components contributing to the composition lateral tibiofemoral joint reaction force. BW, body weight; GRF, ground-reaction force. (Reproduced with permission from Shelburne KB, Torry MR, Pandy MG. Contributions of muscles, ligaments, and the ground-reaction force to tibiofemoral joint loading during normal gait. *J Orthop Res* 2006;24:1983–1990.)

stance. The medially directed ground-reaction force created an external moment that acted to adduct the knee in the frontal plane.[17,18]

The adduction moment is considered a key determinant of the distribution of tibiofemoral load between the medial and lateral sides of the knee (Fig. 17.7A). The external knee adductor moment was resisted by a combination of muscle and ligament forces.[19] The quadriceps provided most of the resistance in the first half of stance, while the gastrocnemius contributed most of the resisting muscular moment thereafter (Fig. 17.7B).[19]

Ligaments provided significant resistance to the external knee adductor moment immediately after heel strike and during midstance (Fig. 17.7C). Schipplein and Andriacchi[18] found that the adductor moment was resisted by the passive lateral supporting structures of the knee for nearly 60% of the stance phase of gait. The contribution of ligament to resist adduction moment during walking was highest when muscle force (and muscular flexion-extension moment) was lowest.

The posterior lateral capsule (PLC), which was represented by the lateral collateral ligament and the popliteofibular ligament, provided the primary passive restraint to lateral joint opening in the model (Fig. 17.7C).[19] Peak forces borne by the lateral collateral ligament and poplite-

ofibular ligament were 167 and 15 N, respectively. Although the peak force borne by the ACL in the model was much higher than that calculated for the PLC, the ability of the ACL to resist the external adductor moment at the knee was much less.[19]

The pattern of force calculated for the PLC was similar to that obtained for the external adductor moment at the knee. PLC force was highest at times when the external adductor moment was high and the resistance provided by the muscles was low. This is consistent with results obtained from cadaveric experiments, which show that the PLC plays an important role in resisting adductor moments applied at the knee.[19]

Functional Adaptations in the Anterior Cruciate Ligament-Deficient Knee

The study of gait in ACL-deficient knees is important because it is difficult to predict from clinical examinations which patients will be functionally impaired and which patients may have only limited symptoms. Clinical studies suggest that some (approximately one third) individuals who have ACL-deficient knees will adapt well to their ligament loss, another one-third will modify their activities to accommodate their knee instability, and another one-third will report poor functional status even after reducing their activity level.[20] Loss of the ACL has been shown to influence the passive mechanics of the knee joint by decreasing the overall knee stiffness and increasing knee instability. However, it is possible that muscles can compensate for the loss of the ACL and individuals can use "muscular substitution" to aid in knee stability.[21]

Kinematically and electromyographically, there is a general consensus that individuals with ACL-deficient knees walk with a more flexed knee pattern and with elevated or prolonged duration of hamstring muscular activity.[22–24] Kinetically, however, there is disagreement as to the existence and functional consequence of the knee extensor and flexor joint torque patterns. Berchuck et al.[25] in 1990 described a "quadriceps avoidance pattern" in subjects with ACL-deficient knees as depicted by the complete elimination of the external knee flexor torque during the stance phase. Since the report by Berchuck et al.,[25] the quadriceps avoidance gait pattern has been noted by others[26–28] and the presence of this pattern has been suggested to be a learned response and a function of time from the initial injury.[21,29,30]

Torry et al.[23] however, recorded no significant changes in the knee torque patterns in ACL-deficient knees and reported no association of time from injury to knee kinetic gait patterns, suggesting ACL deficiency does not always lead to the quadriceps avoidance gait pattern. Other researchers have noted a change in the torque phase transition periods and/or a reduction in the magnitude of the knee torque profiles, but not the complete elimination of knee joint torque transition phases between the knee extensors and flexors during gait.[31,32]

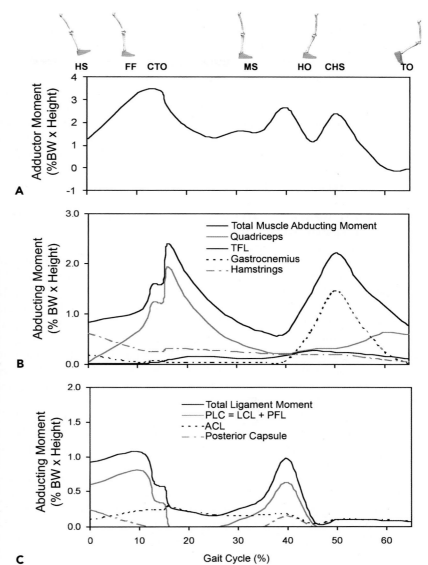

Figure 17.7 **A:** External adductor moment during the stance phase of walking. The external adductor moment is the moment produced by the ground-reaction force about the center of the knee in the frontal plane and acts to abduct the knee joint. Resistance to the external adduction moment is provided by muscles and ligaments. **B:** Composition of the frontal plane abduction moment provided by muscles. The quadriceps followed by the hamstrings provides much of the *abduction* moment to stabilize the knee in the fontal plane during early stance phase (0% to 30% stance). The gastrocnemius muscle provides the majority of abduction support in later stance. **C:** Composition of the frontal plane abduction moment provided by ligaments. HS, heel strike; FF, foot flat; CTO, contralateral toe-off; MS, midstance; CHS, contralateral heel strike; TO, toe-off; TFL, tensor facia latae; PLC, posterior lateral corner, which is composed of the lateral collateral ligament (LCL) and the posterior fibular ligament (PFL); ACL, anterior cruciate ligament. (Reproduced with permission from Shelburne KB, Torry MR, Pandy MG. Contributions of muscles, ligaments, and the ground-reaction force to tibiofemoral joint loading during normal gait. *J Orthop Res* 2006;24(10):1983–1990.)

Torry et al.[23] suggested multiple mechanisms of coping with ACL deficiency during gait exist and the pooling of group mean data can mask important kinematic and kinetic adaptive strategies across select individuals. Indeed, results from their work established that the quadriceps avoidance gait pattern may not be as common in ACL-deficient knees as previously described.[21] Moreover, the hip, knee, and ankle kinematics and kinetics were not different between groups when pooled data were analyzed. However, nine subjects with ACL-deficient knees demonstrated a normal biphasic knee moment pattern, whereas seven subjects demonstrated an all knee extensor pattern. This indicated different adaptive mechanisms are present within select ACL-deficient cohorts. Furthermore, stratifying the pooled subject data according to biphasic or all knee extensor torque parameters yielded two distinct gait strategies: (i) a *hip strategy* that

increased hip extensor output, decreased knee extensor output, and allowed normal knee kinematics; and (ii) a *knee strategy* that increased the stiffness of the joint and used a flexed knee gait pattern.

The hip strategy is exemplified by a near-normal lower extremity kinematic pattern and is kinetically characterized by an increase in hip extensor torque in compensation for a decrease in knee extensor angular impulse. Similar strategies were identified by Ferber et al.,[32] and Devita et al.[29] speculated that the increased extensor hip moment may change the length-tension curve of the hip extensor, potentially reducing anterior tibial translation. Notably, the knee torque pattern remained a biphasic pattern in this group, transitioning between extensor and flexor torques at nearly the same instant as the control group and this is consistent with patterns reported for "copers" by Rudolph et al.[33] Torry et al.[23] suggested that an increased hip extensor torque in conjunction with a slightly reduced knee extensor torque pattern may be considered beneficial as it has been shown that anterior tibial translation and ACL strain depends on the magnitude and timing of the peak knee extensor torque during the gait cycle.[3] Thus, a slight reduction in knee extensor torque may act to reduce anterior tibial translation.[34,35] One method of accomplishing this task would be to increase hip extensor torque (thereby increasing hamstring force) acting to stabilize the net forces acting on the knee by countering the anterior drawer force applied by the net extensor torque during the early periods of the stance phase and this could be accomplished by maintaining a normal knee kinematic profile.[34,35] Given this *hip adaptive strategy*, we would expect hamstring EMG values to be larger compared with controls at this time period; indeed, these values are typically higher in most *in vivo* reports.

Alternatively, the knee strategy employs a flexed knee kinematic pattern characterized by a slight increase in peak knee extensor torque, and dominated by an all extensor knee torque and increased knee extensor angular impulse. At first, this adaptive mechanism seems counterintuitive, as an all extensor knee torque would seemingly induce anterior tibial translation throughout the gait cycle.[36] Recently, however, Shelburne et al.[36] have shown that, in an ACL-deficient knee, a small amount of anterior tibial translation can effectively decrease the angle of the patellar tendon relative to the tibia and this, in turn, decreases the anterior shear force at the knee. Thus, an all extensor knee moment (independent from other coexisting adaptations) may in fact be another appropriate means of reducing anterior shear force during gait. Others have observed these changes in anterior tibial translation in the ACL-deficient knee during gait.[5,7] Another explanation for the flexed knee adaptation is that it increases the angle between the tibia and hamstrings and thus improves their ability to pull backward on the tibia.[36] Indeed, biceps femoris EMG activity and the medial hamstring EMG values typically increase during the second-fourth quartiles of the stance phase.[23]

Torry et al.[23] established the important need to evaluate ACL-deficient gait patterns on a case-by-case basis as pooling the data may mask subtle adaptive strategies that are consistent and distinct in some patients; and, after examining individual performance differences, Torry et al.[23] have identified two distinctive gait patterns that persist long term in subjects with ACL-deficient knees, which were significantly different from each other, and a control group. Understanding the subtle adaptive strategies that may occur within the ACL-deficient population may lead to differentiated rehabilitation efforts that could promote the emergence and maximize the presence of favorable adaptations within each subgroup. However, the identification of the specific mechanical advantages (or disadvantages) of these neuromuscular adaptations must be determined prior to making such clinically focused recommendations.

Shelburne et al.[34] compared the ACL loading patterns of normal walking with those observed in ACL-deficient knees using modeling and simulation techniques. This analysis assumed normal kinematics and muscle forces, consistent with the kinematics and kinetics reported for copers by Rudolph et al.[33] and Torry et al.[23] Loss of the ACL caused MCL force to increase significantly, so much so that it became the primary restraint to anterior tibial translation in the ACL-deficient knee (Fig. 17.8B,C). The peak force borne by the MCL in the ACL-deficient knee was nearly four times greater than that calculated for the intact knee. Peak force borne by the MCL in the ACL-deficient knee was less than half that estimated for the ACL in the intact knee. In contrast, peak force calculated for the PLC in the ACL-deficient knee was roughly the same as that predicted for the intact knee. Even though the peak force transmitted to the MCL increased by a factor of 4 when the model ACL was removed (Fig. 17.8C), this value was still significantly less than the breaking strength reported for the MCL.[37] This is because the magnitude of the resultant anterior shear force acting at the knee decreased when the ACL was removed (Fig. 17.8A). Anterior shear force decreased because the patellar tendon angle was smaller in the ACL-deficient knee. The patellar tendon angle was smaller because anterior tibial translation increased when the model ACL was removed. As a result, the patellar tendon applied a smaller anterior shear force to the tibia, which caused the resultant anterior shear force to be lower.

Peak patellofemoral joint reaction force was 14% lower at contralateral toe-off in the ACL-deficient knee compared with that calculated for the ACL-intact knee. An increase in anterior tibial translation in the ACL-deficient knee caused the quadriceps tendon and patellar tendon to become less steeply inclined to the long axis of the patella, which decreased the contact force acting between the patella and femur. Peak tibiofemoral joint reaction force was 5% lower in the ACL-deficient knee than in the intact knee. Tibiofemoral joint reaction force was lower in the ACL-deficient knee because the component of ACL tension acting to pull the tibia and femur together was nonexistent. In the frontal plane, the location of the center of pressure on the medial side of the knee did not change much when the model ACL was removed. In the sagittal plane, the location of tibiofemoral load on the medial and lateral sides of the tibial plateau shifted posterior because anterior tibial translation increased, as previously noted. The role of the PLC was the same in the ACL-deficient knee as in the intact knee: it contributed most of the passive resistance to the external adductor moment applied to the leg during stance. PLC force increased only a small amount in the ACL-deficient knee.

Some *in vivo* studies have suggested that a reduction in the knee extensor moment, brought about by a decrease in quadriceps muscle activation, is an effective strategy for limiting anterior tibial translation during ACL-deficient gait.[25] To test this hypothesis, Shelburne et al.[35,38] reduced

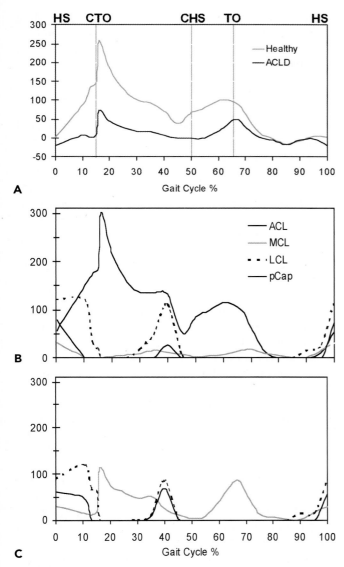

Figure 17.8 A: Total anterior shear force applied to the tibia and the resultant shear forces applied by the various soft tissues in and around the healthy and anterior cruciate ligament (ACL)-deficient (ACLD) knee; knee shear goes down on the ACLD knee because the tibia translates forward. Ligament forces calculated for the ACL-intact knee **(B)** and for the ACLD knee **(C)** for one complete cycle of gait. HS, heel strike; CTO, contralateral toe-off; CHS, contralateral heel strike; TO, toe-off; MCL, medial collateral ligament; LCL, lateral collateral ligament; pCap, posterior capsule. (Reproduced with permission from Shelburne KB, Pandy MG, Torry MR. Comparison of shear forces and ligament loading in the healthy and ACL-deficient knee during gait. *J Biomech* 2004;37:313–319.)

quadriceps force in the model and anterior tibial translation was recalculated to determine whether a change in quadriceps force alone could reduce anterior tibial translation in the ACL-deficient knee to the amount calculated for the intact knee. The model simulation results showed that it was not entirely possible to restore anterior tibial translation in the ACL-deficient knee to the amount calculated for normal gait merely by reducing the magnitude of quadriceps

force. There were periods near heel strike and in midstance when the lower limit of quadriceps force (zero force) was reached, and yet anterior tibial translation in the ACL-deficient knee was still greater than that obtained for the intact knee.[3] The calculated decrease in quadriceps force resulted in complete elimination of the knee extensor moment (a quadriceps avoidance pattern).

Reducing the force in the quadriceps meant that less force was transmitted between the femur and tibia in the model. Although the peak force in the medial compartment decreased by 313 N at contralateral toe-off, practically all of the contact force acting between the femur and tibia was transmitted on the medial side of the knee. As a consequence, the ligaments were required to provide even greater resistance to the external adductor moment than that calculated for the intact knee; peak force borne by the PLC in the ACL-deficient knee was two times greater than that predicted for the intact knee when the quadriceps muscles were deactivated.

Reducing quadriceps force is one method that has been suggested to limit the adductor moment; hamstring facilitation is another. To evaluate the effect of hamstrings muscle compensation on anterior tibial translation during ACL-deficient walking, hamstrings force was increased in the model and anterior tibial translation recalculated to determine whether a change in hamstrings force alone could reduce anterior tibial translation in the ACL-deficient knee to the amount calculated for the intact knee. The calculations showed that it was possible to reduce anterior tibial translation to the level calculated for the intact knee merely by increasing the magnitude of hamstrings force. As expected, an increase in hamstrings force led to a decrease in the knee extensor moment, but the drop in extensor moment was much less dramatic than that obtained for simulated quadriceps avoidance.

An increase in hamstrings force caused an increase in the resultant force acting at the tibiofemoral joint during ACL-deficient gait; the peak force transmitted on the medial side of the knee increased by 307 N. Although an increase in hamstrings force meant that the leg muscles provided more resistance to the adductor moment acting about the knee, this did not significantly alter the peak force borne by the PLC. The PLC force remained about the same because hamstrings force was not increased substantially near foot-flat and prior to heel-off, when PLC resistance to adductor moment was highest.

Although the results of Shelburne et al.[38] support the contention that either isolated quadriceps or hamstrings muscle action can stabilize the ACL-deficient knee during walking, they also suggest that the latter is more effective in reducing anterior tibial translation during ACL-deficient gait. Given that quadriceps avoidance is usually accompanied by quadriceps muscle weakness, which has been associated with medial compartment joint degeneration,[39,40] a hamstrings facilitation pattern would appear to be more effective on these grounds as well. Importantly, both compensatory strategies change not only the resultant force at the tibiofemoral joint, but also the way this load is shared between the soft tissues and the medial and lateral sides of the knee.

Summary of Normal versus Anterior Cruciate Ligament-Deficient Gait Adaptations

The forces transmitted to the knee ligaments during the stance phase of normal walking are explained mainly by the patterns of anterior shear force and varus moment applied to the leg. The pattern of force in the ACL is explained almost entirely by the anterior pull of the patellar tendon, while that in the posterior lateral corner results mainly from a medially directed ground-reaction force, which applies an adductor moment to the leg. When the ACL is absent, the maximum force transmitted to the MCL increases, but it nevertheless remains well below the failure strength of the ligament. The magnitude of force transmitted to the MCL remains limited in the ACL-deficient knee because the magnitude of the resultant anterior shear force decreases significantly relative to that present in the intact joint. This suggests that while the MCL acts as the primary restraint to anterior tibial translation in the ACL-deficient knee, it may still function safely in activities like walking.

The model calculations also indicate that the forces acting at the tibiofemoral and patellofemoral joints are not very different in normal and ACL-deficient walking. The reason is that the ACL does not act to resist much of the varus moment applied by the external ground-reaction force. However, the location of tibiofemoral force on the medial and lateral sides of the tibial plateau is moved posterior by the increase in anterior tibial translation in the ACL-deficient knee. Hamstrings facilitation is more effective than quadriceps avoidance in reducing anterior tibial translation during ACL-deficient gait. However, both forms of muscle compensation can potentially alter the distribution of load across the tibiofemoral joint and quadriceps avoidance gait patterns may increase the force transmitted to the PLC.

Functional Adaptations in the Anterior Cruciate Ligament-Reconstructed Knee

Similar to understanding functional adaptations in the ACL-deficient knee, understanding net muscle forces and their effects on intra-articular loads in ACL-reconstructed knees of individuals is equally important because this information can provide the ground work for the prescription of weightbearing exercises and insight as to why knee joint degeneration often follows ACL-reconstruction, even in the event of successful surgery.

DeVita et al.[29] measured the lower extremity kinematic and kinetic changes before (2 weeks) and after (3 and 5 weeks) bone-patellar tendon-bone (BTB) ACL reconstruction. The primary result was the existence of an extensor moment in the injured knee in both pre- and postsurgical time points. This pattern was in contrast to the final adaptive patterns of a net flexor torque observed in the fully rehabilitated ACL-deficient knees of patients[22] and the ACL-reconstructed knees of patients[23] who exhibit a reduced knee extensor moment.

In a survey of the ACL Study Group, Campbell[41] reported that 76% of the surgeons chose the BTB graft as their primary graft source, and 17% prefer the hamstring (semitendinosus tendon with or without the gracilis tendon). In order to construct viable physical therapy protocols, it is essential to know the developmental processes that lead to final adaptive strategies in BTB and hamstring groups. Torry et al.[42] compared the kinematic and kinetic gait patterns of individuals repaired with either the double-loop semitendinosus plus gracilis graft (DLSTG) or the BTB grafts at 3, 6, 9, and 12 weeks postreconstruction with a healthy control group. Compared with the control group, the DLSTG group contacted the ground and maintained greater average hip and knee joint flexion angles at all test periods. At 3 and 6 weeks, the DLSTG group was 46.5% and 50% more flexed at the hip joint but returned to within 14.5% and 9.8% of normal values at 9 and 12 weeks, respectively. At the knee, the DLSTG group was 65.7% and 37.2% more flexed at heel contact at 3 and 6 weeks, and returned to within 18.5% and 8.9% of the control group by 9 and 12 weeks, respectively. The DLSTG group maintained a 41.5%, 28.8%, and 20.6% more flexed average knee position throughout stance at 3, 6, and 9 weeks; and returned to within 8.3% of the control group at 12 weeks. At the knee, the joint torque remained extensor at 3 and 6 weeks, but showed trends toward the normal biphasic pattern at 9 and 12 weeks post-reconstruction for both groups. Statistically, the knee extensor angular impulse was different from the control group at all test periods and was 27.0%, 56.1%, 30.4%, and 29.9% greater than the control group at 3, 6, 9, and 12 weeks. Collectively, the results showed that the DLSTG group achieved a more normal gait pattern much earlier (patterns were nearly normal by 6 weeks postoperation) compared with the BTB group; but both groups obtained similar kinematic patterns by 12 weeks postsurgery. However, the BTB group exhibited very different underlying kinetics and energetics and associated extensor muscle function through 12 weeks postsurgery.

The findings of Torry et al.[42] combined with the results of DeVita et al.[29] and Torry et al.[23] show that the final adaptive gait patterns often exhibited by ACL-deficient and ACL-reconstructed groups 2 years after surgery (either BTB or DLSTG) are not present at the early postinjury and postoperative periods. This suggests that the adaptations are most likely learned over a long period and thus can then be influenced with training. Based on this theory, Decker et al.[43] applied a post-ACL-reconstructed gait training program to knees of BTB-reconstructed patients and compared the changes in gait patterns to a matched ACL-reconstructed cohort. The protocol emphasized the return of normal gait patterns by training the patients to walk at a harmonic frequency that was based on their own anthropometric measures. The force-driven harmonic oscillator theory suggests individuals use a gait pattern that is metabolically optimized based on stride length and stride frequency. After applying the force-driven harmonic oscillator gait retraining regimen for 3 weeks, the data showed that, in fact, gait patterns can be purposely manipulated and influenced to be more normal (at both the kinematic and kinetic levels) much earlier in the postoperative period than if traditional gait training protocols are used.

Landing

Landing from a Drop Jump

Numerous studies have found females to possess a higher rate of noncontact ACL injury compared with males during athletic competition. The theory for this gender disparity proposes that females perform high-demand athletic maneuvers differently than males and in a manner that predisposes them to higher knee joint stress. Kirkendall and Garrett[44] reported ACL injuries occurring in basketball and soccer were most often noncontact in nature (64 of 72 injuries, 89%) and a result of a deceleration type of movement (landing from a jump was reported in 30 of the 72 injuries, 42%). In light of these observations, controlled laboratory experiments have investigated the performance of females during cutting and landing tasks. Consensus of these studies indicate that the female knee is in a more extended position at ground contact, and thus predisposed to greater ACL loads, and that knee stabilizing muscle force, particularly from the hamstring musculature, is lower in females than in males.

Decker et al.[45] used an inverse dynamics approach to estimate lower extremity joint kinematics, kinetics, and energetic profiles for 12 male and female athletes performing a 60-cm drop landing. Kinematically, both groups also demonstrated similar maximum knee flexion angles (males, 93.0; females 98.4). The females, however, demonstrated greater knee extension and ankle plantar-flexion angles at initial ground contact compared with the male group. Females use greater knee and ankle range of motion compared with males, and females exhibit greater peak angular velocities at all lower extremity joints compared with males. Kinetically, Decker et al.[43] noted that the peak hip extensor moment and the peak ankle plantar-flexor moment was larger for females compared with males and there were significant differences between genders regarding the temporal occurrence of peak knee extensor moment. For females, the time to the peak knee extensor moment occurred 0.063 seconds after ground contact, which corresponded in time with the F2 peak of the vertical ground-reaction force. Conversely, the peak knee extensor moment for the males occurred 0.038 seconds after ground contact, which corresponded in time with the F1 peak of the vertical ground-reaction force. Thus, it appears females activate their quadriceps and thus generate their peak knee extensor torque much later in the contact phase than males.

Although it is generally accepted that external and internal forces can be mediated by manipulating the lower extremity joint kinematics during landing, no consensus has been reached regarding gender differences in the primary energy-absorption strategy. Decker et al.[43] showed that the peak, negative hip power was larger than the peak negative ankle and knee powers for the male group. Compared with the female group, the male group exhibited smaller values for the second peak, negative knee power and peak negative ankle power. Comparisons of negative joint work for the female group demonstrated greater energy absorption from the knee and ankle compared with the hip; whereas the male group demonstrated no energy-absorption differences between the lower extremity joints. Both groups used the knee as the primary joint to absorb energy; however, the female group performed 34% less negative hip work, and 30% and 52% more negative knee and ankle work compared with the male group. Under certain landing conditions, this shock-absorption strategy is proposed to provide a greater potential risk for noncontact ACL injury for females compared with males and increased knee flexion at initial ground contact was advocated to be part of future ACL injury-prevention programs.

Sagittal plane analyses of landing performance provides valuable insights into the noncontact injury mechanisms, but more recent *in vivo, in vitro,* and theoretical studies have shown the varus-valgus (frontal plane) knee motion to be vital in identifying those at risk for ACL injury. Kernozek et al.[46] studied the frontal plane landing characteristics of females compared with those of males. Females demonstrated greater peak knee valgus angles compared with males during the first 30% to 50% of the landing phase. It is important to note that the increased knee valgus motion is apparent in females across a variety of sporting movements that includes landing from a jump, cutting, and side-stepping,[45,47,48] and suggests that a common mechanism of the noncontact ACL injury for females may exist across a wide range of movements. The practical merit of this observation is supported by epidemiologic and clinical annotations that cite aberrant knee kinematic movements in the frontal plane as key elements to the noncontact ACL injury mechanism.[49,50] Kinetically, females exhibited significantly lower peak internal knee varus moments compared with the males, who demonstrated 42% increase in the mean peak internal knee varus moment. Because a high internal knee varus moment would serve to resist valgus knee excursion, this finding suggests that females are at a greater knee valgus position at a time when they also generate low internal varus moment.

Additionally, the timing of the peak valgus knee angle, the peak knee varus-valgus moments, and the peak knee extensor knee moment suggests coupling of these knee kinetics, which may further predispose individuals to noncontact ACL injury. Collectively, we interpret the timing relationships in the peak knee varus-valgus and the peak knee extension moment magnitudes to suggest that females are more prone to higher ACL loads during the drop landing because of the greater valgus knee position combined with a low varus moment at the same time a high knee extensor moment is being applied to the joint.

There are also functional adaptations that occur during landing after the ACL is repaired. Decker et al.[51] measured the landing performance of knees of ACL-reconstructed (DLSTG) individuals. Compared to controls, the ACL-reconstructed-DLSTG group exhibited a more erect landing posture and a reduced loading strategy from the hip extensors that was transferred to the ankle plantar flexors, which did more work. The reduction in the peak hip and knee extensor joint moments and negative powers represent a selective decreased effort in the hamstring ability to dissipate the energy from the land. The ACL-reconstructed group showed a 12% difference in hip extensor energy absorption, which suggests that the harvest of the hamstring tendon for reconstruction had some effect on the neuromuscular function and caused a shift from the hip to the ankle in an effort to accommodate the energy dissipation, which would also serve to protect the hamstring donor site from increased loads.

The *in vivo* experiments discussed here noted several factors that may be related to ACL loading during landing. Yet, these methods cannot describe actual ACL loading patterns. Although many of these studies suggest that the impact on landing may predispose athletes to ACL knee injuries, a detailed analysis of the internal forces acting at the knee has seldom been undertaken. This is because difficulties associated with the measurement and calculation of muscle and knee-ligament forces *in vivo* have hindered progress in evaluating the internal state of the joint during high-impact, functional activities. Using computational modeling and simulation techniques, Pflum et al.[52] sought to calculate and explain the pattern of force transmitted to the ACL during a soft-style drop landing. Results showed that the model ACL was loaded only in the first 25% of the landing phase as the knee flexed from 33 to 48 degrees. ACL force decreased to zero shortly after initial impact and then increased quickly to reach a maximum of 253 N (approximately 0.4 BW) at 40 ms. The total shear force applied to the lower leg was directed anteriorly in the first 70 ms of the landing phase, except for the period shortly after initial impact when the ground reaction applied a large posterior shear force to the lower leg (Fig. 17.9). Peak total anterior shear force was 220 N (approximately 0.3 BW) and occurred at precisely the same instant (40 ms) as the maximum force transmitted to the ACL.

The analysis presented by Pflum et al.[52] indicates that three factors contribute most significantly to the total shear force applied to the lower leg during landing: (i) the anterior shear force supplied by the patellar tendon, (ii) the anterior shear force induced by the compressive force acting at the tibiofemoral joint, and (iii) the posterior shear force applied by the ground reaction (Fig. 17.9). Immediately

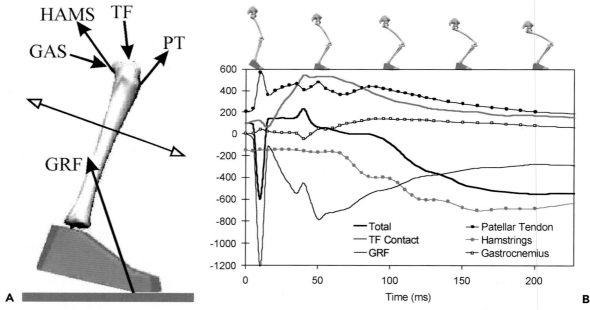

Figure 17.9 **(A)** Free body diagram of shear forces acting on the lower leg (shank +foot) during **(B)** the simulated drop-landing. Positive shear forces are directed anteriorly; negative shear forces are directed posteriorly. Total shear force is the shear force due to the muscle forces, ground-reaction forces, and joint contact forces. Hamstrings always applied a posterior shear force. The ground-reaction force applied a posterior shear force to the lower leg because the line of action of the resultant ground force passed behind the knee. The tibiofemoral contact force applied an anterior shear force to the lower leg because the tibial plateau in the model sloped posteriorly in the sagittal plane. HAMS, hamstrings; TF, tibiofemoral; PT, patellar tendon; GAS, gastrocnemius muscle; GRF, ground-reaction force; TF Contact, TF contact force, (Reproduced with permission from Pflum M, Shelburne KB, Torry MR, et al. Model prediction of anterior cruciate ligament force during drop-landings. *Med Sci Sports Exerc* 2004;36:1949–1958.)

after initial impact, ACL force dropped to zero for a very short period of time. Even though the anterior shear force supplied by the patellar tendon was maximum at this time, ACL force decreased to zero because of the much larger increase in the posterior shear force applied by the ground reaction. The posterior shear force induced by the ground reaction was large shortly after impact because of the direction of the resultant ground-reaction vector. The resultant ground reaction passed far behind the knee because the fore-aft component of the ground reaction pointed posteriorly at this time. The anterior shear force supplied by the patellar tendon was maximum immediately after initial impact, even though quadriceps force did not peak until much later in the landing movement. The peak in patellar tendon shear force at this time was caused by the relatively large angle between the patellar tendon and the long axis of the tibia, which in turn was due to the posterior shift of the tibia relative to the femur brought about by the large posterior shear force applied by the ground reaction.

The anterior shear force induced by the tibiofemoral contact force also peaked around 40 ms after initial impact. There were two reasons for this: (i) vasti force was relatively large at this time, and this force was transmitted directly through the condyles of the knee in the model; and (ii) the magnitude of the resultant ground reaction was highest at this time and its direction was more closely aligned with the long axis of the tibia (i.e., it passed closer to the knee) because the fore-aft component was directed anteriorly. We note here that the vertical component of the ground reaction always passes behind the knee because the tibia is angled anteriorly relative to the ground. Thus, the ground force contributed significantly to the tibiofemoral contact force at around 40 ms after initial impact.

Tibiofemoral contact force results in an anterior shear force at the knee because the articular surface of the model tibia is sloped, on average, 8 degrees posteriorly. This slope, coupled with a large tibiofemoral contact force, creates an anterior drawer of the tibia relative to the femur. The results of Pflum et al.[52] suggest that tibial slope is an important contributor to the anterior shear force applied to the knee during landing.

Much has been written about the intrinsic and extrinsic factors responsible for noncontact ACL injuries in sports. One commonly held belief is that landing with an extended knee increases the anterior pull of the quadriceps, which in turn strains the ACL. The reasoning is as follows. If the knee is more fully extended during ground contact, the patellar tendon will be more anteriorly inclined relative to the long axis of the tibia. This, combined with a large quadriceps force developed in eccentric contraction, causes a large anterior shear force to be applied to the lower leg. Thus, quadriceps force is often implicated in ACL injury, as these muscles are thought to pull the tibia anteriorly with such vigor as to overstrain the ACL. The model calculations of Pflum et al.[52] in agreement with others,[53] revealed that the pattern of ACL force in landing cannot be explained by the mechanism of

quadriceps force alone. The maximum force transmitted to the model ACL resulted from a complex interaction between the patellar tendon force, the compressive force acting at the tibiofemoral joint, and the force applied by the ground to the lower leg. Although the role of the patellar tendon was significant in determining peak ACL loading in landing, the contributions of the shear forces induced by the tibiofemoral contact force and the ground-reaction force were just as important and cannot be discounted. The latter two mechanisms have received less attention in the literature, and future studies ought to be directed at understanding the relationship between knee flexion angle and the anterior and posterior shear forces induced by tibiofemoral contact and the ground-reaction force, respectively.

Landing Performance with Muscular Fatigue

Several intrinsic and extrinsic factors have been debated and attached to the noncontact ACL injury disparity between genders.[54] As previously noted, biomechanical performance differences between males and females during cutting and landing have emerged as significant risk factors that can be reliably measured in controlled laboratory situations.[43,46,55,56] The findings of these studies have contributed to the development of performance-based, ACL injury-prevention training programs that have been effective in identifying individuals who may be predisposed to ACL injury based on their execution of a landing motion. The subsequent implementation of these training programs has shown some success in reducing the noncontact ACL injury in female athletes in competitive arenas.[5,57,58] Despite these efforts, the overall occurrence of the noncontact ACL injury remains one of the more common knee injuries in athletics, and both men and women are still rupturing their ACLs. This suggests that other factors that are not incorporated into the current ACL injury-prevention protocols may contribute to the occurrence of the noncontact ACL injury in both genders.

Bradley et al.[59] have shown that in the (American) National Football League, 68% of noncontact ACL injuries occur during game play and the remaining occur at both the beginning and later months of the competitive season. Hawkins and Fuller[60] and Hawkins et al.[61] have shown that the majority of noncontact injuries occur during the last 15 minutes of the first half and the final 30 minutes of the second half of regulation soccer matches, with knee injuries accounting for up to 17% of these events. Collectively, these findings suggest that muscular fatigue may be a causative factor in the development of the observed noncontact, ACL injury trends.[59-61]

Kernozek et al.[62] sought to determine gender differences in lower extremity joint kinematics and kinetics between age- and skill-matched male and female recreational athletes pre- and postexercise-induced fatigue. The authors employed an inverse dynamic solution that estimated the lower extremity flexion-extension and varus-valgus kinematics and kinetics for 14 females and 16 males performing a 60-cm drop landing. All subjects performed landings pre- and postfatigue, with fatigue induced via a 60% of their one-repetition maximum parallel squat exercise conducted until physical failure of the squat motion. In general, fatigue caused males and females to land with more hip flexion. Males also exhibited greater peak knee flexion angles, while females did not alter knee flexion after fatigue. Males exhibited larger peak knee varus angles, while females demonstrated larger peak valgus angles. Fatigue caused each gender to land with approximately 9% lower peak knee compression force. There were no differences between genders, and each gender responded similarly with a reduction in knee compression force due to the fatigue protocol. Muscular fatigue caused all subjects to adopt a landing style that effectively reduced the peak magnitude of the knee shear force by an average of 29%.

Fatigue, however, affected the knee shear force pattern within each gender differently. Males were able to reduce the magnitude of this force by 38% compared with the females, who were only able to reduce this force by 20%. Muscular fatigue also caused each gender to land with about 22% less knee extensor torque. In the frontal plane, both genders demonstrated an average 11% reduction in the peak knee abduction moment postfatigue. Although the females did reduce the magnitude of this moment approximately 6% more than the males, there were no differences between genders and each group responded similarly to the fatigue protocol with regard to this parameter.

The results of Kernozek et al.[62] suggest that landing characteristics of *both* male and female subjects are significantly altered from muscular fatigue, and the postfatigue landing characteristics resemble landing profiles that resemble the proposed noncontact ACL injury mechanisms. Specifically, females exhibited a 65% increase in the peak valgus knee angles compared with males, an increase in peak knee shear force and a reduction in the varus moment that serves to resist valgus angulation. Moreover, females also showed greater postfatigue affects with a 65% larger peak valgus knee angle compared with their male counterparts. This finding suggests that females may exhibit performance changes that are more conducive (i.e., larger valgus knee angle) to noncontact ACL injury compared with males when muscular fatigue is taken into account. Yet, even the males showed an increase in the stiffness by which they landed; making them also more susceptible to injury in postfatigue conditions. The specific intra-articular loads due to muscle fatigue have yet to be determined.

SUMMARY AND CONCLUSION

The contents of this chapter represent a compilation of research studies that sought to combine *in vivo* data with computational biomechanics techniques. These methods have allowed investigators to explore knee function under normal and pathologic conditions. The application of computational modeling to human movement has allowed for advances in our understanding of intra-articular loads during functional movements that would not otherwise be possible *in vivo*, and not technically feasible using *in vitro* procedures. For instance, in this chapter it was shown that the quadriceps muscle provided most of the resistance to the adductor moment in the first half of stance, while the gastrocnemius muscle contributed most of the resisting muscular moment thereafter; and, the PLC provided the primary passive restraint to lateral joint opening. This identification of "individual tissue contributions" to resisting knee moments during functional exercises and their associated loads is not feasible with *in vivo* or *in vitro* techniques.

ACKNOWLEDGMENTS

Much of the work provided in this chapter was supported by grants to the contributing authors. MG Pandy was supported in part by the National Science Foundation, Engineering Research Centers Grant EEC-9876363, and by Sulzer Orthopedics Inc., Austin, Texas. MR Torry and KB Shelburne were supported by grants from Ossur, National Football League Charities, and Innovation Sports, Inc.

REFERENCES

1. Shelburne KB, Pandy MG. A musculoskeletal model of the knee for evaluating ligament forces during isometric contractions. *J Biomech* 1997;30:163–176.
2. Pandy MG, Shelburne KB. Dependence of cruciate-ligament loading on muscle forces and external load. *J Biomech* 1997;30:1015–1024.
3. Shelburne KB, Pandy MG, Anderson FC, et al. Pattern of anterior cruciate ligament force in normal walking. *J Biomech* 2004;37:797–805.
4. Shelburne KB, Pandy MG. A dynamic model of the knee and lower limb for simulating rising movements. *Comput Methods Biomech Biomed Engin* 2002;5:149–159.
5. Kvist J, Gillquist J. Anterior positioning of tibia during motion after anterior cruciate ligament injury. *Med Sci Sports Exerc* 2001;33:1063–1072.
6. Li XM, Liu B, Deng B, et al. Normal six-degree-of-freedom motions of knee joint during level walking. *J Biomech Eng* 1996;118:258–261.
7. Zhang LQ, Shiavi RG, Limbird TJ, et al. Six degrees-of-freedom kinematics of ACL deficient knees during locomotion-compensatory mechanism. *Gait Posture* 2003;17:34–42.
8. Morrison JB. The mechanics of the knee joint in relation to normal walking. *J Biomech* 1970;3:51–61.
9. Harrington IJ. A bioengineering analysis of force actions at the knee in normal and pathological gait. *Biomed Eng* 1976;11:167–172.
10. Stapleton TR, Waldrop JI, Ruder CR, et al. Graft fixation strength with arthroscopic anterior cruciate ligament reconstruction. Two-incision rear entry technique compared with one-incision technique. *Am J Sports Med* 1998;26:442–445.
11. Shelburne KB. *Modeling the Mechanics of the Intact and Reconstructed Knee* [dissertation]. Austin: University of Texas at Austin; 1997.
12. Shelburne KB, Pandy MG. Determinants of cruciate-ligament loading during rehabilitation exercise. *Clin Biomech.* 1998;13:403–413.

13. Fleming BC, Renstrom PA, Ohlen G, et al. The gastrocnemius muscle is an antagonist of the anterior cruciate ligament. *J Orthop Res* 2001;19:1178–1184.
14. Giffin JR, Vogrin TM, Zantop T, et al. Effects of increasing tibial slope on the biomechanics of the knee. *Am J Sports Med* 2004;32: 376–382.
15. Tibone JE, Antich TJ, Fanton GS, et al. Functional analysis of anterior cruciate ligament instability. *Am J Sports Med* 1986;14:276–284.
16. Torg JS, Barton TM, Pavlov H, et al. Natural history of the posterior cruciate ligament-deficient knee. *Clin Orthop Relat Res* 1986;246: 208–216.
17. Hurwitz DE, Sumner DR, Andriacchi TP, et al. Dynamic knee loads during gait predict proximal tibial bone distribution. *J Biomech* 1998;31:423–430.
18. Schipplein OD, Andriacchi TP. Interaction between active and passive knee stabilizers during level walking. *J Orthop Res* 1991;9: 113–119.
19. Shelburne KB, Torry MR, Pandy MG. Contributions of muscles, ligaments, and the ground-reaction force to tibiofemoral joint loading during normal gait. *J Orthop Res* 2006;24:1983–1990.
20. Noyes FR, Mooar PA, Matthews DS, et al. The symptomatic anterior cruciate-deficient knee. Part I: the long-term functional disability in athletically active individuals. *J Bone Joint Surg Am* 1983;65:154–162.
21. Andriacchi TP, Birac D. Functional testing in the anterior cruciate ligament-deficient knee. *Clin Orthop Relat Res* 1993;288:40–47.
22. Hurwitz DE, Andriacchi TP, Bush-Joseph CA, et al. Functional adaptations in patients with ACL-deficient knees. *Exerc Sport Sci Rev* 1997;25:1–20.
23. Torry MR, Decker MJ, Ellis HB, et al. Mechanisms of compensating for anterior cruciate ligament deficiency during gait. *Med Sci Sports Exerc* 2004;36:1403–1412.
24. Wexler G, Hurwitz DE, Bush-Joseph CA, et al. Functional gait adaptations in patients with anterior cruciate ligament deficiency over time. *Clin Orthop Relat Res* 1998;348:166–175.
25. Berchuck M, Andriacchi TP, Bach BR, et al. Gait adaptations by patients who have a deficient anterior cruciate ligament. *J Bone Joint Surg Am* 1990;72:871–877.
26. Andriacchi TP. Dynamics of pathological motion: applied to the anterior cruciate deficient knee. *J Biomech* 1990;23:99–105.
27. Hewett TE, Blum KR, Noyes FR. Gait characteristics of the anterior cruciate ligament-deficient varus knee. *Am J Knee Surg* 1997;10: 246–254.
28. Noyes FR, Schipplein OD, Andriacchi TP, et al. The anterior cruciate ligament-deficient knee with varus alignment. An analysis of gait adaptations and dynamic joint loadings. *Am J Sports Med* 1992;20:707–716.
29. Devita P, Hortobagyi T, Barrier J, et al. Gait adaptations before and after anterior cruciate ligament reconstruction surgery. *Med Sci Sports Exerc* 1997;29:853–859.
30. Wexler G, Hurwitz DE, Bush-Joseph CA, et al. Functional gait adaptations in patients with anterior cruciate ligament deficiency over time. *Clin Orthop Relat Res* 1998;348:166–175.
31. Chmielewski TL, Rudolph KS, Fitzgerald GK, et al. Biomechanical evidence supporting a differential response to acute ACL injury. *Clin Biomech (Bristol, Avon)* 2001;16:586–591.
32. Ferber R, Osternig LR, Woollacott MH, et al. Gait mechanics in chronic ACL deficiency and subsequent repair. *Clin Biomech (Bristol, Avon)* 2002;17:274–285.
33. Rudolph KS, Axe MJ, Buchanan TS, et al. Dynamic stability in the anterior cruciate ligament deficient knee. *Knee Surg Sports Traumatol Arthrosc* 2001;9:62–71.
34. Shelburne KB, Pandy MG, Torry MR. Comparison of shear forces and ligament loading in the healthy and ACL-deficient knee during gait. *J Biomech* 2004;37:313–319.
35. Shelburne KB, Torry MR, Pandy MG. Muscle, ligament, and joint-contact forces at the knee during walking. *Med Sci Sports Exerc* 2005;37:1948–1956.
36. Shelburne KB, Torry MR, Yanagawa T, et al. Theoretical analysis of the flexed knee pattern in ACL-deficient gait. In: Proceedings of the American Society Mechanical Engineering (ASME) Summer Bioengineering Conference; June 12–15, 2003; Key Biscayne, FL, S122.
37. Butler DL, Noyes FR, Grood ES. Ligamentous restraints to anterior-posterior drawer in the human knee. A biomechanical study. *J Bone Joint Surg Am* 1980;62:259–270.
38. Shelburne KB, Torry MR, Pandy MG. Effect of muscle compensation on knee instability during ACL-deficient gait. *Med Sci Sports Exerc* 2005;37:642–648.
39. Lewek MD, Rudolph KS, Snyder-Mackler L. Quadriceps femoris muscle weakness and activation failure in patients with symptomatic knee osteoarthritis. *J Orthop Res* 2004;22:110–115.
40. Torry MR, Pflum MA, Shelburne KB, et al. The effect of quadriceps weakness on the adductor moment during gait. *Med Sci Sports Exerc* 2004;36(Suppl):S46.
41. Campbell JD. The evolution and current treatment trends with anterior cruciate ligament, posterior cruciate and collateral ligament injuries. *Am J Knee Surg* 1998;11:128–135.
42. Torry MR, Wilson J, Decker MJ, et al. Longitudinal gait adaptations of ACL-injured individuals reconstructed with the hamstring graft. Medicine & Science in Sports & Exercise, 31(5) Supplement: S130, May 1999.
43. Decker MJ, Torry MR, Noonan TJ, Sterett WI, Steadman JR. Gait retraining after anterior cruciate ligament reconstruction. *Arch Phys Med Rehabil* 2004;85:848–856.
44. Kirkendall DT, Garrett WE. The anterior cruciate ligament enigma. Injury mechanisms and prevention. *Clin Orthop Relat Res* 2000;372:64–68.
45. Decker MJ, Torry MR, Wyland DJ, Sterett WI, Steadman JR. Gender differences in lower extremity kinematics, kinetics and energy absorption during landing. *Clin Biomech (Bristol, Avon)* 2003;18: 662–669.
46. Kernozek TW, Torry MR, Van Hoof H, Cowley H, Tanner S. Gender differences in frontal and sagittal plane biomechanics during drop landings. *Med Sci Sports Exerc* 2005;37:1003–1013.
47. Chappell JD, Yu B, Kirkendall DT, Garrett WE. A comparison of knee kinetics between male and female recreational athletes in stop-jump tasks. *Am J Sports Med* 2002;30:261–267.
48. McLean SG, Lipfert SW, van den Bogert AJ. Effect of gender and defensive opponent on the biomechanics of sidestep cutting. *Med Sci Sports Exerc* 2004;36:1008–1016.
49. Hutchinson MR, Ireland ML. Knee injuries in female athletes. *Sports Med.* 1995;19:288–302.
50. Ireland ML. The female ACL: why is it more prone to injury? *Orthop Clin North Am* 2002;33:637–651.
51. Decker MJ, Torry MR, Noonan TJ, Riviere A, Sterett WI. Landing adaptations after ACL reconstruction. *Med Sci Sports Exerc* 2002;34:1408–1413.
52. Pflum M, Shelburne KB, Torry M, Decker MJ, Pandy MG. Model prediction of anterior cruciate ligament force during drop-landings. *Med Sci Sports Exerc* 2004;36:1949–1958.
53. McLean SG, Huang X, Su A, Van Den Bogert AJ. Sagittal plane biomechanics cannot injure the ACL during sidestep cutting. *Clin Biomech (Bristol, Avon)* 2004;19:828–838.
54. Arendt E, Agel J, Dick R. Anterior cruciate ligament injury patterns among collegiate men and women. *J Athletic Training* 1999;34:86–92.
55. Hewett TE, Lindenfeld TN, Riccobene JV, Noyes FR. The effect of neuromuscular training on the incidence of knee injury in female athletes. A prospective study. *Am J Sports Med* 1999;27:699–706.
56. Yu BS, McClure B, Onate JA, et al. Age and gender effects on lower extremity kinematics of youth soccer players in a stop-jump task. *Am J Sports Med* 2005;33:1356–1364.
57. Griffin FM. *Prevention of Non-contact ACL Injuries*. Chicago: American Academy of Orthopaedic Surgeons; 2001:45–76.
58. Hewett TE, Myer GD, Ford KR. Reducing knee and anterior cruciate ligament injuries among female athletes: a systematic review of neuromuscular training interventions. *J Knee Surg* 2005;18:82–88.
59. Bradley JP, Klimkiewicz JJ, Rytel MJ, Powell JW. Anterior cruciate ligament injuries in the National Football League: epidemiology and current treatment trends among team physicians. *Arthroscopy* 2002;18:502–509.
60. Hawkins RD, Fuller CW. A prospective epidemiological study of injuries in four english professional football clubs. *Br J Sports Med* 1999;33:196–203.
61. Hawkins RD, Hulse MA, Wilkeinson C, Gibson M. The association football medical research programme: an audit in professional football. *Br J Sports Med* 2001;35:43–47.
62. Kernozek TW, Torry MR, Wallace BJ, Miller EJ. Biomechanics of a failed single legged landing due to fatigue. *Med Sci Sports Exerc* 2006;38(Suppl):S23–24.

The Pursuit of the Crucial Principles

Principle I. Three-dimensional anatomic diagnosis

Principle II. Treatment program aimed at optimizing function

Principle III. Surgery maximizing the body's potential

Principle IV. Rehabilitation aimed at return to activity within the envelope of realistic function

Principle V. Communication between patient and team

Principle VI. Maintenance of a database that validates the crucial principles

When we first entered the field of knee surgery and care of the knee (circa 1967), there was not much science, but "giants roamed the earth" and anecdotal experience was there to guide our generation. Drs. O'Donoghue, Slocum, Hughston, Larson, Trillat, and others were giants of their generation. For our generation, the challenge was to add the science. Fortunately, the aforementioned giants left us a platform, a podium, and an infrastructure that facilitated and encouraged science in the care of the knee. The Sports Medicine Committee of the American Academy of Orthopaedic Surgeons, The American Orthopaedic Society of Sports Medicine, and their teaching, texts, and publications served as our infrastructure. Our responsibility was clear and our generation heard the call and responded with the best science we could muster. The contributions of Drs. Noyes, De Haven, Daniel, Grood, Jackson, Johnson, Steadman, Warren, Bergfeld, Clancy, Andrews, Arnoczsky, Woo, Fu, and a host of others brought science to our surgery. The contributions of the International Knee Documentation Committee (IKDC) and our colleagues from across the oceans brought us to where we are today: well advanced in the science of care of the knee. This progress has opened many doors. Much lies ahead: prevention, better rehabilitation, better bracing, navigated surgery, cellular manipulation, and a better understanding of arthritis and prostheses. The future is dawning, not diminishing.

The Crucial Principles sets the tone for where we are circa 2007. The joy of this book, which for me follows *The Crucial Ligaments*, has been to combine with Dr. Steadman and our coauthors to bring the latest and best of knee care together in one volume, to guide the student and to challenge the master. Thank you for sharing your time, energy, and thoughts with us as we move forward in the application of science to the care of the knee. To each of you, our fond wishes for success in the care of the knee and in your career.

John A. Feagin, Jr., MD
J. Richard Steadman, MD

Index

Note: Page numbers followed by f indicate figure; t indicate table; and b indicate box.

A

AAOS. *See* Academy of Orthopaedic Surgeons
Abduction moment, during walking, 237f
Ablation, of hypertrophic synovium, 178–179, 180f
Academy of Orthopaedic Surgeons (AAOS), prophylactic bracing position of, 69
ACL. *See* Anterior cruciate ligament
ACL nodules, 164, 165f, 167
ACL reconstruction, 59–60, 99, 117–127
  complications of, 126
  degeneration after, 154
  envelope of function after, 55, 55f–56f
  functional adaptations after, 240–242
  graft malposition in, 164–166, 165f
  kinematic competence of, 8–9
  knee biomechanics after, 229–245
  outcomes of, 125–126
  patient selection for, 117–118
  postoperative management of, 124–125, 127
  rehabilitation of, 124–125, 127, 217
  stiffness with, 164, 207
  surgical technique for, 118–124, 119f–124f
ACL-deficient knee, 52. *See also* Surgical knee care
  biomechanics of, 229–245
  case studies of, 27–50
    acute dislocation of patella in skeletally mature competitive male athlete, 41–43, 41f–42f, 42b
    "isolated" ACL injury, 29–33, 29b, 29f–30f, 32f
    multiligament-injured knee, 33–37, 33f–37f, 34b
    subluxation of patella in adolescent female athlete, 38–41, 38f–40f, 40b
  function return of, 8–9
  functional adaptations in, 236–240, 239f
  kinematic competence of, 8–9
  natural history of, 3–4
  patient selectivity for surgical repair of, 3
  physical examination of, 72–81
  prevention of injury of, 59–71
  principles for care of, 7–10
  prognosis of, 8
  realistic expectations for, 8–9
  rehabilitation for, 3–4, 9, 59–60, 85

  surgical methodology for, 3, 4, 9
  thoughts on, 3–4
  three-dimensional anatomic diagnosis of, 8–9
  treatment program for, 8–9
Activities of daily living, knee function and loads during, 230–244, 232f, 234f–237f, 239f, 242f
  flexion and extension, 231–233, 232f
  knee bends and squatting, 122
  landing, 241–244, 242f
  walking, 233–241, 234f–237f, 239f
Activity. *See also* Tegner activity score
  desired v. current levels of, 187–188, 188f
  meniscus loss effect on, 200–201
  return to, 32–33, 41, 125, 145, 148, 158–159, 205–206, 211–212, 213f–216f
Activity preservation. *See* Joint preservation
Acute cartilage lesion, 129, 131f
Acute chondral injury, 188–189
  microfracture for, 134–140, 136f–142f
    imaging of, 135–137, 137f–139f
    indications and contraindications for, 134–135, 136f–137f
    preoperative planning of, 135, 137f
    surgical technique for, 137–140, 139f–142f
Adaptations
  in ACL-deficient knee, 236–240, 239f
  in ACL-reconstructed knee, 240–242
Adduction moment, during walking, 236, 237f, 239
Adhesions
  with immobilization, 207
  lysis of, 170–171, 170f, 217–218
  of multiligament-injured knee, 37
Adjunct tests, in physical examination, 18
Administrative assistant, role of, 10
Adolescent female athlete, subluxation of patella in, 38–41, 38f–40f, 40b
Advanced rehabilitation, 210–211, 211f–212f
Aerobic conditioning, during rehabilitation, 207, 209
Age. *See* Patient
Aggrecan expression, after microfracture, 134, 134f–135f, 223, 225
Agility, rehabilitation of, 24
Alae, examination of, 77
Alignment, 186–187, 186f–187f. *See also* Malalignment
  axial, 134, 137f, 140–141

  of lower extremities, ACL injury with, 61, 61f
  varus, 186–187, 186f, 189, 189b, 193
Allograft, 31, 35–36, 118, 121f, 125–126
  magnetic resonance imaging of, 95
  of menisci, 189
Anabolic processes, of chondrocytes, 130–132
Analgesia, for arthrofibrosis treatment, 169
Anatomic diagnosis, 16, 73
  of ACL deficiency or rupture, 8–9
Anatomic restoration, of ACL-deficient knee, 9
Anderson Knee Stabler, 67
Anesthesia
  for arthrofibrosis treatment, 169
  examination under, 20, 35, 41
Animal models, selection of, 222
Ankle plantar-flexor moment, during landing, 241
Ankle, rehabilitation of, 85
Antalgic sway, 79, 80f
Anterior cruciate ligament (ACL)
  bracing of, 67–70
  in central pivot, 73–75, 73f–75f
  examination of, 12, 16, 18, 73, 75–76
  forces induced in
    during knee bends and squatting, 233
    during knee flexion and extension, 231–233, 232f
    during landing, 241–243
    during walking, 233–236, 234f, 237f, 238, 239f
  magnetic resonance imaging of, 98–99, 100f–101f, 157f
  prevention of injury of, 59–71
    bracing for, 67–70
    noncontact injury in female athlete, 60–67, 60f–61f, 62t–66t, 67f, 241–244, 242f
    role of coach and athletic trainer in, 69–70, 70t
    studies of, 61–67, 62t–66t
  release of, 173
  tear of, 12, 29–37, 29b, 29f–30f, 32f, 33f–37f, 34b, 41, 59–60, 89, 91f, 97f, 99, 101f–102f, 106, 111f–112f, 157f, 217–218
    healing response for, 153–162
    prevention studies of, 61–67, 62t–66t
Anterior drawer test, 74
Anterior forces, during walking, 238, 239f

Anterior interval
  arthroscopic treatment of, 171, 171f
  release of, 181–182, 181f, 217–218
  restoration of, 37
  scarring of, 166–167, 167f, 171, 171f,
    179, 181f
Anterior knee pain, 54, 124, 126, 164
Anterior tibial translation, 233, 238–239
Anterolateral bundle of PCL, magnetic
    resonance imaging of, 99, 104f
Anteromedial bundle of ACL, magnetic
    resonance imaging of, 98, 100f,
    102f
Anteroposterior (AP) glide, of injured
    knee, 14–15, 15f
Antibiotics, for infection causing
    arthrofibrosis, 167, 169
Antiembolic hose, for "isolated"
    ACL-injured knee, 32
Anti-inflammatory medications, 167.
    See also Nonsteroidal anti-
    inflammatory drugs
AP glide. *See* Anteroposterior glide
Apprehension test, 78, 79f. *See also*
    Patellar apprehension
Aquatic therapy, 208
Arcuate complex, examination of, 14, 16,
    75–76
Arcuate ligament, magnetic resonance
    imaging of, 105
Arthritis, after knee repair, 51–57
Arthrocentesis, 167, 169
Arthrofibrosis, 163–176
  with ACL reconstruction, 118
  diagnosis of, 166–167, 166f–167f
  in "isolated" ACL-injured knee, 33
  outcomes of, 174
  pathophysiology of, 163–166, 164t,
    165f
  postoperative management of,
    173–174, 176
  prevention of, 174
  treatment of, 167–173, 168f–173f
Arthrometers, 24, 24f
Arthroplasty, activity after, 188
Arthroscopic microfracture awl, 157, 158f
Arthroscopic treatment
  for arthrofibrosis, 169–171, 169f–171f
  of degenerative knee, 177–184
    initial evaluation for, 177–178
    package of, 178–182, 178b,
      178f–182f
    patient selection for, 178
  open surgery combined with, 171,
    171f–172f
  outcomes of, 182–183, 183f
  postoperative care of, 182, 184
Arthroscopy
  for ACL reconstruction, 118f, 119
  in horse, 221
  of injured knee, 22
  for microfracture of acute chondral
    injury, 137–138, 139f
  of multiligament-injured knee, 34
  for patella dislocation, 42
Arthrosis, patellofemoral, 174
Arthrotomy, 171, 171f, 172, 172f

Articular cartilage
  calcification of, 133, 133f, 138, 140f,
    142–143, 222–223, 225f
  degeneration of, 130, 131f, 143f–144f,
    148f, 149
  future of repair of, 226–227
  horse studies of, 221–227
    of chondrocyte transplantation,
      225–226, 226f–227f
    of gene therapy with microfracture,
      224–225
    as model of human articular defects,
      222
  immobilization effects on, 207
  injury of, 129–134, 130f–135f, 154
  loss of, 177, 186–187
  magnetic resonance imaging of, 89–95,
    92f–99f
  microfracture for repair of, 129–151,
    130f
    acute chondral injury, 134–140,
      136f–142f
    chronic chondral injury, 140–144,
      143f–144f
    complications of, 145
    outcomes of, 145–147, 146t
    rehabilitation of, 144–145, 150–151,
      216
    results of, 147–149, 147f, 148t
  separation of, 129, 130f
Athletic trainer, ACL injury prevention by,
    69–70, 70t
Atrophy, prevention of, 207
Augmentation grafting, of multiligament-
    injured knee, 35
Autograft, 118
  magnetic resonance imaging of, 95, 112
  of patellar tendon, 119–120, 119f–121f,
    124–125
Autologous chondrocyte implantation,
    microfracture v., 147–148
Autologous chondrocyte transfer, 188
Autologous chondrocyte transplantation,
    horse models of, 225–226,
    226f–227f
Avulsion fracture, 87, 93–94
  with ACL tear, 30f, 99, 101f
  with lateral collateral ligament tear,
    105, 109f
  with patellar tendon tear, 112, 114f
  with posterior cruciate ligament tear,
    99–103
  with retinacular ligament tear, 112, 114f
  Segond, 106–107, 112f
Awl, for microfracture, 139, 141f,
    154–155, 157, 158f, 222
Axial alignment, for microfracture, 134,
    137f, 140–141

B

Backward running, for rehabilitation, 211,
    211f, 213f, 215f–216f
Baker's cyst, 79
Balance board training, 67f
Balance, rehabilitation of, 24
Basic fibroblast growth factor, 130–132
Biceps femoris

magnetic resonance imaging of, 109f,
    115f
  tear of, 115f
  walking forces in, 238
Big Ten Conference, knee bracing studies
    of, 69
Biochemical changes, with healing
    response, 156–157
Biologic transmission, by knee, 52
Biology, of articular cartilage injury,
    130–132
Biomechanical paradigm, of knee repair, 51
Biomechanics
  of knee, 229–245
    computer simulation of, 230, 231f
    function and loading during
      activities of daily living, 230–244,
      232f, 234f–237f, 239f, 242f
    in vivo measurement of, 230, 231f
  of noncontact ACL injury in female
    athlete, 60–67, 60f–61f, 62t–66t,
    67f, 241–244, 242f
  of prophylactic knee bracing, 67–68
Bleeding, with microfracture, 140, 142,
    142f–143f
Bone
  heterotopic formation of, 87, 109–112
  magnetic resonance imaging of, 88–95,
    92f–99f
  radiographic imaging of, 87
Bone blocks, harvest and preparation of,
    120–121, 120f
Bone-patellar tendon-bone graft, 31,
    117–118, 124–126, 240
Bracing
  after ACL reconstruction, 125
  after arthrofibrosis treatment, 174
  after healing response, 157–159
  of intact native ACL, 67–70
  for joint preservation, 188
  after microfracture, 144–145
  during rehabilitation, 208–209
Bruise. *See* Contusion
Burmester curve, 36, 37f

C

Calcification
  of cartilage, 133, 133f, 138, 140f,
    142–143, 222–223, 225f
  magnetic resonance imaging of, 89
Canine studies, of healing response,
    154–157, 154f–156f
Capsular distension, 178, 178b,
    178f–179f
  for arthrofibrosis treatment, 169, 169f
  during rehabilitation, 206
Capsular release, 173
Capsuloligamentous contracture, with
    acute dislocation of patella, 42
Cardiopulmonary conditioning, during
    rehabilitation, 207, 209
Carpet drags, for rehabilitation, 210, 210f
Cartilage. *See* Articular cartilage
Case studies, 27–50
  acute dislocation of patella in skeletally
    mature competitive male athlete,
    41–43, 41f–42f, 42b

"isolated" ACL-injured knee, 29–33, 29b, 29f–30f, 32f
  multiligament-injured knee, 33–37, 33f–37f, 34b
  subluxation of patella in adolescent female athlete, 38–41, 38f–40f, 40b
Catabolic processes, of chondrocytes, 130–132
Central pivot, examination of, 73–75, 73f–75f
Change of direction, injury with, 12
Cheerleader, subluxation of patella in, 38–41, 38f–40f, 40b
Chondral defects, 143f
  ACL reconstruction with, 118
  magnetic resonance imaging of, 88, 90–95, 92f–99f
Chondral imaging technique, 90–95, 92f–99f
Chondral lesions, 41, 188–189. See also Osteochondral fracture
  acute, 134–140, 136f–142f, 188–189
  chronic, 93, 94f, 129–130, 140–144, 143f–144f
  microfracture for repair of, 129–151, 130f
    articular cartilage injury and, 129–134, 130f–135f
    complications of, 145
    outcomes of, 145–147, 146t
    rehabilitation of, 144–145, 150–151, 216
    results of, 147–149, 147f, 148t
  of multiligament-injured knee, 36
  rehabilitation of, 216
Chondral resurfacing, 95, 188–189, 190–191, 193
Chondrocyte, anabolic and catabolic processes of, 130–132
Chondrocyte transplantation
  horse models of, 225–226, 226f–227f
  magnetic resonance imaging of, 95
Chondro-Gide, 226
Chondroitin sulfate, 188, 207
Chronic chondral injury, microfracture for, 140–144, 143f–144f
  contraindications of, 141, 143f
  nonoperative treatment of, 140–141, 143f
  postoperative management of, 143–144
  procedure for, 141–143, 143f–144f
Chronic chondral loss, 129–130
Chronic grade 4 chondral loss, 93, 94f
Chronic pain, investigation of, 185–186
Cine-MRI, of injured knee, 22
Clinical application
  of envelope of function, 54–55
  of healing response, 157–160, 157f–159f
  of knee bracing, 68–69
Clinical studies, of collagen meniscus implant, 199–201, 199f
Closed chain exercise, open chain exercise v., 208

Closure
  of patellar tendon, 124, 124f
  of peritenon, 124
CMI. See Collagen meniscus implant
Coach, ACL injury prevention by, 69–70, 70t
Cold therapy, for microfracture, 144–145
Collagen
  immobilization effects on, 207
  typing of, 132f, 133–134, 134f–135f
Collagen meniscus implant (CMI), 197–201, 198f–199f
  clinical studies of, 199–201, 199f
  fabrication of, 198, 198f
  indications and contraindications for, 198
  surgical technique for, 198–199, 199f
Collateral ligaments. See also specific ligaments, e.g., Lateral collateral ligament
  examination of, 14, 14f, 75–76, 75f–76f
  magnetic resonance imaging of, 103–105, 105f–109f
Communication, with patient, 9–10, 31, 72, 80, 204–206
Compartmentalization
  of quadriceps tendon, 179b
  of suprapatellar pouch, 182, 182f
Competition, return to, 32–33, 41, 125, 145, 148, 158–159, 205–206, 211–212, 213f–216f
Competitive male athlete, acute dislocation of patella in, 41–43, 41f–42f, 42b
Complete tear
  of ACL, 99, 101f
  of lateral collateral ligament, 109f
  of medial collateral ligament, 106f–107f
  of posterior cruciate ligament, 99
  of quadriceps, 108
  of secondary restraints, 107
Compliance, of patient, 205–206
Complications
  of ACL reconstruction, 126
  of collagen meniscus implant, 199–201
  of high tibial osteotomy, 192
  of "isolated" ACL-injured knee, 32–33
  management of, 205
  of microfracture, 145
  of multiligament-injured knee, 37
Compression
  of joint, 179
  of patella, 37, 79, 135, 137f, 179
Compressive dressing, 32, 36
Compressive force
  during landing, 242–243, 242f
  during normal walking, 235–236
Computed tomography, 40, 89, 94
Computer simulation
  of knee biomechanics, 230, 231f
  of walking, 234f
Conduct, of knee examination, 72–73
Conformity, examination of, 73
Contact ACL injury, bracing against, 68

Containment test, 78, 79f
Continuity of care, 31
Continuous passive motion (CPM)
  for ACL reconstruction, 124
  for acute dislocation of patella, 42
  after arthrofibrosis treatment, 173
  after arthroscopic treatment, 182
  of "isolated" ACL-injured knee, 32
  after microfracture, 144–145
  for multiligament-injured knee, 37
  after osteotomy, 191–192
  during rehabilitation, 207, 209
Contraindications
  for collagen meniscus implant, 198
  for microfracture of acute chondral injury, 134–135, 136f–137f
  for microfracture of chronic chondral injury, 141, 143f
Contributing factors, of arthrofibrosis, 163–164, 164t
Contusion
  of lateral condyle, 29, 34
  of lateral femoral condyle, 91f
  of subchondral bone, 93
  of tibia, 29, 89, 89f, 92f, 94f
Coronary ligaments, magnetic resonance imaging of, 106f
Costs, of ACL tear, 59–60
CPM. See Continuous passive motion
Crepitus, 77, 78f, 166
Cruciate ligaments. See also specific ligaments, e.g., Anterior cruciate ligament
  examination of, 14–15, 15f, 80
  magnetic resonance imaging of, 98–103, 100f–104f
  primary repair of, 153–154
  walking forces in, 234–235, 234f
Cryotherapy, for multiligament-injured knee, 36–37
Curette, for calcified cartilage removal, 138, 140f
Cyclops lesion. See ACL nodules
Cystic degeneration, 77f

D

Database, maintenance of, 10
Debridement, for arthrofibrosis, 171–172
Deceleration, injury with, 12, 60–61
Decision-making, in physical examination, 22–24, 80
Degeneration
  after ACL reconstruction, 154
  of articular cartilage, 130, 131f, 143f–144f, 148f, 149
  cystic, 77f
  of ligaments, 98
Degenerative joint disease
  collagen meniscus implant effect on, 199–201
  microfracture for, 140–143, 143f–144f
Degenerative knee, arthroscopic treatment of, 177–184
  initial evaluation for, 177–178
  package of, 178–182, 178b, 178f–182f
  patient selection for, 178

Diagnosis. *See also* Anatomic diagnosis
  of ACL deficiency or rupture, 8–9
  of acute patella dislocation, 41, 42b
  of arthrofibrosis, 166–167, 166f–167f
  of effusion, 13
  of "isolated" ACL-injured knee, 29b
  of multiligament-injured knee, 34, 34b,
    34f
  of pain, 12
  principles of, 11–25, 72–75, 73f–75f
Dislocation, of patella, 41–43, 41f–42f,
  42b
Disuse, of knee joint, 52, 53f
DLSTG. *See* Double-loop semitendinous
  plus gracilis graft
Double-loop semitendinous plus gracilis
  graft (DLSTG), 240, 242
Drawer test, 14–15, 15f, 73–74
  with acute patella dislocation, 42b
  of multiligament-injured knee, 34b,
    35f
  of patella subluxation, 40b
Drop jump, landing from, 241–243, 242f
Dynamic cine tomographic scan, 80

E

Early degenerative arthritis, after knee
  repair, 51, 55
Edema
  in "isolated" ACL-injured knee, 30f
  magnetic resonance imaging of, 88–89,
    89f, 91f–92f, 93, 93f–99f, 96,
    101f–104f, 107–109, 107f,
    111f–112f, 115f
Effusion, 166–167
  with acute patella dislocation, 42b
  diagnosis of, 13
  of "isolated" ACL-injured knee, 29b
  after microfracture, 145
  of multiligament-injured knee, 34b
  with osteochondral fracture, 41
  of patella subluxation, 40b
  during rehabilitation, 205–206, 209
Elastic stocking
  for "isolated" ACL-injured knee, 32
  for multiligament-injured knee, 36
Electrocautery, for adhesion lysis,
  170–171, 170f
Energy-absorption strategy, 241–243,
  242f
Envelope of function, 51–57, 52f–53f,
  55f–56f
  clinical application of, 54–55
  factors determining, 53–54
  indicators of, 54
Envelope of motion, 16, 18, 74
Epidural analgesia, for "isolated"
  ACL-injured knee, 32
Epiphyseal injury, with ACL
  reconstruction, 117
Equine studies. *See* Horse studies
Etiology, of sports injury, 60, 60f
Examination
  of ACL-deficient knee, 72–81
  of acute patella dislocation, 42b
  adjunct tests of, 18
  of alae, 77

  of anterior cruciate ligament, 12, 16,
    18, 73, 75–76
  of arcuate complex, 14, 16, 75–76
  of collateral ligaments, 14, 14f, 75–76,
    75f–76f
  of cruciate ligaments, 14–15, 15f, 80
  of fat pad, 17f, 18, 20f, 77–78, 78f–79f
  of femoral trochlea groove, 18, 22f
  of function, 72, 79, 80f
  of gait, 73, 79, 80f
  of history, 72–73
  in hyperextension, 75, 75f
  of inferior capsular ligaments, 17f, 18,
    20f, 78f
  of inferior lateral ligament, 18, 22f, 78f
  of inferior medial ligament, 18, 22f,
    78f
  of infrapatellar tendon, 77–78
  of "isolated" ACL-injured knee, 29b,
    30–31
  of knee, 72–81
    central pivot, 73–75, 73f–75f
    conduct of, 72–73
    decision making in, 22–24, 80
    functional, 79, 80f
    imaging, 79–80
    menisci, 76, 77f
    patellofemoral joint, 76–79, 78f–79f
    philosophy of, 72
    secondary restraints, 75–76, 75f–76f
  of lateral capsuloligamentous
    structures, 13, 15, 75
  of lateral collateral ligament (LCL), 16,
    75–76, 75f–76f
  of lateral meniscus, 76
  of laxity, 75–76
  of medial capsuloligamentous
    structures, 13–15, 75
  of medial collateral ligament (MCL),
    12, 16, 18, 74–76, 75f–76f
  of medial meniscus, 76
  of menisci, 18, 23f, 76, 77f, 80
  of multiligament-injured knee, 34, 34b
  of patella, 15, 16f–17f, 18, 20, 20f, 22,
    22f, 76–79, 78f–79f
  of patella subluxation, 39–40, 39f,
    40b, 40f
  of patellofemoral joint, 18, 76–80,
    78f–79f
  of posterior cruciate ligament (PCL),
    13–15, 73, 75–76
  of posterior lateral ligament, 75–76,
    75f–76f
  of posterior medial ligament, 75–76,
    75f–76f
  of posterior oblique ligament, 16, 76
  principles of, 13–15, 72–75, 73f–75f
  of retinacular ligaments, 18, 22f, 78f
  of secondary restraints, 75–76,
    75f–76f, 80
  tests of, 15–18
Examination under anesthesia (EUA), 20
  for multiligament-injured knee, 35
  of patella dislocation, 41
Exercise
  of injured limb, 85
  open chain v. closed chain, 208

Extension
  function and loading during, 231–233,
    232f
  of injured knee, 13–14
  loss of, 164, 164t
Extensor mechanism
  in ACL absence, 233
  arthrofibrosis of, 164
  magnetic resonance imaging of, 108,
    113f
  release of, 172–173, 173f
  scarring of, 166
Extensor tendons, magnetic resonance
  imaging of, 108, 113f
External rotation, of injured knee, 15, 15f

F

Fabrication, of collagen meniscus
  implant, 198, 198f
Facility, for rehabilitation, 218
Failure, of microfractures, 149
Fat droplets, with microfracture, 140,
  141f–142f
Fat pad
  examination of, 17f, 18, 20f, 77–78,
    78f–79f
  magnetic resonance imaging of, 109,
    114f
  scarring of, 166–167, 172–173, 173f,
    179, 181f
Fat-suppression MRI, 88, 90–91, 90f,
  91f–93f, 93, 95f–96f, 98f
Feasibility studies, of collagen meniscus
  implant, 199–201
Female athlete, noncontact ACL injury in,
  60–67, 60f–61f, 62t–66t, 67f,
  241–244, 242f
Femoral condyle
  adhesions to, 170
  magnetic resonance imaging of, 91
  microfracture of, 130f, 144–145,
    151, 216
  point tenderness over, 135
Femoral metaphysis, exposure of, 122,
  122f
Femoral nerve block, 124, 169, 173
Femoral peel, 173
Femoral screw, placement of, 123, 123f
Femoral torsion, with patella
  subluxation, 40
Femoral trochlea groove
  examination of, 18, 22f
  magnetic resonance imaging of, 90
Femoral tunnel placement, for grafting,
  122–123, 122f, 165–166, 165f
Femorotibial angle, 187
Femur, tibia placement on, 28
Fentanyl citrate, 169
Fibrillation, chondral, 90–91, 130
Figure 4 position, for physical testing of
  knee, 18, 21f, 23f, 76, 77f
Finochietto lesion, 34, 35f
Fissuring, chondral, 90–91, 92f–93f,
  99f, 130
Fixation
  of graft, 123–124, 123f
  of plate, 191, 192f–193f, 193

Flaps, chondral, 90–91, 93f
Flexed knee gait pattern, 236–237
Flexion
    function and loading during, 231–233, 232f
    of injured knee, 13–14
    loss of, 164, 164t
Follow-up
    of "isolated" ACL-injured knee, 32–33
    of multiligament-injured knee, 37
Force-displacement curve, of knee, 74, 74f
Force-driven harmonic oscillation theory, 241
Forward running, for rehabilitation, 211, 211f, 213f, 215f
Fracture. See also Microfracture; Stress fracture
    avulsion, 30f, 87, 93–94, 99–103, 101f, 105–107, 109f, 112, 112f, 114f
    chondral, 92f, 129, 130f
    magnetic resonance imaging of, 88–89, 93–94, 94f–95f
    osseous, 87
    osteochondral, 13, 41
    of patella, 40
    of subchondral bone, 93
    of tibia, 53, 85, 95f, 106–107, 112f
Function
    of ACL-deficient knee after surgery, 8–9
    during activities of daily living, 230–244, 232f, 234f–237f, 239f, 242f
        knee bends and squatting, 233
        knee flexion and extension, 231–233, 232f
        landing, 241–244, 242f
    envelope of, 51–57, 52f–53f, 55f–56f
    examination of, 72, 79, 80f
    of knee after microfracture, 148t
    meniscus loss effect on, 200–201

G
Gadolinium contrast agent, 115
Gait
    with acute patella dislocation, 42b
    examination of, 73, 79, 80f
    flexed knee pattern of, 236–238
    of "isolated" ACL-injured knee, 29b
    knee function and loading during, 233–241, 234f–237f, 239f
    of multiligament-injured knee, 34b
    of patella subluxation, 40, 40b
    quadriceps avoidance in, 166–167, 236–239
Gait cycle, shear forces acting on leg during, 235f
Gait training, 210, 240–241
Gas pedals, for rehabilitation, 210, 211f
Gastrocnemius muscle
    forces of, 232, 232f, 235–236, 237f
    magnetic resonance imaging of, 111f
Gastrocnemius tendon, magnetic resonance imaging of, 110f
Gender. See Patient
Gene therapy, microfracture combined with, 224–225
Glucosamine, 188

Goals
    of joint preservation, 185–186
    of rehabilitation, 205, 208–210
    of sport-specific training, 211
Gracilis tendon
    grafting with, 118
    magnetic resonance imaging of, 110f
Grade 4 chondral loss, 93, 94f
Gradient echo MRI, 90
Grading, of pivot shift test, 74–75
Graft
    for articular cartilage repair, 226
    choice of, 118
    fixation of, 123–124, 123f
    harvesting of, 119–120, 119f–121f
    impingement of, 118–119, 121–122, 122b, 164–166, 165f
    of "isolated" ACL injury, 31
    magnetic resonance imaging of, 95, 98f–99f, 112
    malposition of, 164–167, 165f
    of menisci, 189
    of multiligament-injured knee, 35
    passage of, 123, 123b
    at patellar tendon harvest site, 124, 124f
    preparation of, 120–121, 120f–121f
    tunnel positioning for, 118, 121–123, 121f–122f, 165–166, 165f
    two-incision bone-tendon-bone patellar tendon, 117–118, 124–125
Graft passer, 123, 123b
Ground-reaction force
    during landing, 242–243, 242f
    during walking, 235–236
Growth factors, microfracture promotion of, 129, 130f, 156–157
Guide wires, for graft fixation, 123
Gutters, arthroscopic treatment of, 170, 170f

H
Halting gait, with patella subluxation, 40
Hamstring graft, 31, 240
Hamstring muscle
    forces in
        during knee bends and squatting, 233
        during knee flexion and extension, 232, 232f
        during landing, 241
        during walking, 235, 237f, 238–239
    strengthening of, 188
Hamstring tendons, 112
Hanging position, for physical testing of knee, 23f, 76, 77f
Harvesting, of graft, 119–120, 119f–121f
Healing
    maximization of, 9
    overstressed tissues during, 206
Healing response, 118, 153–162
    basic science studies of, 154–157, 154f–156f
    clinical use and outcome studies of, 157–160, 157f–159f
    of "isolated" ACL injury, 31

Heel walking, examination of, 79, 80f
Hemarthrosis, 166–167
Hemorrhage
    in "isolated" ACL-injured knee, 30f
    magnetic resonance imaging of, 88–89, 93, 96, 101f–104f, 107–108, 107f, 109f, 111f–115f
Heterotopic bone formation, 87, 109–112
High tibial osteotomy (HTO), 189
    complications of, 192
    microfracture with, 189–191, 190f–193f, 193
    postoperative management and rehabilitation for, 191–192, 195
Hip extensor moment, during landing, 241–242
Hip rotation, with patella subluxation, 39, 39f
Hip strategy, for walking with ACL-deficient knee, 237–238
Histologic measurements
    of cartilage repair, 222, 223f, 225f–226f
    of ligament repair, 156, 156f
History, 12–13. See also Natural history
    of ACL injury, 28
    of acute patella dislocation, 41
    examination of, 72–73
    of injury, 12, 72–73
    of "isolated" ACL-injured knee, 29
    of multiligament-injured knee, 33
    of patella injuries, 38
    of patella subluxation, 39
    of previous injury, 12
Home exercise, weight machines v., 208
Home therapy, supervised therapy v., 208
Homeostasis. See Tissue homeostasis
Hop tests, for return to activity, 212
Horse studies
    of articular cartilage repair, 221–227
    of chondrocyte transplantation, 225–226, 226f–227f
    of gene therapy with microfracture, 224–225
    of microfracture, 132–134, 132f–135f, 222–223, 223f–224f
    as model of human articular defects, 222
Hostile knee environment, 186–187
Howard Head Sports Medicine Return-to-Sports Test, 213f–216f
HTO. See High tibial osteotomy
Human-horse relationship. See Horse studies
Hyalograft C, 226
Hyaluronic acid, 188
Hyperextension
    examination in, 75, 75f
    of injured knee, 13–14, 14f
Hyperlaxity, ACL injury with, 69
Hypertrophic synovium, ablation of, 178–179, 180f

I
IGF-1. See Insulinlike growth factor-1
IL-1. See Interleukin-1

Iliotibial band
  incision of, 122
  magnetic resonance imaging of, 105,
    107, 112f
Imaging
  of articular cartilage, 89–95, 92f–99f
  of knee, 20–22, 79–80, 87–116
    current expectations and future
      developments in, 112–115
    magnetic resonance, 20–22, 80,
      87–112, 88f–115f
    radiographic, 87
  of ligaments, 96–107, 100f–112f
    collateral, 103–105, 105f–109f
    posterolateral corner, 105–107,
      110f–112f
    secondary restraints, 105–107,
      110f–112f
  of meniscus, 88f–91f, 89
  of microfracture for acute chondral
    injury, 135–137, 137f–139f
  of multiligament-injured knee, 34b
  of patella subluxation, 40
  of tendon and muscle, 107–112,
    113f–115f
Immediate postoperative care, of
  "isolated" ACL-injured knee, 32
Immediate rehabilitation, 208–209, 209f
Immobilization
  arthrofibrosis with, 166
  prevention of detrimental effects of,
    206–207
  weightbearing with, 85
Impact Safety Factor (ISF), of knee braces,
    68
Impingement, of graft, 118–119,
    121–122, 122b, 164–166, 165f
Implantation
  of collagen meniscus implant,
    197–201, 198f–199f
  of menisci, 189
In vivo measurement, of knee
    biomechanics, 230, 231f
Incision
  for ACL reconstruction, 118–119,
    119f–120f, 122, 122f
  for collagen meniscus implant,
    198–199
  for high tibial osteotomy with
    microfracture, 191, 191f
  of medial collateral ligament, 172, 173f
  of peritenon, 119, 120f, 172
  of semimembranosus tendon, 172,
    173f
Indications
  for collagen meniscus implant, 198
  for microfracture of acute chondral
    injury, 134–135, 136f–137f
Induration
  of injured knee, 13, 73
  of menisci, 76–77
Infection, arthrofibrosis with, 166–167,
    169
Inferior capsular ligaments, examination
    of, 17f, 18, 20f, 78f
Inferior lateral ligament, examination of,
    18, 22f, 78f

Inferior medial ligament, examination of,
    18, 22f, 78f
Inflammation
  with ACL reconstruction, 118
  magnetic resonance imaging of, 88, 109
  during rehabilitation, 208–209
Infrapatellar contracture syndrome, 166
Infrapatellar plica, removal of, 179, 179b,
    180f
Infrapatellar tendon, examination of,
    77–78
Initial evaluation, for arthroscopic
    treatment of degenerative knee,
    177–178
Injection, of saline solution, 178, 178b,
    178f–179f
Injury
  history of, 12, 72–73
  mechanism of, 12–13
Insertion
  of collagen meniscus implant, 199,
    199f
  of osteotome, 191, 192f
Inspection, of injured knee, 13
Insufflation, 178, 178b, 178f–179f
Insulinlike growth factor-1 (IGF-1),
    130–132, 156–157, 224–225
Intercondylar notch, 31
  exposure of, 122
  magnetic resonance imaging of, 90f,
    100f
Interference screw, placement of, 123,
    123f
Interleukin-1 (IL-1), in cartilage repair,
    224–225
Intermediate rehabilitation, 209–210,
    210f–211f
Intermeniscal ligament, 182b
Intermuscular septum, dissection of, 122,
    122b
Internal rotation, of injured knee, 15, 15f
International Knee Documentation
    Committee (IKDC)
  knee examination criteria of, 73
  physical examination principles of, 15
  pivot shift grading system of, 74–75
Interventions, for joint preservation,
    188–191, 190f–193f
Intra-articular anesthesia, for "isolated"
    ACL-injured knee, 32
Intra-articular drain, 140
Intra-articular ligament healing. *See*
    Healing response
ISF. *See* Impact Safety Factor
Isokinetic strength testing, for return to
    activity, 212
"Isolated" ACL-injured knee, 29–33, 29b,
    29f–30f, 32f
  complications and follow-up of, 32–33
  history of, 29
  physical examination of, 29b, 30–31
  postoperative care and rehabilitation
    of, 32
  surgery of, 29–32
  treatment plan for, 31–32
Isometric knee extension, ACL load
    during, 232–233, 232f

J
Jakob test, 18
Joint compression, 179
Joint preservation, 185–195
  complications in, 192
  desired v. current activity levels in,
    187–188, 188f
  goals of, 185–186
  interventions for, 188–191, 190f–193f
  of joint alignment, 186–187,
    186f–187f
  outcomes in, 192–193
  with postmeniscectomy knee, 186
  postoperative management and
    rehabilitation for, 191–192, 195
Joint surface, shape of, 140, 142f
Joint-space narrowing, 87, 135
Jumper's knee, 78, 109

K
Kinematic competence, of ACL
    reconstruction, 8, 9
Kinematic factors, of envelope of
    function, 54
Kirschner wires, placement of, 191, 191f
Knee. *See also* ACL-deficient knee;
    Degenerative knee; Surgical
    knee care
  biomechanics of, 229–245
    computer simulation of, 230, 231f
    function and loading during
      activities of daily living, 230–244,
      232f, 234f–237f, 239f, 242f
    in vivo measurement of, 230, 231f
  force-displacement curve of, 74, 74f
  imaging of, 20–22, 79–80, 87–116
    current expectations and future
      developments in, 112–115
    magnetic resonance, 20–22, 80,
      87–112, 88f–115f
    radiographic, 87
  injury of
    crucial principles for and care of,
      7–10
    diagnosis and treatment principles
      for, 7–10
  postmeniscectomy, 186
Knee bends
  knee function and loading during, 233
  for rehabilitation, 210–211, 210f,
    212f–214f
Knee copers, 54
Knee extensor moment
  during landing, 241–242
  during walking, 238–240
Knee strategy, for walking with ACL-
    deficient knee, 237–238
Knee transmission, 38, 52
KT-1000 arthrometer, 24, 24f
KT-1000 manual maximum difference
    testing, after healing response,
    159–160

L
Laceration, chondral, 129, 130f
Lachman test, 14–17, 15f, 73–74
  with acute patella dislocation, 42b

of "isolated" ACL-injured knee, 29b
of multiligament-injured knee, 34b
of patella subluxation, 40b
Landing
from drop jump, 241–243, 242f
knee function and loading during, 241–244, 242f
during muscular fatigue, 243–244
Lateral agility exercise, for rehabilitation, 211, 212f–215f
Lateral alae, examination of, 77
Lateral capsular ligament, of multiligament-injured knee, 34
Lateral capsuloligamentous structures, examination of, 13, 15, 75
Lateral collateral ligament (LCL)
bracing of, 68
examination of, 16, 75–76, 75f–76f
forces induced in, during walking, 234f, 236, 237f, 239f
magnetic resonance imaging of, 105–107, 108f–109f, 112f
release of, 173
tear of, 105, 109f
Lateral condyle
contusion of, 29, 34
in patella dislocation, 41
Lateral femoral condyle, 89, 91f
Lateral geniculate vessels, 173
Lateral gutters, arthroscopic treatment of, 170, 170f
Lateral meniscus
examination of, 76
magnetic resonance imaging of, 88f, 89, 110f–111f
of multiligament-injured knee, 34
tear of, 89, 91f, 93f, 111f
Lateral patella ligaments, 78
Lateral release
of multiligament-injured knee, 37
for patella dislocation, 42
of patella subluxation, 41
Lateral retinacula, 138
magnetic resonance imaging of, 114f
release of, 172, 173f
Lateral retinacular decompression, 124
Lateral tibial condyle, injury of, 91f
Lateral tibial margin, Segond avulsion fracture of, 106–107, 112f
Lateral tibial plateau, magnetic resonance imaging of, 93f–94f
Laxity
with acute patella dislocation, 42b
examination of, 75–76
of "isolated" ACL-injured knee, 29b
of multiligament-injured knee, 34b
of patella subluxation, 40b
as risk factor for ACL injury, 69
LCL. See Lateral collateral ligament
Lennox Hill Brace, 68
Ligaments
loading of, 230, 233–236, 234f–237f, 239f
magnetic resonance imaging of, 96–107, 100f–112f
collateral, 103–105, 105f–109f
cruciate, 98–103, 100f–104f

posterolateral corner, 105–107, 110f–112f
secondary restraints, 105–107, 110f–112f
release of, 171, 171f, 173
Linea aspera, of multiligament-injured knee, 34, 35f, 41
Load acceptance, of injured knee. See Envelope of function
Loading
during activities of daily living, 230–244, 232f, 234f–237f, 239f, 242f
knee bends and squatting, 233
knee flexion and extension, 231–233, 232f
landing, 241–244, 242f
of ligaments, 230, 233–236, 234f–237f, 239f
Loading to structural failure, of knee, 53, 53f
Long standing radiographs
for high tibial osteotomy with microfracture, 189–190, 190f
of joint alignment, 187, 187f
of microfracture for acute chondral injury, 135, 137f
Long-term rehabilitation, of "isolated" ACL-injured knee, 32
Losee test, 18, 19f, 74, 75f
Lower extremity alignment, ACL injury with, 61, 61f
Lysholm score, 187
after arthrofibrosis treatment, 174
after arthroscopic treatment, 183
after healing response technique, 159–160
after high tibial osteotomy with microfracture, 193
after microfracture, 146–147, 149
Lysis of adhesion, 170–171, 170f, 217–218

M

MACI. See Matrix-induced autologous chondrocyte implantation
MacIntosh test, 18
Magnetic resonance imaging (MRI), 54
of anterior cruciate ligament, 98–99, 100f–101f, 157f
for arthrofibrosis diagnosis, 167, 167f
of articular cartilage, 89–95, 92f–99f
chondral technique, 90–95, 92f–99f
of bone, 88–95, 92f–99f
of fracture, 88–89, 93–94, 94f–95f
of "isolated" ACL-injured knee, 29, 30f
of knee, 20–22, 80, 87–112, 88f–115f
of ligaments, 96–107, 100f–112f
collateral, 103–105, 105f–109f
cruciate, 98–103, 100f–104f
posterolateral corner, 105–107, 110f–112f
secondary restraints, 105–107, 110f–112f
of menisci, 76, 88f–91f, 89
of microfracture, 95, 96f–97f, 135–137, 139f

of multiligament-injured knee, 34, 34f
of patella dislocation, 41–42, 42f
of patella injuries, 38
of patella subluxation, 40
of tendon and muscle, 107–112, 113f–115f
of torn medial meniscus, 52f
Malalignment, 177, 186–187, 186f–187f, 189, 189b, 193
Malposition, of graft, 164–167, 165f
Marrow clot
for articular cartilage healing, 129, 130f, 138, 141–142, 142f–144f, 144
for healing response technique, 154, 156–157
Matrix-induced autologous chondrocyte implantation (MACI), 225–226
McDavid Knee Guard, 67
MCL. See Medial collateral ligament
McMurray position, for knee examination, 76
Measures, for microfracture outcomes, 146–147
Medial alae, examination of, 77
Medial capsuloligamentous structures
examination of, 13–15, 75
repair of, 36
Medial collateral ligament (MCL)
bracing of, 68–69
examination of, 12, 16, 18, 74–76, 75f–76f
forces induced in, 233, 234f, 235, 238, 239f
incision of, 172, 173f
magnetic resonance imaging of, 103–105, 105f–107f
rehabilitation of, 85
release of, 173
tear of, 33–37, 33f–37f, 34b, 103–105, 106f–107f
Medial compartment
of ACL-reconstructed knee, 56f
arthritis of, 57
arthrosis of, 186
Medial femoral condyle
articular defect of, 222
magnetic resonance imaging of, 93f–94f, 96f–98f, 106f
Medial femoral epicondyle, in patella subluxation, 39
Medial gutters, arthroscopic treatment of, 170, 170f
Medial intermuscular septum, of multiligament-injured knee, 34, 35f
Medial meniscectomy, 56f
Medial meniscus
examination of, 76
magnetic resonance imaging of, 88f–89f, 89, 106f, 110f
tear of, 12, 33–37, 33f–37f, 34b, 52f, 89, 89f–90f, 93f
Medial parapatellar arthrotomy, 172, 172f
Medial patella ligaments, 78
Medial patellofemoral ligament, of multiligament-injured knee, 34, 35f

Medial release, 172, 172f–173f
Medial retinacula, magnetic resonance imaging of, 114f
Medial tibial plateau, magnetic resonance imaging of, 93f–94f
Medial translation test, 17
Meniscectomy, preservation of meniscus tissue during, 200–201
Menisci, 52. *See also specific meniscus, e.g.*, Medial meniscus
  collagen implant of, 197–201, 198f–199f
  examination of, 18, 23f, 76, 77f, 80
  loss of, 186
  magnetic resonance imaging of, 88f–91f, 89
  repair of, 36
  replacement of, 189
  tear of, 88, 113, 118, 178, 186–187
Meniscocapsular junction, magnetic resonance imaging of, 105
Meniscofemoral ligaments, magnetic resonance imaging of, 105, 105f–106f
Meniscofemoral ligaments of Humphrey, magnetic resonance imaging of, 102f
Meniscofemoral ligaments of Wrisberg, magnetic resonance imaging of, 102f
Meniscopopliteal fascicles, magnetic resonance imaging of, 110f–111f
Meniscosynovial junction, tear of, 89
Meniscotibial ligaments
  magnetic resonance imaging of, 105, 105f
  repair of, 36
Mepivacaine hydrochloride, 169
Merchant view, of patella, 20, 40, 80
Metabolic factors, of envelope of function, 54
Metabolism, of musculoskeletal system, 51
Microfracture, 129–151, 130f
  for ACL reconstruction, 118
  for acute chondral injury, 134–140, 136f–142f
    imaging of, 135–137, 137f–139f
    indications and contraindications for, 134–135, 136f–137f
    preoperative planning of, 135, 137f
    surgical technique, 137–140, 139f–142f
  articular cartilage injury and, 129–134, 130f–135f
  autologous chondrocyte implantation v., 147–148
  basic science of, 132–134, 132f–135f
  basic science studies of, 154–157, 154f–156f
  for chronic chondral injury, 140–144, 143f–144f
    contraindications of, 141, 143f
    nonoperative treatment of, 140–141, 143f
    postoperative management of, 143–144
    procedure for, 141–143, 143f–144f

complications of, 145
gene therapy combined with, 224–225
healing response with, 153–162
with high tibial osteotomy, 189–191, 190f–193f, 193
horse studies of, 132–134, 132f–135f, 222–223, 223f–224f
magnetic resonance imaging of, 95, 96f–97f, 135–137, 139f
outcomes of, 145–147, 146t
preparation for, 136f, 138, 139f, 142, 142f–143f
rehabilitation of, 144–145, 150–151, 216
results of, 147–149, 147f, 148t
Microfracture holes, creation of, 139–142, 141f–142f, 154, 155f, 157, 158f
Micropicking. *See* Microfracture
Midsubstance tears
  of ACL, 99, 101f
  of medial collateral ligament, 106f
  of posterior cruciate ligament, 103f
Mobility
  after ACL reconstruction, 124–125
  after microfracture, 144–145
Monitored Rehabilitation Systems, 218
Morselized cartilage-fibrin-polydioxanone membrane technique, 226, 226f–227f
Motion
  computer simulation and *in vivo* measurement of, 230, 231f
  loss of, 163–166, 164t, 165f, 168f
Motivation, of patient, 205
Motorized burr, for microfracture preparation, 142, 143f
MRI. *See* Magnetic resonance imaging
Multiligament-injured knee, 33–37, 33f–37f, 34b
  complications and follow-up of, 37
  diagnostic studies of, 34, 34b, 34f
  history of, 33
  physical examination of, 34, 34b
  postoperative care and rehabilitation of, 36–37
  surgical procedure for, 35–36
  treatment plan for, 35
Muscle, magnetic resonance imaging of, 107–112, 113f–115f
Muscular fatigue, landing performance during, 243–244
Musculoskeletal function, restoration of, 51

N

Natural history
  of ACL injury, 28
  of ACL-deficient knee, 3–4
  of patella injuries, 38
Neuromuscular factors, of envelope of function, 54
Neuromuscular training, for ACL injury prevention, 61–67, 67f
Neurovascular system
  with acute patella dislocation, 42b
  of "isolated" ACL-injured knee, 29b

of multiligament-injured knee, 34b
of patella subluxation, 40b
Nodules, of anterior cruciate ligament, 164, 165f, 167
Noncontact ACL injury
  bracing against, 68
  in female athlete, 60–67, 60f–61f, 62t–66t, 67f, 241–244, 242f
  prevention training program for, 70, 70t
Nonoperative treatment
  for arthrofibrosis, 167
  for chronic chondral injury, 140–141, 143f
  for joint preservation, 188
Nonsteroidal anti-inflammatory drugs, 54, 140, 188, 209
Notch preparation, for ACL reconstruction, 118f, 119
Noyes test, 18

O

Observation, of injured knee, 13
O'Donoghue triad, 12, 33, 68
Older athlete, joint preservation in, 185–195
  complications in, 192
  desired v. current activity levels in, 187–188, 188f
  goals of, 185–186
  interventions for, 188–191, 190f–193f
  of joint alignment, 186–187, 186f–187f
  outcomes in, 192–193
  with postmeniscectomy knee, 186
  postoperative management and rehabilitation for, 191–192, 195
Open chain exercise, closed chain exercise v., 208
Open debridement, for arthrofibrosis, 171–172
Open medial parapatellar approach, for patella dislocation, 42
Open release, for arthrofibrosis, 171–172
Open surgery
  for arthrofibrosis, 171–173, 172f–173f
  arthroscopic treatment combined with, 171, 171f–172f
  for multiligament-injured knee, 36
Osgood-Schlatter disease, 78, 112
Osseous fracture, 87
Osseous homeostasis, 51, 55, 56f, 57
Osseous remodeling, 87, 94f, 109
Osteoarthritis
  arthroscopic treatment of, 177–184
  in horse, 221
  malalignment in, 186
  measurement of, 146
  posttraumatic, 55
  prevention of, 222
Osteochondral fracture, 13, 41
Osteochondral graft, magnetic resonance imaging of, 95, 98f–99f
Osteophytectomy, 178
Osteophytes, 87, 178, 180f
Osteotome, insertion of, 191, 192f

Osteotomy
  complications of, 192
  high tibial, 189
  outcomes of, 192–193
  postoperative management and
    rehabilitation for, 191–192, 195
Outcomes
  of ACL reconstruction, 125–126
  of arthrofibrosis treatment, 174
  of arthroscopic treatment, 182–183,
    183f
  of healing response, 159–160
  of high tibial osteotomy, 192–193
  of microfracture, 145–147, 146t
Overstress, of healing tissue, 206
Overuse
  of knee joint, 53–55, 53f, 73, 80
  magnetic resonance imaging of, 94

P

Pain
  in anterior knee, 54, 124, 126, 164
  after arthrofibrosis surgery, 169
  diagnosis of, 12
  investigation of, 185–186
  management of, 124
  after microfracture, 145
  during rehabilitation, 205, 208–209
Palpitation, of injured knee, 13, 73,
  76–77, 77f, 79f
Partial tear
  of ACL, 99, 102f
  of patellar tendon, 113f
  of posterior cruciate ligament, 99, 104f
  of quadriceps, 108
Partial-thickness closure, of patellar
  tendon, 124, 124f
Passage, of graft, 123, 123b
Patella
  acute dislocation of, 41–43, 41f–42f, 42b
    considerations for, 42
    diagnosis of, 41, 42b
    history of, 41
    physical examination of, 42b
    rehabilitation of, 42
    treatment plan for, 42
  compression of, 37, 79, 135, 137f, 179
  examination of, 15, 16f–17f, 18, 20,
    20f, 22, 22f, 39–41, 39f, 40b, 40f,
    76–79, 78f–79f
  history of, 38
  magnetic resonance imaging of, 91,
    92f, 109, 112, 114f
  microfracture of, 118
  stress fracture of, 40
  subluxation of, 38–41, 38f–40f, 40b
  in trochlear groove, 39–41, 77, 78f
Patellar apprehension, 29b, 34b, 40b,
  42b, 78
Patellar bone block, harvest and
  preparation of, 120–121
Patellar capture, in "isolated" ACL-injured
  knee, 33
Patellar eversion, 172–173, 173f
Patellar mobility, 166, 166f
  after ACL reconstruction, 124
  after arthroscopic treatment, 182

immobilization effect on, 207
loss of, 177
  during rehabilitation, 209, 209f
Patellar tendon, 78, 172
  closure of, 124, 124f
  forces of, 232–233, 235, 242–243,
    242f
  graft harvest of, 119–120, 119f–121f
  magnetic resonance imaging of,
    108–109, 112, 113f–114f
  during rehabilitation, 209, 209f
  shortening of, 174
  tear of, 109, 112, 113f–114f, 135
Patellar tendon bone-tendon-bone graft,
  31, 117–118, 124–126, 240
Patellofemoral arthrosis, 174
Patellofemoral joint, 38, 52
  examination of, 18, 76–80, 78f–79f
  mobility of, 37
Patellofemoral lesions, rehabilitation for,
  145, 150
Patellofemoral loads, 54, 233, 235, 238
Patellofemoral mechanism, of
  multiligament-injured knee,
  34, 35f
Patellofemoral overloading, 54
Patellotibial tendon interval, 42
Pathokinetic chain, 61
Pathophysiology, of arthrofibrosis,
  163–166, 164t, 165f
Patient
  age of
    in ACL reconstruction, 117–118
    in microfracture, 134, 147–148
    in repair of "isolated" ACL-injured
     knee, 31
    in repair of patella subluxation, 40
  communication with, 9–10, 31, 72, 80,
    204–206
  compliance of, 205–206
  gender of
    ACL injury risk and, 60–61, 60f,
     241–244, 242f
    in repair of patella subluxation, 40
  motivation of, 205
  rehabilitation influence on, 85
  reinforcement of, 205
  safety of, 205–206
  satisfaction of, 125–126
    after arthrofibrosis treatment, 174
    after arthroscopic treatment, 183
    after healing response technique,
     159–160
    after high tibial osteotomy with
     microfracture, 193
    after microfracture, 146–147
  selection of, 3, 117–118, 178
PCL. See Posterior cruciate ligament
PDS membrane. See Polydioxanone
  membrane
Peritenon
  closure of, 124
  incision of, 119, 120f, 172
Pes anserinus, magnetic resonance
  imaging of, 105, 107f
Pes tendons, magnetic resonance imaging
  of, 105, 107f, 112

Philosophy
  of knee care, 85–86
  of knee examination, 72
Physical examination. See Examination
Physical stimulation, of chondrocytes,
  132
Physical therapy, for symptomatic joints,
  54
Physiologic loading, of knee, 53, 53f
Physiological factors
  of envelope of function, 54
  in regaining knee function, 51
Physiology, of articular cartilage injury,
  130–132
Physis, microfracture and, 157, 159f
Pick, for microfracture, 139
Pivot shift, 8, 16, 28, 89, 159–160
Pivot shift test, 15–16, 16f, 18, 19f,
  73–74
  with acute patella dislocation, 42b
  grading of, 74–75
  of "isolated" ACL-injured knee, 29b
  of multiligament-injured knee, 34,
    34b
  of patella subluxation, 40b
PKB. See Prophylactic knee bracing
Plate fixation, for osteotomy, 191,
  192f–193f, 193
Plicae, 138, 139f, 179, 179b, 180f, 182
Plyometric neuromuscular training, 67f
Polydioxanone (PDS) membrane, 226,
  226f–227f
Pop, with ACL tear, 12
Popliteal nerve, 171
Popliteofibular ligament
  forces induced in, during normal
    walking, 236, 237f
  magnetic resonance imaging of, 105,
    111f
Popliteus hiatus, magnetic resonance
  imaging of, 91f, 110f–111f
Popliteus muscle, magnetic resonance
  imaging of, 111f
Popliteus tendon, magnetic resonance
  imaging of, 105, 110f–111f
Portals
  for arthroscopic evaluation of ACL
    reconstruction, 119, 139f, 199f
  for arthroscopic evaluation of
    microfracture, 139f
  for arthroscopic treatment of
    arthrofibrosis, 169, 169f, 171
  for arthroscopic treatment of
    degenerative knee, 178
Positioning
  of graft tunnels, 118, 121–123,
    121f–122f, 165–166, 165f
  of interference screw, 123, 123f
  of Kirschner wires, 191, 191f
Posterior capsule
  forces induced in, during walking,
    234f, 239f
  release of, 171, 171f
Posterior collateral ligament
  magnetic resonance imaging of,
    102f
  release of, 173

Posterior cruciate ligament (PCL)
    ACL fall onto, 31, 32f
    ACL scarring to, 153
    in central pivot, 73–75, 73f–75f
    examination of, 13–15, 73, 75–76
    forces induced in, 231–233, 234f, 235
    magnetic resonance imaging of, 90f,
        99, 102f–104f
    marrow stimulation of, 154–157,
        154f–156f
    of multiligament-injured knee, 34
    tear of, 99–103, 103f–104f, 154, 154f
Posterior horn of lateral meniscus, of
        multiligament-injured knee, 34
Posterior lateral ligament, examination
        of, 75–76, 75f–76f
Posterior medial ligament, examination
        of, 75–76, 75f–76f
Posterior oblique ligament
    examination of, 16, 76
    of multiligament-injured knee, 34, 36
    release of, 171, 171f
Posterolateral arthrotomy, 171, 172f
Posterolateral bundle of ACL, magnetic
        resonance imaging of, 98,
        100f–102f
Posterolateral capsule
    magnetic resonance imaging of, 105,
        110f–111f
    walking forces in, 236, 237f, 238–239
Posterolateral corner
    magnetic resonance imaging of,
        105–107, 110f–112f
    walking forces in, 237f
Posteromedial bundle of PCL, magnetic
        resonance imaging of, 99, 104f
Posteromedial capsule, magnetic
        resonance imaging of, 110f
Posteromedial corner, magnetic
        resonance imaging of, 107, 110f
Posteromedial limited arthrotomy, 171,
        171f
Postmeniscectomy knee, 186
Postoperative analgesia, for arthrofibrosis
        treatment, 169
Postoperative care
    of ACL reconstruction, 124–125, 127
    of arthrofibrosis treatment, 173–174,
        176
    of arthroscopic treatment, 182, 184
    of healing response, 157–159, 162
    of "isolated" ACL-injured knee, 32
    for joint preservation, 191–192, 195
    of microfracture of chronic chondral
        injury, 143–144
    of multiligament-injured knee,
        36–37
Posttraumatic osteoarthritis, 55
Preoperative planning
    of healing response, 157, 157f
    for high tibial osteotomy with
        microfracture, 189–191, 190f–191f
    for microfracture of acute chondral
        injury, 135, 137f
Preparation
    for ACL reconstruction, 118f, 119
    of graft, 120–121, 120f–121f

for microfracture, 136f, 138, 139f, 142,
        142f–143f
Preservation, of joint, 185–195
    complications in, 192
    desired v. current activity levels in,
        187–188, 188f
    goals of, 185–186
    interventions for, 188–191, 190f–193f
    of joint alignment, 186–187,
        186f–187f
    outcomes in, 192–193
    with postmeniscectomy knee, 186
    postoperative management and
        rehabilitation for, 191–192, 195
Pretibial recess, arthroscopic treatment of,
        171, 171f
Prevention
    of ACL injury, 59–71
        bracing for, 67–70
        noncontact injury in female athlete,
            60–67, 60f–61f, 62t–66t, 67f,
            241–244, 242f
        role of coach and athletic trainer in,
            69–70, 70t
        studies of, 61–67, 62t–66t
    of anterior knee pain, 124
    of arthrofibrosis, 167, 174
    of atrophy, 207
    of immobilization effects, 206–207
    of osteoarthritis, 222
Primary repair
    of cruciate ligament injury, 153–154
    of "isolated" ACL injury, 31
Primary restraints, 8
Principles
    of diagnosis and treatment, 11–25
        adjunct tests, 18
        arthroscopy, 22
        decision-making, 22–24
        examination under anesthesia, 20
        history and trauma mechanism,
            12–13
        imaging, 20–22
        physical examination, 13–15, 72–75,
            73f–75f
        physical tests, 15–18
        rehabilitation, 24
    for knee-injured patient, 7–10
        evolution and application of, 7–10
        pursuit of, 246
        validation of, 10
    of rehabilitation, 203–206
        communication, 205
        compliance, 205
        goals, 205
        managing complications, 205
        motivation, 205
        optimizing results, 205–206
        reinforcement, 205
        teamwork, 204–205
Prognosis
    of ACL deficiency or rupture, 8
    medial translation test in, 17
Progression, of rehabilitation, 208–212,
        209f–216f
Prone Lachman test, 16–17, 17f
Prone medial translation test, 17, 18f

Prone position
    for patella subluxation examination,
        40f
    testing in, 16–18, 17f–18f, 20f, 77–79,
        78f
Prophylactic knee bracing (PKB), 67–70
Proprioception
    immobilization effect on, 207
    rehabilitation of, 24
Proprioceptive training, for ACL injury
        prevention, 61
Protocols, for rehabilitation, 206
Pulmonary embolus, with "isolated"
        ACL-injured knee, 32

Q

Quadriceps
    contraction of, 12, 79, 178
    forces in, 232–233, 235–236, 237f,
        243
    strengthening of, 188
Quadriceps avoidance gait pattern,
        166–167, 236–239
Quadriceps tendon, 170, 170f
    compartmentalization of, 179b
    grafting with, 108, 118
    tear of, 108

R

Radial extrusion test, 23f, 76, 77f
Radiographs
    for arthrofibrosis diagnosis, 167
    for arthroscopic treatment, 177–178
    for high tibial osteotomy with
        microfracture, 189–190, 190f
    of joint alignment, 187, 187f
    of knee, 87
    for knee examination, 79–80
    of microfracture for acute chondral
        injury, 135, 137f–138f
    of osteophytes, 180f
    of reconstructed knee, 56f
    standard views of, 20
Range of motion
    after ACL reconstruction, 124
    with acute patella dislocation, 42b
    after arthroscopic treatment, 182
    after healing response, 157
    of injured knee, 13, 77–79, 78f
    of "isolated" ACL-injured knee, 29b
    after microfracture, 144
    of multiligament-injured knee, 34b, 37
    after osteotomy, 191–192
    of patella subluxation, 40b
    during rehabilitation, 207–210
    of secondary restraints, 75
Realistic expectations, for ACL-deficient
        knee, 8–9
Reconstruction, of ACL, 59–60, 99,
        117–127
    complications of, 126
    degeneration after, 154
    envelope of function after, 55, 55f–56f
    functional adaptations after, 240–242
    graft malposition in, 164–166, 165f
    kinematic competence of, 8–9
    knee biomechanics after, 229–245

outcomes of, 125–126
patient selection for, 117–118
postoperative management of, 124–125, 127
rehabilitation of, 124–125, 127, 217
stiffness with, 164, 207
surgical technique for, 118–124, 119f–124f
Re-examination, of injured knee, 73
Rehabilitation
    of ACL reconstruction, 124–125, 127, 217
    for ACL-deficient knee, 3–4, 9, 24, 59–60, 85
    of acute dislocation of patella, 42
    of adhesion lysis, 217–218
    of ankle, 85
    of anterior interval release, 217–218
    of arthrofibrosis treatment, 173–174, 176
    of arthroscopic treatment, 177, 182, 184
    biomechanics of, 231–232
    current research in, 207–208
    future of, 218
    of healing response, 157–159, 162
    of "isolated" ACL-injured knee, 32
    for joint preservation, 191–192, 195
    of medial collateral ligament, 85
    of microfracture, 144–145, 150–151, 216
    of multiligament-injured knee, 36–37
    pain during, 205, 208–209
    patient attitude toward, 85, 205
    preventing immobilization effects during, 206–207
    principles of, 203–206
    progression of, 208–212, 209f–216f
    protocols for, 206
    stress on healing tissue during, 206
Reinforcement, of patient, 205
Reinjury, of "isolated" ACL-injured knee, 32–33
Release
    of anterior interval, 181–182, 181f, 217–218
    for arthrofibrosis, 171–172
    capsular, 173
    of extensor mechanism, 172–173, 173f
    lateral, 37, 41–42
    of lateral retinacula, 172, 173f
    of ligaments, 171, 171f, 173
    medial, 172, 172f–173f
    of posterior capsule, 171, 171f
    of retinacula, 170
    of suprapatellar pouch, 182, 182f
Relocation, of patella, 41–43, 41f–42f, 42b
Remodeling, osseous, 87, 94f, 109
Removal, of calcified cartilage, 223, 225f
Repair. See also Primary repair
    of multiligament-injured knee, 36, 37f
Repair tissues
    of healing response, 155–157, 156f
    of microfracture, 132f, 133–134, 134f–135f, 222–223, 223f–224f, 225

Repetitive stress injury, magnetic resonance imaging of, 94
Resistance exercise
    after arthroscopic treatment, 182
    after microfracture, 144–145
    during rehabilitation, 209–211
    type of, 208
Restoration
    of ACL-deficient knee, 9
    of musculoskeletal function, 51
Results
    of microfracture, 147–149, 147f, 148t
    optimization of, 205–206
Resurfacing, chondral, 95, 188–191, 193
Retinacula, release of, 170
Retinacular ligaments
    examination of, 18, 22f, 78f
    magnetic resonance imaging of, 112, 113f–114f
    tear of, 112, 113f–114f
Return to activity, 32–33, 41, 125, 145, 148, 158–159, 205–206, 211–212, 213f–216f
Risk factors, for ACL injury, 60–67, 60f–61f, 69–70
Roentgenography, 80
Rosenberg x-ray, 54–55
Rotation, of injured knee, 15, 15f, 74
Rotatory laxity, 8
Rotatory osteotomy, 40
Running, for rehabilitation, 211, 211f, 213f, 215f–216f

S
Safety, of patient, 205–206
SAID principle, 32
Saline solution, injection of, 178, 178b, 178f–179f
Saphenous nerve, 36f
Satisfaction. See Patient
Scarring. See also Arthrofibrosis
    after ACL reconstruction, 124
    of anterior interval, 166–167, 167f, 171, 171f, 179, 181f
    of extensor mechanism, 166
    of fat pad, 166–167, 172–173, 173f, 179, 181f
    with immobilization, 207
    of ligaments, 96
    of patellar tendon, 109
    of suprapatellar pouch, 170, 170f, 182, 182f
Sciatica, 79
Sclerosis, 87, 94f, 97f, 143f
Screw. See Interference screw
Secondary restraints, 8
    examination of, 75–76, 75f–76f, 80
    magnetic resonance imaging of, 105–107, 110f–112f
    tear of, 106–107
Secondary trabecular pattern, 79–80
Segond avulsion fracture, 106–107, 112f
Selection
    for ACL surgery, 3, 117–118
    of animal models, 222
    for arthroscopic treatment, 178

Semimembranosus tendon
    grafting with, 118
    incision of, 172, 173f
    magnetic resonance imaging of, 110f
    repair of, 36
Semitendinosus tendon
    grafting with, 118, 240
    magnetic resonance imaging of, 110f
Separation, from subchondral bone, 129, 130f
Sinding-Larsen-Johansson syndrome, 112
Skeletally immature patient
    ACL reconstruction in, 117–118
    healing response in, 159
Skin incision, for ACL reconstruction, 119, 119f
Slocum test, 18
SMPFL. See Superomedial patellofemoral ligament
Soft tissue
    magnetic resonance imaging of, 88–89
    radiographic imaging of, 87
Spin echo MRI, 90–91
Sport Cord, for rehabilitation exercises, 210–211, 210f–212f
Sports injury etiology, 60, 60f
Sport-specific training, during rehabilitation, 211–212, 213f–216f
Sprain
    of ACL, 99, 102f
    of lateral collateral ligament, 105
    of ligaments, 96
    of medial collateral ligament, 103
    of posterior cruciate ligament, 99, 104f
    of secondary restraints, 106
Spurring, 80
Squatting, knee function and loading during, 233
Steadman Hawkins Research Foundation, 86, 145, 204
Steadman Sports Medicine Foundation, 86
Stem cells, microfracture promotion of, 129, 130f
Stiffness
    after ACL reconstruction, 124, 164
    with arthrofibrosis, 166
    of degenerative knee, 177
    with immobilization, 207
    of multiligament-injured knee, 37
Strain
    of gastrocnemius, 111f
    of patellar tendon, 109
    of popliteus, 111f
    of quadriceps muscle, 108
Strength training
    after arthroscopic treatment, 182
    after microfracture, 144–145
    during rehabilitation, 209–211
    type of, 208
Stress fracture
    magnetic resonance imaging of, 88, 94, 95f
    of patella, 40
    of tibia, 53
Stress, of healing tissue, 206
Stress radiographs, of injured knee, 20
Stress roentgenography, 80

Structural failure, loading to, 53, 53f, 55f
Structural paradigm, of knee repair, 51
Subchondral bone
    contusion of, 93
    injury of, 93, 96f
    separation from, 129, 130f
Subchondral plate, 142f
    maintenance of integrity of, 138, 140, 140f, 223
    thickening of, 140
Subluxation, of patella, 38–41, 38f–40f, 40b
Subperiosteal, dissection of, 173f
Subphysiologic loading, of knee, 53, 53f
Superclot, for articular cartilage healing, 129, 130f, 138
Superomedial patellofemoral ligament (SMPFL), 39–41
Supervised therapy, home therapy v., 208
Suprapatellar plica, removal of, 179, 179b, 180f
Suprapatellar pouch
    arthroscopic treatment of, 170, 170f
    compartmentalization of, 182, 182f
    release of, 182, 182f
    saline injection into, 178, 178b, 178f–179f
    scarring of, 170, 170f, 182, 182f
Supraphysiologic loading, of knee, 53–55, 53f, 55f
Surgery. See also Open surgery
    for ACL reconstruction, 118–124, 119f–124f
        arthroscopic evaluation and notch preparation, 118f, 119
        femoral tunnel placement, 122–123, 122f, 165–166, 165f
        fixation, 123–124, 123f
        graft choice, 118
        graft harvest, 119–120, 119f–121f
        graft passage, 123, 123b
        graft preparation, 120–121, 121f
        tibial tunnel placement, 121–122, 121f, 165, 165f
        two-incision technique, 118, 122
    for arthrofibrosis, 167–169, 171–173, 172f–173f
    arthrofibrosis after, 164
    arthroscopic treatment combined with, 171, 171f–172f
    for collagen meniscus implant, 198–199, 199f
    of healing response, 157, 158f–159f
    for high tibial osteotomy with microfracture, 190–191, 191f–193f
    for "isolated" ACL-injured knee, 29–32
    for joint preservation, 188–189
    for microfracture of acute chondral injury, 137–140, 139f–142f
    for microfracture of chronic chondral injury, 141–143, 143f–144f
    for multiligament-injured knee, 35–36
    for patella dislocation, 42
    for patella subluxation, 41
Surgical knee care, 83–245
    ACL reconstruction, 117–127
    for arthrofibrosis, 163–176

arthroscopic treatment of degenerative knee, 177–184
collagen meniscus implant, 197–201, 198f–199f
healing response, 153–162
horse models of, 221–227
joint preservation in, 185–195
knee biomechanics with, 229–245
knee imaging for, 57–116
microfracture, 129–151, 130f
philosophy of, 85–86
rehabilitation after, 203–219
Surgical methodology, 9
    for ACL-deficient knee, 3–4
Survivorship
    after arthroscopic treatment, 183, 183f
    after healing response technique, 159
    after osteotomy, 193
Suturing
    of collagen meniscus implant, 199, 199f
    of graft, 123, 123f
Swelling
    after microfracture, 145
    onset of, 13
    during rehabilitation, 205, 209
Sympathic dystrophy, of multiligament-injured knee, 37
Synovium, ablation of, 178–179, 180f

T
Taylor gap, 53
Team, communication with, 9–10, 204–206
Teamwork, in rehabilitation, 204–205
Tear
    of ACL, 12, 29–37, 29b, 29f–30f, 32f, 33f–37f, 34b, 41, 59–60, 89, 91f, 97f, 99, 101f–102f, 106, 111f–112f, 157f, 217–218
        healing response for, 153–162
        prevention studies of, 61–67, 62t–66t
    of biceps femoris, 115f
    of lateral collateral ligament, 105, 109f
    of lateral meniscus, 89, 91f, 93f, 111f
    of ligaments, 96
    of medial collateral ligament, 33–37, 33f–37f, 34b, 103–105, 106f–107f
    of medial meniscus, 12, 33–37, 33f–37f, 34b, 52f, 89, 89f–90f, 93f
    of menisci, 88, 113, 118, 178, 186–187
    of meniscosynovial junction, 89
    of patellar tendon, 109, 112, 113f–114f, 135
    of posterior cruciate ligament, 99–103, 103f, 104f, 154, 154f
    of quadriceps muscle, 108
    of retinacular ligaments, 112, 113f–114f
    of secondary restraints, 106–107
    of trochlea, 135
TEC scan, of patella subluxation, 40
Technetium bone scan, 51, 53, 55, 56f, 80
Technology, for rehabilitation, 218
Tegner activity score, 187–188, 188f
    after arthrofibrosis treatment, 174

after arthroscopic treatment, 183
after collagen meniscus implant, 200–201
after healing response technique, 159
meniscus loss effect on, 200–201
after microfracture, 146, 149
Teleradiology practice model, 114
Templating, for high tibial osteotomy with microfracture, 189–190, 190f
Tenderness
    with acute patella dislocation, 42b
    of "isolated" ACL-injured knee, 29b
    of menisci, 76–77
    of multiligament-injured knee, 34b
    of patella subluxation, 40b
Tendinosus, of patellar tendon, 109, 113f
Tendon, magnetic resonance imaging of, 107–112, 113f–115f
Tendon of linea aspera, in patella subluxation, 39
Tendonitis, during rehabilitation, 205
Testing
    of injured knee, 15–18
    for return to sports, 212, 213f–216f
"The Use of Knee Braces" (AAOS), 69
Therapy
    aquatic, 208
    location of, 208
    for symptomatic joints, 54
Thermal ablation, for adhesion lysis, 171
Thinning, chondral, 90, 95, 99f, 130
Three-dimensional anatomic diagnosis, of ACL deficiency or rupture, 8–9
Tibia
    contusion of, 29, 89, 89f, 92f, 94f
    fracture of, 53, 85, 95f, 106–107, 112f
    placement of, 28
    Segond avulsion fracture of, 106–107, 112f
Tibial bone block, harvest and preparation of, 120–121, 120f
Tibial plateau
    magnetic resonance imaging of, 91, 92f
    microfracture of, rehabilitation for, 144–145, 151
    point tenderness over, 135
Tibial screw, placement of, 123
Tibial torsion, with patella subluxation, 39–40, 39f
Tibial tubercle
    alignment of, with patella subluxation, 39
    magnetic resonance imaging of, 112, 113f
Tibial tunnel placement, for grafting, 121–122, 121f, 165, 165f
Tibiofemoral loads, 233, 235, 236f, 238, 242–243
Timing, of surgery
    for ACL reconstruction, 118
    for "isolated" ACL-injured knee, 29–30
    for multiligament-injured knee, 34–35
    for patella dislocation, 42
Tissue engineering
    for articular cartilage injury, 225–226, 226f–227f
    of meniscuslike tissue, 197–201, 198f–199f

Tissue homeostasis, 51–57, 52f–53f, 55f–56f
TKA. *See* Total knee arthroplasty
Toe walking, examination of, 79, 80f
Total knee arthroplasty (TKA), activity after, 188
Tourniquet time, 36
Training, for ACL injury prevention, 61–67, 67f, 70, 70t
Transforming growth factor-β, 130–132, 156–157
Translation, of injured knee, 74
Transmission, by knee, 38, 52
Transplantation, of chondrocyte, 95, 225–226, 226f–227f
Trauma mechanism, 12–13
Treatment factors, of envelope of function, 54
Treatment program. *See also* Nonoperative treatment; Surgical knee care
    for ACL-deficient knee, 8–9
    for acute dislocation of patella, 42
    for arthrofibrosis, 167–173, 168f–173f
    for "isolated" ACL-injured knee, 31–32
    for multiligament-injured knee, 35
    for overloaded knee, 55
    for patella subluxation, 40–41
    principles of, 11–25, 72–75, 73f–75f
Trochlea
    microfracture of, 118
    tear of, 135
Trochlear groove, patella in, 39–41, 77, 78f
Tumors, of leg, 79

Tunnel positioning, for graft, 118, 121–123, 121f–122f, 165–166, 165f
Tunnel view, of injured knee, 20, 23f
Turbo/fast spin echo MRI, 90–91
Two-incision technique, 118, 122
    for bone-tendon-bone patellar tendon operation, 117–118, 124–125
Type I fibers, atrophy of, 207
Type II collagen, after microfracture, 132f, 133–134, 134f–135f, 222–223, 224f, 225
Type II fibers, atrophy of, 207

V
Valgus alignment, ACL injury with, 61, 61f
Valgus angulation, 14, 75–76, 241–242, 244
Valgus laxity
    with acute patella dislocation, 42b
    examination of, 75–76
    of "isolated" ACL-injured knee, 29b
    of multiligament-injured knee, 34b
    of patella subluxation, 40b
Varus alignment, 186–187, 186f, 189, 189b, 193
Varus angulation, 14, 75–76, 244
Varus deformity, 78
Varus laxity
    with acute patella dislocation, 42b
    examination of, 75–76
    of "isolated" ACL-injured knee, 29b
    of multiligament-injured knee, 34, 34b
    of patella subluxation, 40b
Varus-valgus moments, during landing, 241–242
Vasti forces, 235, 243

Vastus lateralis muscle, dissection of, 122, 122f
Vastus medialis oblique (VMO), 39–41
VMO. *See* Vastus medialis oblique

W
Walking. *See also* Gait
    ACL-deficient knee adaptations of, 236–240, 239f
    ACL-reconstructed knee adaptations of, 240–241
    knee function and loading during, 233–241, 234f–237f, 239f
    ligament loading during, 233–236, 234f–237f
WBL. *See* Weightbearing line
Weight machines, home exercise v., 208
Weightbearing
    after arthrofibrosis treatment, 174
    after arthroscopic treatment, 182
    with cast immobilization, 85
    after healing response, 157
    after microfracture, 144–145
    after osteotomy, 192
    during rehabilitation, 206, 208–210
Weightbearing line (WBL), 187, 187f
Weightbearing tunnel view, of injured knee, 20, 23f, 80
West Point athletes, knee bracing studies of, 69
Western Ontario and McMaster University Osteoarthritis Index, after microfracture, 146–147

Z
Zones, of envelope of function, 53f